Environmental Social Work

Social work has been late to engage with the environmental movement. Often working with an exclusively social understanding of environment, much of the social work profession has overlooked the importance of environmental issues. However, recently, the impact of and worldwide attention to climate change, a string of natural disasters, and increased understanding of issues around environmental justice has put the environment, sustainability, and well-being in the spotlight.

Divided into three parts, this field-defining work explores what environmental social work is, and how it can be put into practice. The first section focuses on theory, discussing ecological and social justice, as well as sustainability, spirituality, and human rights. The second section comprises case studies of evolving environmental social work practice. The case studies derive from a range of areas from urban gardens and community organizing to practice with those affected by climate change. The final section – relevant to students and lecturers – looks at learning about environmental issues in social work.

Environmental Social Work provides an integrated theoretical and practical overview of why and how social work might respond to environmental factors affecting the societies and people they work with at international, national, local and individual levels.

Mel Gray is Professor of Social Work and Research Professor in the Research Institute for Social Inclusion and Wellbeing (RISIW), in the School of Humanities and Social Science at University of Newcastle, Australia.

John Coates was Professor and Director of the School of Social Work at St Thomas University in New Brunswick, Canada, and is Chair and a founding member of the Canadian Society for Spirituality and Social Work.

Tiani Hetherington is a Lecturer in Social Work at Griffith University, Australia.

Environmental Social Work

Edited by Mel Gray, John Coates, and
Tiani Hetherington

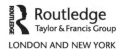

Routledge
Taylor & Francis Group

LONDON AND NEW YORK

First published 2013
by Routledge
2 Park Square, Milton Park, Abingdon, Oxon, OX14 4RN

Simultaneously published in the USA and Canada
by Routledge
711 Third Avenue, New York, NY 10017

Routledge is an imprint of the Taylor & Francis Group, an informa business

British Library Cataloguing in Publication Data
A catalogue record for this book is available from the British Library

Library of Congress Cataloging in Publication Data
Gray, Mel, 1951-
Environmental social work / Mel Gray, John Coates, and Tiani
Hetherington. – 1st ed.
p. cm.
1. Social service–Environmental aspects. 2. Environmentalism–Social
aspects. I. Coates, John, 1948- II. Hetherington, Tiani. III. Title.
HV40.G6973 2012
363.7'053–dc23
2012011456

ISBN13: 978-0-415-67811-7 (hbk)
ISBN13: 978-0-415-67812-4 (pbk)
ISBN13: 978-0-203-09530-0 (ebk)

Typeset in Baskerville
by Saxon Graphics Ltd, Derby

Contents

List of figures and tables

Figures

Tables

List of contributors

Editors

Mel Gray is Professor of Social Work in the School of Humanities and Social Science and Research Professor in the Research Institute for Social Inclusion and Wellbeing, University of Newcastle, New South Wales, Australia. She has published extensively on social work and social development. Recent books include *Indigenous Social Work around the World* (with Coates and Yellow Bird, Ashgate, 2008), *Social Work Theories and Methods* (with Webb, Sage, 2008), *Evidence-based Social Work* (with Plath and Webb, Routledge, 2009), *Ethics and Value Perspectives in Social Work* (with Webb, Palgrave, 2010), *International; Social Work – 4 vols* (with Webb, Sage, 2010), *Sage Handbook of Social Work* (with Webb and Midgley, 2012), *Decolonizing Social Work* (with Coates, Hetherington, and Yellow Bird, Ashgate, 2012), *Social Work Theories and Methods* (2nd ed., with Webb, Sage, 2012), and *New Politics of Critical Social Work* (with Webb, Palgrave, 2012). Mel is Associate Editor of the *International Journal of Social Welfare* and also a keen photographer.

John Coates, PhD was Professor and Director, School of Social Work, St Thomas University, Fredericton, New Brunswick, Canada. He is Chair and a founding member of the Canadian Society for Spirituality and Social Work. His recent publications include *Ecology and Social Work* (Fernwood Press, Halifax, 2003); *Spirituality and Social Work: Selected Canadian Readings* (with Graham, Swartzentruber, and Ouellette, Canadian Scholars Press, 2007); *Indigenous Social Work around the World* (with Gray and Yellow Bird, Ashgate, 2008); and *Decolonizing Social Work* (with Gray, Hetherington, and Yellow Bird, Ashgate, 2012). He has co-edited several journal issues in the area of spirituality and social work, and on environmental social work, most recently *Critical Social Work*, *11*(3), 2010 (with Fred Besthorn) and *International Journal of Social Welfare*, *21*(3), 2011 (with Mel Gray). Recent journal articles include 'The spirituality of justice: Bringing together the eco and the social' (with Arielle Dylan), *Journal of Religion and Spirituality in Social Work*, *31*(1–2), 1-22; and 'Environmental ethics for social work: Social work's responsibility to the non-human world' (with Mel Gray), *International Journal of Social Welfare, 21.*

Tiani Hetherington, PhD, is a Lecturer in Social Work at Griffith University, Queensland, Australia, where she is currently working on environmental social work curriculum development for BSW students. Tiani is a graduate of the University of Newcastle where she recently completed her PhD on a *Comparative Study of Indigenous Social Work in New Brunswick, Canada and Alice Springs, Australia.* She worked closely with Mel Gray and John Coates as a research assistant on *Indigenous Social Work around the World* (Ashgate, 2008) and attended the Writer's Workshop in New Brunswick which preceded this publication. Tiani has published with Gray and Coates, 'An "Eco-spiritual" perspective: Finally a place for Indigenous Approaches' (2006), *British Journal of Social Work, 36,* 1–19 and 'Hearing Indigenous voices in mainstream social work' (2007), *Families in Society, 88*(1), 53-64.

Contributors (alphabetical by first name)

Arielle Dylan, PhD, is Assistant Professor of Social Work at St Thomas University in Fredericton, New Brunswick, Canada. Her scholarly and research areas include First Nations realities, Roma issues, transnational practices, mental health and addictions, complementary and alternative ontological understandings and wellness approaches, and environmental and social justice. She was recently awarded a Social Sciences and Humanities Research Council of Canada grant to develop further her postdoctoral work examining effects of Impact Benefit Agreements in a northern First Nation community. She is also currently conducting research on the effectiveness of meditation, yoga, and self-awareness practices as an intervention for women living with addictions challenges. She has published in the area of environmental social work, ecosocial justice and spirituality, transnational social work, groupwork, empathic direct practice, and First Nations realities.

Barbara Holguin received her Bachelor of Science and Master of Science in Sociology from the University of Houston, Clear Lake in 2003 and 2011 respectively. She served as Criminal Justice Coordinator for the Great Plains Restoration Council and assisted with programming and data collection for the new *Restoration Not Incarceration* program, offering her extensive knowledge on Law Enforcement from her experience as a probation officer for Harris County Corrections in Houston, Texas. Ms Holguin continues to conduct research in the field of Sociology and Criminal Justice, with a particular interest in innovative approaches to offender reintegration. She is a faculty member at the University of Phoenix as well as San Jacinto Community College in Houston, Texas, where she currently resides with her husband and son.

Benjamin Shepard, PhD, is an Assistant Professor of Human Service at New York School of Technology/City University of New York. He received his Masters at the University of Chicago School of Social Service Administration and PhD at the Graduate Center of the City University of New York. As a social worker he has worked with community gardens and environmental activism for a number of years. He is the author or editor of several books including: *Queer political performance and protest* (Routledge, 2010), *Play, creativity, and the new community organizing* (Routledge, 2011), *The beach beneath the streets: Exclusion, control, and play in public space* (co-written with Greg Smithsimon, SUNY Press, 2011), and *From ACT UP to the WTO: Urban protest and community building in the era of globalization* (co-edited with Ron Hayduck, Verso, 2002). The latter work was a non-fiction finalist for the Lambda Literary Awards in 2002. His forthcoming work is *Community projects as social activism* (Sage).

Cathryne L. Schmitz, MSW, PhD, is a Professor in the Department of Social Work and the Program in Conflict and Peace Studies at the University of North Carolina Greensboro. She has extensive experience in the fields of community change and leadership development. Much of her scholarship focuses on organizational and community change, critical multiculturalism, privilege or oppression, leadership, multidisciplinary education and practice, global engagement, and environmental sustainability. She has numerous publications, including a co-authored book on *Critical Multicultural Social Work*. She is actively engaged in global and environmental education and scholarship, having presented nationally and internationally on these issues.

Channelle D. James, PhD, is a Lecturer in the Department of Business Administration at the University of North Carolina in Greensboro. Her research interests include sustainability, social entrepreneurship, and community support for entrepreneurship related to vulnerable communities. Dr James engages an interdisciplinary approach to research and teaching sparked by her dissertation on African American women activists. She has developed courses in innovation and creativity, social entrepreneurship, and environmental sustainability. Dr James also directs the Triad Women's Entrepreneurial Initiative. In Greensboro, she consults with microenterprises, many of which are community-based ventures, social enterprises, and nonprofit organizations.

Christine Lynn Norton, PhD, LCSW, is Assistant Professor of Social Work at Texas State University-San Marcos. She received her PhD in Social Work from Loyola University Chicago. With over 15 years' experience working with adolescents in a variety of practice settings, using innovative interventions, including therapeutic wilderness, juvenile justice, family counselling, and youth mentoring and educational empowerment programs, Dr Norton is a specialist in child and adolescent mental health. Her edited book *Innovative Interventions in Child and Adolescent Mental Health* (Routledge, 2010) includes chapters on wilderness and animal-assisted therapy.

Daniela Stehlik, PhD, was Foundation Director of The Northern Institute and is currently Professor of Sociology at Charles Darwin University. She also holds Adjunct Professorial appointments at the School of Sociology at the Australian National University and the Cairns Institute at James Cook University. In 2008 she was a member of the Expert Panel for the Review of Social Impacts of Drought on Farm Families and Rural Communities. She is the Ministerial appointed Chair of the Rural Industries Research and Development Corporation and has published on matters associated with social sustainability, community capacity building, and evidence-based policy. She is particularly interested in the generative capacity of women's energy and enthusiasm as the foundation of community flourishing and how practice builds community (social) capital.

Dyann Ross, PhD, is a mental health clinical educator for the Mental Health Service on the Sunshine Coast in Queensland and is an adjunct Senior Lecturer at the University of the Sunshine Coast. Dyann's social work experience was highly relevant in the case study research which underpins her most recent publication *Under Corporate Skies: A Struggle between People, Place and Profits* (with Dr Martin Brueckner, Fremantle Press, 2010). The book has been shortlisted for the Blake Dawson Business Literary Award.

Frank Tester is a Professor of Social Work at the University of British Columbia where he teaches social and international development theory and practice. Since graduating with a Master's Degree in Environmental Design, based on his work in Arctic Bay, Nunavut, he has worked in the eastern Arctic documenting its colonial history and dealing with contemporary social and environmental matters affecting Inuit. Frank also has degrees in medical research, social work, and a doctoral degree in human geography. He has worked internationally with indigenous populations in Latin America, New Zealand, the Republic of Vanuatu, Tanzania and Mozambique. A former board member of CUSO and Chair of the City of Vancouver's Family Court/Youth Justice Committee, he is a founding member of the Vancouver Association for Restorative Justice. Frank is a recipient of the 1995 Erminie Wheeler-Voeglin Prize for his work on the ethnohistory of Canadian Inuit, and the 1998 Gustavus Myers Award for his work on human rights in North America.

Fred H. Besthorn, PhD, LMSW, M. Div., is Associate Professor of Social Work at Wichita State University. He has written extensively on the development of a framework for integrating deep ecological awareness with social work policy and strengths-based practice and is the creator of The Global Alliance for a Deep-Ecological Social Work (http://

ecosocialwork.org/). Dr Besthorn brings experiences in the faith community, higher education, psychotherapy, criminal justice, community advocacy, and environmental activism to his writing and research interests in the application of spirituality, deep ecological, and ecofeminist thought to social work theory, practice, and curriculum development, as well as to the development of transpersonal models of personal and social transformation. He has authored published works in numerous national and international professional journals on issues of spiritual awareness, eco-justice, and curriculum development.

Jarid Manos is the Founder and CEO of the Great Plains Restoration Council based in Houston, Texas. As an author, philanthropic leader, activist, and empowerment speaker, he leads national conversations regarding the new ecological health movement that weave a common thread between the destruction and preservation of Earth and self. Manos was selected as a member of the Obama administration's new Relevancy Committee, through the National Park Service, to help diverse communities connect to wild nature as a matter of our own public health. He also serves on the Board of Directors of the Black Vegetarian Society of Texas.

Jennifer Boddy, PhD, is a Lecturer in Social Work at Griffith University, Queensland, Australia where she is working at embedding environmental social work issues into core courses on the sociopolitical context of social work practice, research methods, and social work theory. Much of her scholarship is focused around feminism, community development, and social activism. Jennifer is particularly interested in the impacts of the environmental fallout of climate change on disadvantaged populations, especially women. She works with a number of community groups to promote community awareness about climate change.

Lacey M. Sloan, PhD, MSSW, is Associate Professor and Director of the Social Work Program at the College of Staten Island (CUNY). Across her career, she has focused on issues of social, political, economic, and environmental justice and the dismantling of oppression. Her area of research is violence and social injustice, with a particular focus on violence against women, LGBT people, and people with disabilities. Recently her research has examined the ways in which distance education might be used to facilitate international student exchanges. Dr Sloan teaches human rights, policy, macro practice, and research.

Lena Dominelli, Chair in Applied Social Sciences and Associate Director at the Institute of Hazards, Risk and Resilience Research at Durham University, has two major research projects on environmental issues and climate change and has a wealth of experience as an educator, researcher, and practitioner. She has published widely, including several classics that have been translated into other languages. Her most recent books are:

Introducing Social Work; Social Work in a Globalising World; and Green Social Work. A leading figure in social work education internationally, Lena was elected President of the International Association of Schools of Social Work from 1996–2004. She currently chairs its Committees on Disaster Interventions and Climate Change and attended the UNFCCC discussions in Cancun and Durban. Lena has also received various honours for her work

Mishka Lysack, PhD, RSW, is Associate Professor in Social Work and adjunct assistant professor in Psychiatry at the University of Calgary, where he teaches social work and ecosocial work. He was the Coordinator for a Social Sciences and Humanities Research Council funded project *Alberta Acts on Climate Change.* In 2008, he organized the first Teach-In on Global Warming at the University of Calgary. Since 2009, he has organized a series of over 20 conferences and workshops with a network of organizations in Ottawa, Toronto, and Calgary on environmental decline and climate change as moral issues and building leadership for environmental advocacy.

Peter Jones is Senior Lecturer in the Department of Social Work and Community Welfare at James Cook University. He has been awarded two Australian Learning and Teaching Council (ALTC) National Citations for his teaching practice, holds a Teaching Fellowship from the Higher Education Research and Development Society of Australasia (HERDSA) and is currently one of four Curriculum Scholars at JCU. He is involved in environmental and community activism and recently co-organized an international conference on ecosocial justice in Kerala, India. His activism, teaching, and research interests are in the areas of environmental social work, ecosocial justice, transformative learning, and social work education.

R. Anna Hayward, MSW, PhD, is an Assistant Professor at Stony Brook University School of Social Welfare, USA, where she teaches Psychopathology and Human Behavior in the Social Environment (HBSE) in the MSW program. Dr Hayward has a BS in Applied Psychology from New York University, MSW from Hunter College, and PhD from the University of Maryland Baltimore. Her primary research interests are children and families living in poverty with a focus on strengthening families and preventing and responding to child maltreatment, juvenile delinquency, and parental incarceration. She conducted a study of social work students' attitudes toward environmental issues and is interested in the integration of environment in social work curriculum.

Shari E. Miller, MSW, PhD, is an Assistant Professor at the University of Georgia School of Social Work, USA. She teaches in the undergraduate and graduate programs, including classes that introduce students to the social work profession, practice with families and groups, and Human

Behavior in the Social Environment. Dr Miller's dissertation was an exploratory study focused on the professional socialization of social workers, including the development of a theoretical framework, exploration of predictors of socialization, and differences between groups. Her primary research interests relate to social work education and the culture of the profession. She has spent the past year developing a service learning course focused on environmental and ecological justice and social work practice. In an interdisciplinary effort, she's worked to develop a school garden initiative in Athens-Clarke County, Georgia with a focus on children's relationships to place and nature, where food comes from, food security, sustainability, and parent and community involvement.

Susan A. Taylor has a PhD in Policy Analysis and Public Administration, and an MSW from Saint Louis University in Saint Louis, Missouri. Dr Taylor's emphasis is in policy and program development, administration, and clinical practice. She is a professor at California State University Sacramento, where she oversees a Mental Health Training program, and campus-wide suicide prevention programming. Her writing and research are in health, psychiatric rehabilitation, and mental health policy. Part of her University service is spent in the education and veterinary science departments of the Marine Mammal Center, a rehabilitation, research, and education facility north of San Francisco.

Terry V. Shaw, MSW, MPH, PhD, is an Assistant Professor at the University of Maryland Baltimore, School of Social Work where he teaches child welfare policy and research. Dr Shaw has an MSW from the University of Missouri-Columbia and an MPH and PhD in Social Welfare from the University of California-Berkeley. His dissertation was an exploratory study that gauged the environmental knowledge and attitudes of professionals in the field of social work in the United States, titled 'Social Workers' Knowledge and Perception of the Ecological Environment'. His research background and interests focus on social justice and the experience of children in the child welfare system. Issues around families, poverty, equity, racial disproportionality, child welfare policy (at the state and federal levels), and methods of accurate statistical analysis have formed the basis of his work.

Thomas Ryan, BSW, PhD, is a social worker with 19 years' continuous practice experience. He has spent most of his life in country communities, and animals have always been part and parcel of the wider Ryan household. His book *Animals and Social Work: A Moral Introduction* (Palgrave, 2011) is a pioneering work that presents cogent arguments for the inclusion of animals within social work's moral and conceptual frameworks, and articulates a revised social work code of ethics that has profound theoretical and practical implications for the discipline and its practitioners. Tom is also an Associate Fellow of the Oxford Centre for Animal Ethics.

Tom Matyók, PhD, is an Assistant Professor in the Conflict Peace Studies
Program at the University of North Carolina in Greensboro. His interests
include the changing nature of war, modern-day slavery, and human and
environmental oppression. He is the convener of TRANSCEND-USA, a
global peace and development network, and has negotiated international
agreements. He has worked with the Center for a Sustainable Coast
(Georgia) and the Glynn Environmental Coalition. His educational and
scholarship expertise involve creating responses to complex, global
issues, including war, poverty, and violence, which result in oppression
and degradation of both the community and the environment.

Preface

A good preface sets the stage for enjoyable reading. I hope to provide some orienting information that will help you better to engage with and apply this new *Environmental Social Work* text. As a practising psychologist, I have worked closely with social work colleagues and know the range and contributions of their efforts. With the social work fields' ethical mandate to address human well-being and basic needs in a societal context – in particular the needs and well-being of those least privileged – it comes as no surprise in our global, ecological age that social work would focus on what social scientists call 'interactions between human and natural systems', that is, people and the planet.

Here briefly are my key points: Be prepared that the selections may apply social work, or may revision the field altogether. The idea of environmental social work is not new; while I can attest that this volume captures the leading edge of practice, its foundations have been maturing for quite some time. This material is based on robust findings in the social and health sciences and not simply on well-meaning environmentalist values and intentions. At the same time, the material cannot be understood apart from values and intentions. Readers should be willing to expand, modify, or let go of their previous conceptions of 'environmentalism' or 'environmental issues'. Finally, as a social worker, or other health care provider, you do not need to change your work, your location, or the people you serve in order to make use of the ideas in this book.

Environmental social work parallels ecologically conscious initiatives occurring in all fields, including other healthcare and social service disciplines. In social work, as in my field of psychology, these eco-initiatives ask two basic questions. The order and relative primacy of these questions is typically a product of the questioner's environmental identity and worldview, and thus their sense of possibility and desired behaviours. The most conventional question is 'What can we apply of our discipline to help us understand and ameliorate environmental issues?' A more fundamental and radical question (in the sense of deep change) is: 'Given our place as natural beings in an earthly ecology, what would our discipline – in this case, social work – look like?' This latter question moves us from a position of application to a place of revisioning. As you survey *Environmental Social Work*, note the relative stress on assimilation of the familiar or accommodation of the new (e.g., in recommendations that the field 'start from scratch' or 'play to its strengths'). How you resolve this tension in your own practice will be a product of your context and your worldview. As a pragmatist, I would say these processes can and indeed must happen simultaneously, as we have no reset button for planet Earth, or our disciplines, and must overcome much inertia on the path to sustainability.

While much is made of this volume as a new endeavor, and rightly so, it is important to take a long view and recognize that an awareness of human ecology and interdependence is perennial in all cultures, as is an age-old debate about humanity's role vis-à-vis the other than human world. More to the point in our current era, there have been initiatives within academia and healthcare fields to address so-called environmental issues since the advent of the modern environmental movement in the mid-1960s. These have included research programs, task forces, and localized attempts at practical application. For recent examples see the Australian Psychological Association position paper on the natural environmental and the American Psychological Association's recent task force on global climate change. Scholarly discourse has evolved from an abstract, implicitly human-centric schema of social ecology or person-in-environment and from a value-neutral approach to human-environment interactions. As this volume ably illustrates, the discourse has given way to explicit consideration of the effects of environmental degradation on health and well-being and of the synergistic benefits of environmental conservation and restoration programs.

As implied above, the material in this book is based on years of solid research and a robust body of evidence in the social, health and natural sciences. We know, for example, that green spaces (i.e., those with some preponderance of organic, self-organizing or wild properties, on a continuum from gardens to wilderness-like areas) offer health benefits. These benefits range from stress management, restored attention, and promotion of creativity to celebration of shared cultural values and transcendent experiences. We are prepared through evolution to experience these benefits and they are mediated and moderated by our culture and identity. Recognition of this core aspect of human health and functioning will enhance the well-being of social workers and those they serve.

Social work also has a role to play in attending to the combined natural and human-made disasters that will plague our increasingly populous, technologically advanced, and interconnected world. There is a growing body of evidence in the field of environmental health on the negative effects of environmental toxins, pollution, and degraded ecosystems, and their impacts on the scale of communities, regions, and nations. Along with ubiquitous opinion polling and calls for behaviour change, research on global climate change is also replete with examples of the physical and mental health impacts of chaotic climate and weather systems, impacts that fall disproportionately on those least privileged (confirming the contention of many contributors to this volume). These impacts range from the obvious effects of climate change-related disasters, to large-scale psychosocial impacts of droughts, displacement and resource conflicts; to more subtle, emotional impacts – even among those that are ostensibly most privileged and shielded from direct harm.

Given the evidence, it is tempting to think of the assertions in this volume as common sense, or as simple as placing your feet on solid ground. However, given humans' flexibility in framing their situations and propensity toward cognitive biases, I think it actually the wisest course to imagine that these findings rest on relatively shaky foundations. By this I mean that, as a rule in modern industrialized nations, societal and educational systems do not promote a clear understanding of the role and value of the natural environment in human health and identity – or teach ways to negotiate the complex social-environmental dilemmas we face in the 21st century. We (as otherwise educated people) lack language to describe the value of commonplace experiences in the outdoors or our affiliation with other species. There is simply no way to approach the 'facts' of environmental social work without the mediating presence of our social and cultural beliefs, and our personal experiences. The recognition of shaky cultural ground is not something to bemoan as much as to own. There are clear benefits to recognizing our cultural assumptions and blind spots (environmentalist or otherwise): It can allow us to humanize and respect the opinions of others who espouse quite different worldviews. It can also provide a validity check on our own assumptions and a place to begin to speculate about our blind spots. Of course, the most important gifts of this text are a language for social workers to express the environmental implications of their models and practices and a new forum for dialogue.

It is important to realize that the worldview and movement known as environmentalism is diverse, constantly evolving, and often contradictory. For those immersed in the literature of environmentalism, it is clear that there are open questions about the movement, debates about its livelihood or 'death', and a stream of new incarnations as ecological paradigms integrate feedback from the perspectives of social equity, healthcare, multiculturalism, technology, business, politics, the arts and humanities, and spirituality and organized religion. To prejudge this text based on environmentalist stereotypes would be to miss the point. The pertinent question implied by this volume is 'How might social work change environmentalism?'

It is important to recognize the potential for self-criticism and judgment that comes with an environmental turn for social work, particularly among more altruistic and ecologically-minded practitioners. The initiative confronts entwined, social systemic 'wicked problems' and leads us head-on into needs, harms, injustice, the intractability of large systems, and quite naturally to feelings of threat, overwhelm, urgency, despair, and recrimination – that are all too easy to direct toward ourselves and others. (For insights into this phenomenon, we can take a few lessons from our psychoanalytic forbears.) Our challenge is as always to move forward with integrity, discipline, and compassion.

A consolation, as I noted at the outset, is that it might not be necessary to change your work, your setting, or the populations that you serve to make use of the ideas in this book. While it is true that the field of social work has been historically reluctant to embrace the environmental movement, it is also the case that social work has had its hands full, and many good people worked to the edge of their abilities to make possible what the field has accomplished. As we break down the artificial, conceptual barriers between 'environmental issues', 'human health issues', and 'social equity issues', we may find that we are working toward a similar, expanded, ecological vision of health. It is at moments like this that a glimpse of a shared vision of what some call the 'great work' provides sufficient information and inspiration needed to move forward.

Be well and good luck on your efforts,

Thomas Joseph Doherty, Psy.D.
Editor in Chief, *Ecopsychology*
Lewis & Clark Graduate School of Education and Counseling
Portland, Oregon, USA

Introduction

Overview of the last ten years and typology of ESW

Mel Gray, John Coates, and Tiani Hetherington

> The environment was born at exactly the moment when it became a problem (Morton, 2007: 141).

This book provides the first concerted overview and analysis of social work's relatively recent engagement with the modern environmental movement. It seeks to extend scholarship in this area beyond hortatory claims of what the profession ought to be doing to address environmental concerns. A recent special issue of the *International Journal of Social Welfare (vol 21)* was a precursor to the issues developed further in this book and reflected the emerging interest in environmental concerns for social work, raising questions about the profession's responsibility to the non-human world. In this introduction, we review the ecological discourse in social work in order to map the terrain of environmental social work and examine the profession's response to environmental concerns over the past ten years. While some positive steps have been taken, remaining challenges include a disconnection between the work of environmentalists and environmentally oriented NGOs, and social workers. Thus we attempt to address this important issue by drawing connections between these overlapping areas of practice.

To date, social work writing in this area tends to have a circular or insular nature in which a small group of scholars reaffirm one another's work, asserting their claims for social work's responsibility (see, for example, Molyneux's (2010) review of the ecosocial work literature), and that of all societies, for the pervasive impact of human activities that are exhausting non-renewable resources, pushing renewable resources to the brink of extinction, and polluting the air, water, and land with toxins that are significantly changing the functioning of the planet and killing and endangering many forms of life. Like broader writing in the field of ecology, social work writing in this area reflects its 'strong gravitational pull to the "new and improved" world' (Morton, 2007: 142) – the 'paradigm shift' or 'new paradigm' (Berry, 1999; Coates, 2003; Korten, 2009; Peeters, 2011; Rifkin, 2009). Typifying this trend is Schmitz *et al.*'s (2011) exhortative claim that 'a paradigm shift is needed to transform unsustainable, unrestrained, and unregulated capitalism into ecologically and socially sustainable economic practices, locally and globally' (p. 2). However, as Molyneux (2010) states:

> Disappointingly, while the [social work] literature did centre on the transactional relationship between people and their environment, it did not explore the practical application of this relationship. Instead, the literature overwhelmingly advocated that social work lead in creating a new vision for practice by critiquing the existing relationship between the natural environment and oppression. Approaches … appeared somewhat abstract, devoid of detail and detached from everyday interaction with service users. Perhaps this is due to the fact that their recommendations appeared to rely mostly on theorizing.
>
> (p. 66)

Calls for a paradigm shift within social work arise in the context of a developing ecological consciousness among social work scholars and practitioners, who see environmental social work as an essential though underdeveloped area of professional scholarship and practice. These scholars and practitioners argue for social work – and other professions – to break free of their academic silos and work in unison, or, at least cooperatively, to better understand and respond to the many dimensions of climate change and environmental destruction (see also Coates and Besthorn, 2010).

Most environmental social work scholars accept the scientific evidence where the predictions of disasters, such as drought, mudslides, floods, hurricanes, and environmental refugees, are seen to be influenced by climate change on a planet substantially altered by human activities, such as globalization, deforestation, pollution, industrial agriculture, habitat destruction, soil problems (acidification, desertification, erosion, salinization, and soil fertility losses), water management problems (including 'water wars' and dam construction interfering with waterways), overhunting, overfishing, effects of introduced species on native species, species decline and species extinction, human population growth, and increased per capita impact of people (Capra, 1982; Diamond, 2005; Godrej, 2001; Hofrichter, 1993; Shiva, 1989, 2003). Environmentalists, overall, call society to respond to the symptoms and causes of climate change and environmental degradation. There is general scientific agreement that we have now reached a period of 'peak oil', where we have now used over half of the world's original oil reserves (extraction has now reached its maximum level) and it is expected there will be a steady decline in the amount of oil available (Bardi, 2009; Hirsch, 2008). The excessive burning of fossil fuels is widely argued as a major source of carbon in the atmosphere as others argue for the significance of agribusiness – industrial agriculture – including monocultures and factory farms (methane production), excessive use of chemicals and packaging, and the transportation of food over thousands of kilometres. Prominent among all these activities is the externalization of the costs of production, such as releasing toxins directly into the environment, and the destruction of habitat in mining and oil extraction. The secondary effects, such as the release of methane as the permafrost thaws in the wake of global warming, will also contribute significantly to the increase in greenhouse gas emissions (Freeman *et al.*, 2004; Giddens, 2009; Jarman, 2007).

Global warming, arguably the most severe crisis facing humanity from an environmentalist's perspective, is occurring and demands that humanity as a whole addresses this problem 'before dangerous thresholds are breached by our unwitting collective activities' (McNeill, 2001: xvi). Despite the well-publicized but scientifically marginalized critiques of climate change (e.g., Durkin, 2007; Lomborg, 2001; Singer and Avery, 2007; Solomon, 2008), the vast majority of scientists are in agreement that climate change is happening and human activity has played a significant role (Gleick, 2011; Intergovernmental Panel on Climate Change (IPCC), 2001, 2007). The only critical debate remaining is a political one (Giddens, 2009) though Lomborg (2001) questions whether global warming is a more pressing issue than AIDS and world poverty. For environmentalists, the question is whether humanity will act in time to mitigate the most serious negative impacts of climate change. Responses to global warming can be as complex and diverse as its causes and consequences. What is at issue for environmental scholars is why there is so much resistance to effective intervention at global, national, and local levels. Some attribute this to the Western way of life with its focus on consumerism, individualism, and corporate market domination supported by adherence to the values and beliefs of what Giroux (2001) labels the 'neoliberal juggernaut' and its deregulation, privatization, and commodification. Urry (2010), too, sees a link between Western consumerism and wastefulness, and global neoliberalism.

With the public media carrying increasingly more stories on climate change and global warming following the Brundtland Commission (1987) and the several international efforts and gatherings addressing climate change, such as the Kyoto Protocol (United Nations, 1998), IPCC (2001, 2007), and Al Gore's *An Inconvenient Truth* (Laurie, Bender, Burns and Guggenheim, 2006), course texts began to give more than a passing mention of the relevance of the natural environment in social work practice in some quarters (see Hoff and McNutt, 1994; Van Wormer and Besthorn, 2011). Environmental social work scholars believe there is little doubt global warming will impact not only on the sociopolitical, economic, and physical environment in which social workers are engaged, but also on the type of work, both mitigating and adaptive, social workers will be called upon to carry out (Coates, 2003; Lysack, 2010; Polack, Wood, and Smith, 2010). The social consequences of climate change include the spread of tropical diseases, malnutrition, relocation and reunification of refugee and immigrant families, housing and food challenges, disaster relief, and changes to employment patterns.

A second front was the environmental justice movement, which focused on the negative consequences of industrial production and waste disposal experienced disproportionately by low-income and racialized groups (Bullard, 1990; Chavis and Lee, 1987). Over time, the focus was absorbed within an expanded environmental movement that now includes industrial pollution and toxic exposure and attention to the overall relationship of people to the physical environment, for example, transportation, and agricultural practices, use of fossil fuels, overharvesting and habitat destruction, alternative energy, urban design, community gardens and community-supported agriculture, environmentally related therapy, and structural inequalities related to the differential benefits and costs of climate change and the responses to it.

In recent years, social work has responded by expanding its theoretical considerations and practice interventions so that the physical environment, and human connectedness to the entire planet and all of life, became more central to social work discourse. A good example is Van Wormer and Besthorn (2011) *Human Behavior and Social Environment: Groups, Communities and Organizations*, which expands the traditional concern of social work texts as it gives serious attention to the environment, as well as spirituality, as central to social work practice. This publication followed closely on a number of other social work books incorporating environmental issues as central to social work practice, and has led some social work scholars to see the need to reconceptualize social work theory and practice (Coates, 2003; Mary, 2008; Zapf, 2009). In this social work discourse, the disregard of the natural environment was attributed to separation of humans from nature through modernization, industrialization, and urbanization. This dualism is foundational to modernist thinking, specifically the scientific paradigm, whereby humans are seen to be separate from and superior to nature. Dryzeck (2005) describes this as a 'promethean' view (associated with Western civilizations). It is also known as 'human exemptionalism' (see Catton and Dunlap, 1980). Environmentalists argue that humanity is part of nature whereby there are limits regarding the use of the world's resources, as each ecosystem has a unique 'carrying capacity'.

Environmental realities have played a significant role in pulling social work to re-evaluate its modernist foundations, and to shift from the primacy of therapy and rehabilitation to recognize humans' essential connection to all of nature, including all people and all life on the planet. Environmental social work scholars argue that effective professional interventions must address not only personal stress and family reactions to climate-related issues, but also significant lifestyle, community, and public policy issues in efforts to shift away from the current 'extractive economy' (Berry, 1999) that is exploiting nature and the majority of humanity toward a sustainable society (Besthorn, 2002; Coates, 2003; Hoff and McNutt, 1994; Mary, 2008).

Public policy issues include the need to prevent the exposure of people and wildlife to toxic chemicals, which are the by-product of industrial progress, and the exploration of the human rights violations and social injustices inherent in ecological degradation.

How then might practical solutions be mobilized? Is it necessary to sacrifice economic well-being for sustainability? The answer to these questions often centres on arguments as to the cause of the environmental crisis. Princen (2010), for example, blames prevailing consumerist norms that motivate overconsumption, believing 'what we take for normal is actually excess' (p. 12). Patel (2009) notes that if we calculated the environmental costs from clearing forests to graze beef, and the huge public health expenditure associated with obesity, the true cost of a McDonald's hamburger would be in excess of US$200 dollars. Consequently, Patel (2009) and Princen's (2010) solution is a 'new normal' around which consumer expectations and aspirations can be formed. Princen (2010) also intimates that a change in focus and tone from conventional environmental discourse is needed if imperatives of sustainability are to be realized.

Not only does the ecologocentric realm accept as problematic the priority of overconsumption and consumerism, but also the goal of 'a restricted economy in which elements of the ecosystem get fed back into it perfectly without excess' (Morton, 2007: 157). In his *Growth Fetish*, Hamilton (2003) argues for an alternative to the dominance of economic growth and consumption, and the consumer spending indicators of economic health and well-being. Likewise, Schor (2010) in *Plentitude* argues that environmentalism needs a 'new narrative' if it is to effectively reorient human behaviour to ensure well-being for all. For Schor (2010), ecological regeneration and restoration have obvious environmental but also salutary social justice and community solidarity benefits.

In much of the environmental scholarship in social work, the centrality and essentiality of nature, especially of 'place', is uncritically celebrated (Zapf, 2005a, 2005b, 2009). As Morton (2007) notes in relation to ecological discourse generally, globalization is said to have 'undermined any coherent sense of place ... Such thinking aims to conserve a piece of the world ... from the ravages of industrial capitalism and its ideologies' (p. 84). Morton (2007) places all ecology and nature writing under the umbrella of 'environmental Romanticism' so, from his perspective, it overlooks the subject embedded within this discourse – the subject from whose position it is written and the subjects about whom it is written:

> Place and the local, let alone nation, entail subject positions – places from which Romantic ideas of place make sense. For this reason, it is all the more important to consider deeply the idea of place, and in general the Romantic attitude to nature prevalent today.
>
> (Morton, 2007: 84)

Environmental writers like Abrams, Dillard, and Thoreau, who uncritically adopt romantic notions of place as best left untouched by human intervention or hark back to a time when humans lived harmoniously with nature, overlooking scientific progress and modern achievements, are, according to Morton (2007), preventing serious engagement with the consequences of environmental damage and climate change. This is where dedicated environmental scholars, such as Berry (1999), Coates (2003), Diamond (2007), Korten (2009), and Spretnak (1990), part company with Morton (2007). Environmental writers appreciate that humans have always exploited (and destroyed) environments (see Diamond, 2007) and would agree with Morton (2007) that it is unrealistic to expect people to return to some other time in history or place unsullied by humans, as the answer to today's problems. Many environmental writers would agree that modern individual identities – subjectivities – are consumerist. People want the modern comforts. People want what progress offers and they want economic development, and few would deny that there are many advantages to modernity (see, for example, Capra, 1982; Coates, 2003; Dylan and Coates, 2012). Perhaps this is highlighted most by the environmental concerns raised between the Global North and South, those that outline concerns between the 'rich' and 'poor', 'victim' and 'perpetrator', 'developed' and 'developing' nations and ultimately lead to a political blame game for global warming. However, what Capra (1982), Coates (2003), and Shiva (2003) challenge, and what Morton (2007) seems not to appreciate, is the inequality and exploitation in the production and distribution of the benefits of technology. Further, as the unregulated use of technology spreads and the population increases, environmental and social injustices become more severe. They also challenge the current dominant belief in the myth of progress and unending economic growth (the challenge to sustainability that the Brundtland Commission (1987) brought into public view).

Connections between social work and broader ecological discourse

While Morton (2007) would entreat environmental social workers to realize that they were writing from within an already existing ecological discourse which is moulding their claims *vis-à-vis* nature and the environment, it is important also not to lose sight of the important alternatives to modernity they propose and the complexity of environmental and social problems. From this enlarged perspective, among the varied themes social work shares with the broader ecological discourse are the following:

Respect for ecological limits: Nature is a scarcity that must be conserved – natural resources are finite and depletable (Peeters, 2011; World Commission on Environment and Development (WCED), 1987). Each ecosystem has a 'carrying capacity' – the population of a specific species that can exist in a given environment – which, if exceeded, may lead to ecological degradation, species decline, and eventually ecosystem collapse (Dryzek, 2005). With the human species reaching unprecedented levels of population and affluence, humans are exceeding the carrying capacity of the planet (WWF, 2010). The activities of industrial societies, especially the creation and release of increasing volumes of carbon dioxide, are believed to be causing massive damage to ecosystems, threatening the entire planet through global warming.

Environmental sustainability: Although the term 'environmental sustainability' has become somewhat of an overused cliché (Fuller, 2010), population growth and the spread of technology must be balanced with a view to the consequences on the limited resources of Earth and its uniquely balanced life-sustaining processes. The WCED (1987) established a strong connection between poverty, food insecurity, social inequality, environmental degradation, sustainability, and development (see Schmitz *et al.*, 2011). Harper (2008) has suggested there seem to be a number of straightforward measures that might be adopted to promote environmental sustainability: stabilizing the human population; putting constraints on excess material consumption; and developing and employing new, efficient technologies that are environmentally benign.

Global ecological justice: In the context of the neoliberal market-oriented consumerist paradigm of exploitation, there is a need for regulation to protect the majority of humans as well as the Earth from anthropogenic destruction or unintended ecological suicide or ecocide (Diamond, 2005). At its heart, environmental justice concerns the just allocation of natural resources (Hoff and Polack, 1993): '[E]nvironmental justice ecocriticism … considers how environmental destruction, pollution, and the oppression of specific classes and races go hand in hand' (Morton, 2007: 10). Early and more recent scholarship on the environment in social work, as outlined above, used frameworks of environmental justice (see, for example, Besthorn, 2003, 2004; Dylan and Coates, 2012; Hoff and Polack, 1993; Hoff and McNutt, 1994).

Environmental preservation: Wilderness must be protected as it provides an antidote to materialism. While earlier environmental writers have written of the environment as wilderness, which humanity should leave alone, more recent scholars recognize the fact that all species impact upon and change the environment (Diamond, 2005; Swimme and Berry, 1992). Humans, plants, and animals change the environment as they live – this is fundamental to evolution. Earth's surface is largely the product of interactions among organisms (soil, rainwater, savannahs, forests, coral reefs, limestone, coal, and oil, to name a few). Rather than being separate from nature, humans have always been involved in their world even as they judge it (Morton, 2007). In light of contemporary knowledge, technology, and the number of humans, the bigger question today is under what conditions will humans live, and what role will they take in establishing those conditions.

The political philosophies of environmental social movements: Place is endangered or made potent by its absence or loss – real or threatened – in notions like 'solastalgia' (Albrecht *et al.*, 2007). The solution lies in ecological awareness and action. Hence educational efforts are very important and must lead to changes in social and political behaviour (Coates, 2003; Besthorn, 2004; Besthorn and Canda, 2002; Lysack, 2011). Today, three component groupings have been identified as comprising the environmental movement: grassroots, community-based groups; formal professionally based organizations with a largely reformist agenda; and radical ecologically focused groups committed to direct action (One World, 2012). Social workers engaged in environmental movements have the opportunity to lead developments in environmental practice and policy. The profession has the responsibility to engage with communities suffering from imminent or current environmental damage. This may take the form of advocating for change, engaging in political activism, or community organizing: 'The main point stressed is that social workers should act as political actors, and that they should have a political agenda and the possibility to guide society in the direction of sustainable development' (Närhi and Matthies, 2001: 33).

Environmental ethics: There is emerging interest in environmental ethics for social work, raising questions about the profession's responsibility to the non-human world. Gray and Coates (2011) asked whether moral or ethical grounds could be established to support claims relating to social workers' duties, obligations, responsibilities, and commitments to the non-human world. They provided an overview of the field of environmental ethics in searching for moral stance to affirm an environmental social work. They asked to what extent social workers should be engaged, and on what basis, in fundamental geopolitical issues concerned with climate change, global warming, environmental degradation, pollution, chemical contamination, sustainable agriculture, disaster management, wilderness protection, and so on.

Deep Ecology: Fred Besthorn has actively promoted the importance of Deep Ecology for social work education and practice, believing it offers an essentially different view of the person–environment construct and a fundamental shift in the way humanity views its relationship with nature. Deep Ecology moves away from anthropocentrism as it sees humans as interdependent and connected to all of nature. Human well-being is only possible in the context of the well-being of all life – a healthy and thriving Earth. In light of this innate connection, Deep Ecology raises questions about the proper role of the human on the planet. Besthorn's most recent contribution is a retrospective on Deep Ecology's contribution to social work over the last decade (Besthorn, 2011).

Religion and spirituality: A re-enchantment of the world is needed to compensate for the rampant materialism and 'spiritual depletion of modernity' (Morton, 2007: 87). Many religious and spiritual writers have noted the decline of religious affiliation (Bibby, 1987; Coates, Gray, and

Hetherington, 2006; Roof, 1999) and the human search for meaning that leads many people toward spiritual paths. Dylan and Coates (2012) argue for the role that spirituality can play in linking ecological and social justice. As Gray (2008) stated: 'We need an outward focussed eco-spiritual social work in which spirituality is "other" rather than self-centred, and not anthropocentric since it embraces all life forms as well as sustainability for the planet' (p. 192). Among others, Coates (2003) and Lysack (2011) have examined ways in which eco-social workers interested in religion and spirituality might play a role through social networks that care and advocate for the Earth, such as faith communities and practices of community engagement and public education.

Biophilia hypothesis: Several writers use Wilson's (1984) biophilia hypothesis about humans' innate need to associate with the natural world and advance this connection as a way to enhance human physical and psychological well-being drawing on research from a wide range of disciplines on the health benefits of nature (Besthorn and Saleebey, 2003; Clinebell, 1996; Heinsch, 2011). As Berry (1999: 98) notes:

> It is the destruction of the world in our own lives that drives us half insane, and more than half. To destroy that which we were given in trust: how will we bear it? To have lost, wantonly, the ancient forests, the vast grasslands is our madness, the presence in our very bodies of our grief.

While this has relevance at the micro level, in seeking to develop an eco-critical perspective, mindful of Morton's (2007) thesis, we need to ensure that social work writing on nature and place does not obstruct engagement with ecological politics.

Indigenous worldviews: Morrissette, McKenzie, and Morrissette (1993) argued that the distinctiveness of Aboriginal worldviews and traditions included their historical development 'involving a symbiotic relationship to the earth and a belief in the delicate balance among all things' (p. 93). They suggested this intimate and respectful relationship had resulted in a spiritual consciousness based on survival needs and a belief in people's responsibility to live in harmony with Earth's resources. This fundamental view of Earth as a sacred living thing is important to many Indigenous Peoples (Baskin, 2011; Holthaus; 2008). Such Indigenous worldviews are in tension with capitalist agendas based on exploiting the Earth, and dominant science perspectives implying human control over nature, because they cultivate harmony between humans and all living things, and see the entire world as interrelated, thriving, and unstable (Baskin, 2002). If social work wishes to continue to cite social justice, human well-being and empowerment as central principles, then, argues Muldoon (2006), the preservation of the natural environment must become of primary importance.

Ecopsychology and ecofeminism: Feminists have long argued that gender inequalities and the feminization of poverty expose women to higher risk with fewer resources for addressing oppressive environmental conditions (Demetriades and Esplen, 2010). Ecofeminist scholars, such as Merchant (1990), Plant (1989), Ruether (1992), Shiva (1989, 2003), and Spretnak (1990), have challenged the patriarchy, capitalism, and economism (to name a few) that have resulted in the exploitation of women and Earth. This complements racist and class analyses that point to the racialized nature of exploitation:

> Ecofeminist criticism ... examines ways in which patriarchy has been responsible for environmental deterioration and destruction, and for sustaining a view of the natural world that oppresses women in the same way it oppresses animals, life in general, and even matter itself.
>
> (Morton, 2007: 9)

Some environmental social work scholars have broadened social work's ecosystems perspective by embracing insights from ecopsychology and ecofeminism relating to the parallel oppressions of women and nature, the concepts of deep empathy and empowerment (Besthorn, 2003; Besthorn and McMillen, 2002; Norton, 2009, 2011).

Interdisciplinarity: Environmental work is inevitably interdisciplinary. It involves a wide array of knowledge from the contested science of global warming; scientific studies on air, water, and soil pollution; habitat destruction and species extinction; sustainable agricultural practices; and globalization and trade policies, to name a few. As noted by McNeill (2001), the 'ecological history of the planet and the socioeconomic history of humanity make sense only if seen together' (p. xxvi). This interdisciplinarity has led some social workers into alliances with a broad range of academic scholars, community educators, faith-based groups, and social activists from many fields – psychology (Norton, 2009), anthropology (Tester, 1983), science, philosophy (Besthorn, 2011), political science, particularly peace and conflict studies (Schmitz *et al.*, 2010, 2011), and corporate social responsibility (Ross, 2009) in their efforts to explore effective responses across levels of theory and practice development. This has resulted in an evolving theory, though one that has yet to be accepted as a consistent, overarching framework for environmental social work practice.

Environmental movement and social work engagement

A review of the recent history of social work's engagement on environmental issues (see Coates and Gray, 2011) essentially reveals three major trends:

1   *From the early 1970s onwards,* a raft of literature from social work scholars who introduced ecological concepts and opened social work to initial conceptualizations of environmental issues (e.g., Germain, 1973; Grinnell, 1973; Meyer, 1970, 1983). These writers helped to move the profession away from the prominence of psychodynamic forces toward consideration of interactions, assets, and limitations among the systems involved with a client's life. The ecological approach and systems' thinking (Pincus and Minahan, 1973) provided a major step forward as social workers now had an effective way to conceptualize the various 'sub-systems' in the social environment.

2   *In the late 1980s and 1990s,* there was a resurgence of interest in environmental issues (e.g., Berger and Kelly, 1993; Besthorn, 1997; Hoff and McNutt, 1994; Hoff and Polack, 1993; Marlow and van Rooyen, 2001; Park, 1996; Rogge, 1994a, 1994b; Soine, 1987). Several of these scholars drew attention to the work of the environmental justice movement (see, for example, Bullard, 1990, 1993; Chavis and Lee, 1987; Hofrichter, 1993; Pulido. 1996; Sachs, 1995). These publications drew attention to the negative impacts of industrial pollution, the dumping of industrial waste and agricultural practices – spraying and run-off – resulting in exposure to toxins in water, soil, and air. These authors first drew attention to racial and class-based injustices in the USA (see Rogge, 1994a), and then to injustices around the globe. Most of this scholarship was general in focus, urging social workers' involvement in environmental issues or sketching broad outlines of how the profession might respond to environmental concerns.

3   *In more recent years,* various authors have again called for social work to embrace a broader view of the 'physical environment', including a focus on 'place' and spirituality, and its impact on human well-being (Besthorn, 2000, 2001; Coates, 2003; Mary, 2008; Zapf, 2009). The website 'Global Alliance for Deep-Ecological Social Work' was developed by Besthorn (2001) to encourage dialogue and interest in Deep Ecology and extend social work practice beyond the social to the natural environment. Environmental social work scholars, like Besthorn (2001, 2002) and Coates (2003), blame the profession's overall reluctance to accept the importance of environmental issues for social work and the profession's failure to see connections between human well-being and environmental issues on the dominance of the therapeutic model in North America for the shallow, exclusively social interpretation of social work's longstanding 'person-in-environment' focus. Much environmental scholarship within social work berates the person-in-environment configuration or ecosystems approach for limiting attention to the connection between individuals and their social environment. It attributes the profession's reluctance to engage in environmental issues and the environmental movement to this narrow or shallow view of the environment, where often the physical

environment is treated simply as a modifier or context (Besthorn, 1997, 2002; Coates, 2003; Zapf, 2005a, 2009). Also, environmental social work scholars argue that Western knowledge systems, ideologies, and social care and development methods are not only inappropriate, but also totally inadequate for addressing the major crises confronting our planet – ecological, spiritual, social, economic, and security (Coates, 2003; Gray, Coates, and Hetherington, 2007).

This history of social work's engagement with the environment reveals some major trends and gaps in environmental social work scholarship that are developed further in the book. First, while social work scholarship is slowly changing, the tendency to berate the narrow person-in-environment and ecosystems perspective for failing to take account of the natural environment persists:

> If the physical environment is consistently dropped from the diagrammed models of practice, it comes as no surprise that the assessment tools offered in mainstream practice textbooks concentrate primarily on aspects of social functioning, social networks, and social roles ... Organizing data for an assessment using genograms and eco-maps limits the view to the social environment.
>
> (Zapf, 2009: 33)

Second, environmental literature in social work calls for a 'new paradigm' – a transition to a sustainable society. Peeters (2011) enumerates the crux of 'new paradigm' thinking in relation to sustainable development as concerning: (1) A dematerialization of the economy, which means a substantial reduction in the input and throughput of natural resources including energy; (2) the fair distribution of wealth; and (3) a new vision of human and planetary well-being. This he says requires

> changes in all aspects of society: ecological, technological, economic, social, political, structural-institutional, and parallel changes in the most important subsystems of society: energy production and consumption, the monetary systems, the mobility pattern of people, food production and distribution, and the organization of labour and care systems.
>
> (Peeters, 2011: 4)

Third, implicit in the call for a 'new paradigm' is a critique of modernity and capitalism (Coates, 2003) though modern notions of 'human rights' and 'social justice' are retained as an essential element of 'ecological justice'. In fact, according to Coates (2003) and Peeters (2011), among others, these modern ideas are central to the new paradigm – hence the tendency to take a rights-based approach to climate change and to attribute environmental degradation to the worst effects of capitalism (Hoff and Polack, 1993).

Fourth, since many social workers value critical theory, environmentalism can be seen as a way to both revive the radicalism that disappeared with the demise of socialism and the entrenchment of neoliberal welfare reform, and renew critiques of capitalism which many critical theorists regard as the root cause of the problems society faces today (Coates, 2003).

Fifth, there is a tendency to link spirituality and place by displacing the exploitation of nature – as resource – with the view of nature as sacred and where human actions fit within the innate rhythms and limits of the Earth reflecting Indigenous connections with space and place (Baskin, 2011; Zapf, 2009).

Sixth, interdisciplinarity, including calls for a broad (interdisciplinary) knowledge base and working in unison with other professions in order to respond effectively to the many dimensions of climate change and environmental degradation, is a major theme in social work discourse on the environment (see below). Hence this discourse claims that responding to the challenges of environmental destruction has opened opportunities for the profession to review its foundational knowledge and obligations to people and environments (see, for example, Dylan and Coates, 2012). The search is on for theoretical frameworks, examples, and case studies of what social workers are doing, or might do, in relation to environmental and educational initiatives.

Issues	Interventions
Destruction of natural resources, including mining and industrial damage	**Issue** Earth's resources are finite and attitudinal and lifestyle changes are needed to curb humans' profligate habits of energy use, environmentally destructive mining and industrial practices, and greed-driven consumerism. **Interventions** *Micro* • Lifestyle counselling and individually oriented mental health and personal growth initiatives aimed at changing consumption-oriented values • Crisis intervention with individuals and families who have lost employment due to mining development or had drinking water contaminated • Direct practice and consultation on sustainable economic development and corporate social responsibility *Mezzo* • Educational programs teaching about scarcity and environmental destruction, e.g., alternative lifestyles (simple living and voluntary simplicity movement), public vs. private transportation) • Development of conservation and recycling programs • Ecosystem restoration programs • Sustainable community development *Macro* • Initiation and monitoring of policy change and enforcement to protect and restore natural resources • Social action and advocacy around patenting of genetic materials (protect biodiversity and reduce corporate commodification of life) • Support for Indigenous rights and control over their lands

Issues	Interventions

Global warming and climate change

Issue

Earth's dependence on fossil fuels – oil, gas, and coal – for energy is widely argued as the major source of carbon in the atmosphere and reducing our dependence on them is imperative for mitigating climate change: 'The debate about the limits of the world's fossil fuel resources is of great consequence for climate change' (Giddens, 2009: 38).

Interventions

Micro
- Health intervention with skin cancer and other diseases
- Crisis intervention and recovery assistance for victims of floods, tornados, and other climate-related disasters (e.g., drought and bush fires)
- Intervention with people affected by solastalgia and psychoterratic illness

Mezzo
- Education programs to raise awareness on the dangers of global warming and climate change and the value and behaviour changes needed
- Integrate low-income housing into urban design that reduces fossil fuel consumption
- Develop organic community gardens, tree planting, and reforestation programs

Macro
- Develop and support bicycle and pedestrian-friendly urban design
- Initiate and monitor enforcement of policy changes on pollution emissions
- Redirect policy toward green energy solutions (wind and solar power development)
- Develop and support public education programs (e.g., Earth Hour)

Toxic materials production and waste disposal

Issue

Exposure of low-income, marginalized and racialized communities, especially children, to toxins

Interventions

Micro
- Crisis intervention for stress issues – individuals, families (especially impacts on children), workers and communities
- Material emergency services (health, housing, and income)
- Case finding for workplace-based illnesses

Mezzo
- Educational programs on the dangers of toxic materials and safety precautions and on the use of alternative, non-toxic materials (i.e., environmentally safe household cleaning products)
- Coordination of health and social interventions around hazards; community relocation and community development for victims of hazardous waste accidents or irremediable sites
- Social Impact Analysis of sites for production facilities

Macro
- Policy development and enforcement of workplace safety standards
- Advocacy for research on development of non-toxic products for workplace and home
- Advocacy for monetary compensation and psychological recovery programs for victims of toxic waste

Issues	Interventions
Air, soil, and water pollution	**Issue** Health-related issues are seen to result directly from or be exacerbated by air, soil, and water pollution **Interventions** *Micro* • Crisis intervention and other mental health intervention for stress caused by exposure (e.g. support groups for asthma sufferers) • Health assessment and interventions aimed at children (e.g. lead levels) *Mezzo* • Health services for persons with acute or chronic illnesses (e.g. asbestos-related diseases) • Development of public education programs about the dangers of air and water pollution and citizen involvement in clean-up campaigns *Macro* • Improve public monitoring and enforcement of air, soil, and water quality standards • Promote and enforce policy change to reduce air, soil, and water pollution • Develop advocacy programs for victims of air, soil, and water pollution (especially in low-income communities) • Support research and social impact analysis
Species extinction	**Issue** When species decline or become extinct, so does biodiversity. Biodiversity is essential to the planet in providing ecosystem health. If species are eliminated this can weaken the ecosystem, reducing both its productivity and its ability to adapt to change. **Interventions** *Micro* • Mental health and personal growth initiatives oriented toward changing consumer-oriented values and consumption patterns endangering species *Mezzo* • Educational initiatives to teach about ecological science (species interdependency) and sustainability • Development of habitat conservation programs • Support Indigenous Peoples' involvement in conservation initiatives on their traditional lands *Macro* • Sustainable economic development initiatives with communities to support species preservation • Community and family-based sustainable agriculture (research and policy on community-based food systems) • Improved policy measures to support endangered species and habitat • Support for preservation of agricultural seed diversity • Advocacy and public education on the dangers and social injustices of corporate patenting of life-forms

Issues	Interventions
Sustainable development and food security	**Issue** Development that meets the needs of the present without compromising that ability of future generations to meet their own needs. Food security exists when sufficient quantities of safe, nutritious foods are available to all peoples, at all times. **Interventions** *Micro* • Community gardens in low-income neighbourhoods • Educational initiatives around food consumption and transportation patterns *Mezzo* • Social and environmental justice efforts to confront the ill effects of globalization • Support for local fresh grown produce and farmers markets *Macro* • Urban agriculture, and community-supported agriculture to create employment, sustainable livelihoods, and food security • Support national and international policies that enable poverty reduction and food security in less developed countries. • Protests against investments by food-deficient, but wealthy countries and corporations in the farming systems of poorer countries
Natural disasters and traumatic events, including drought and floods	**Issue** Disasters, such as drought, mudslides, floods, hurricanes and environmental refugees, are seen to be influenced by climate change on a planet substantially altered by human activities like globalization, deforestation, pollution, industrial agriculture, and dam construction. **Interventions** *Micro* • Crisis intervention with survivors and provision of disaster relief services *Mezzo* • Community educational initiatives around preparing for an emergency, having a safe evacuation plan and the importance of having emergency survival kits *Macro* • Planning for the reception of environmental refugees • Supporting alternatives to dam construction, deforestation and monoculture.

Figure I.1 Typology of social work practice on environmental issues

Environmental themes in social work scholarship

The varied but interrelated themes outlined in Figure I.1 reflect the diversity of areas in which environmentally concerned social workers are or might be engaged. However, this diversity raises questions as to the nature of environmental social work: What role does social work have to play in terms of the social and environmental changes required for a sustainable future?

In what ways can social workers incorporate the natural environment into their direct work with clients? What can the social work profession specifically do in terms of macro, mezzo, and micro environmental social work practice interventions and, moreover, what does environmental social work look like in practice? Anecdotal evidence suggests many environmental social workers are practising on the margins (i.e., they are practitioners who are 'doing' environmental social work in diverse practice contexts but not necessarily 'writing' about these interventions in social work fora).

This book is a first attempt to introduce theoretical frameworks and concrete examples and case studies of what social workers are doing – or might do – in relation to environmental issues and educational initiatives. It brings together several international social work scholars who apply their knowledge and experience to examine the most significant global trends and issues relating to the development of environmental social work, and to share and discuss ways in which environmental concerns are shaping a more inclusive and holistic social work practice. Increased interest in environmental issues and concerns emerging in response to various manifestations of ecological destruction has opened avenues for social work to explore its obligations to people and environments as they experience the impact of globalization and international 'development' efforts. While historically somewhat reluctant to embrace the environmental movement, the profession of social work with its ecosystems or person-in-environment approach is, according to environmental scholars, well placed to contribute to the response to environmental issues at the micro, mezzo, and macro levels of practice. This book is divided into three sections: Part 1: Theory: Mapping the terrain of environmental social work; Part 2: Practice: Case studies of environmental social work practice, and Part 3: Education: Challenging students to respond to environmental issues.

In Part 1, we look at theory and map the terrain of environmental social work. In Chapter 1 *Fred Besthorn* examines ecological and social justice. He outlines deep ecological social work as a foundation to revitalize the profession. The environmental and social justice logic of a deep ecological social work portends nothing short of radical change in the social, political, and economic structures of modern, industrial society. Adopting a new ecological framework would change the identity of conventional social work. It calls for the profession to return to and significantly expand upon its progressive, activist roots. It suggests the profession has an obligation to examine all oppressive political, social, economic, and environmental structures of modern society and the policies which extend them. It requires social workers to become professionally involved and personally committed both within and outside the confines of the office, agency, and academy to implement change to protect the planet and all its inhabitants.

Tiani Hetherington and *Jenny Boddy* (Chapter 2) discuss social work interventions with marginalized populations affected by climate change. There is a paucity of social work commentary in the academic literature on how environmental matters affect disadvantaged populations and on social work responses. The adverse effects of climate change on marginalized people and communities mean that social workers need to respond appropriately for the well-being of current and future generations. This chapter explores the potential effects of climate change on marginalized peoples and proposes a model of social work practice that includes strategies for respecting and promoting environmentally sustainable practices at the micro and macro levels. Despite repeated calls in the literature for social work's unique person-in-environment construct to be reconceptualized to incorporate not only the built and social environments but also the natural environment, mainstream social work has yet to take up this challenge. Yet there are opportunities for social workers to work with disadvantaged communities and participate in environmental movements through interdisciplinary practice opportunities, international collaborations, social activism, and policy development. This chapter provides several examples of successful social work engagement in this area to counteract inequalities resulting from environmentally unsustainable policies inherent in economic rationalist and politically conservative ideologies in an effort to further the discourse on environmental social work scholarship, education, and activism.

In Chapter 3, *Arielle Dylan* explores environmental sustainability and social work and asks what it means to be sustainable and what this implies for social work practice. Sustainable development refers to development meeting the needs of present generations without jeopardizing the ability of future generations to meet their needs. Problems such as poverty, environmental degradation, political unrest, social injustice, and warfare are all interconnected. It follows that solutions must sustain environmental, social, and political systems in the long term. If social work is to continue to be a viable, meaningful profession addressing the problems of our age, then it must consider a paradigm to help secure a sustainable future for us all. Dylan outlines a model for social work practice in a sustainable world and explores opportunities for translating this knowledge into strategies in clinical, community, and policy practice.

Sue Taylor (Chapter 4) examines social work, the environment, and healing, and asks whether the profession can move toward the notion of living in full partnership with a living conscious environment sustaining life and toward which humans have powerful and respectful obligations for mutual survival. She argues the broad notion of spirituality found in the social work literature has the potential to transform social work's limited notion of person and environment, if human beings came to understand themselves as elements of a living environment. When social work moves toward a perspective of 'person as environment', they can begin to see themselves as dynamic components of a living system. Such transformation calls social work to look beyond interpersonal relationships to the very nature of human spiritual connection with the planet – to literally find their 'common ground'.

In Chapter 5, *Frank Tester* advocates climate change as a human rights issue. He positions climate change as a human rights problem and argues the dominant growth–profit model is completely at odds with a perspective taking action to protect the health and welfare of the planet. Drawing on examples from the Canadian Arctic which highlight the current 'moral bankruptcy' over issues of climate change, the author contends climate change must become a discourse and, moreover, an action guided by human rights. Tester argues radical change is needed and a human rights perspective can assist this process with its emphasis on our human collective responsibility for one other. So how can social workers connect human rights to environmental concerns? The profession's value base toward social justice makes it ideally placed to make an important contribution to environmental issues facing the planet. Implications and potential practice actions social workers can take are also discussed.

Part 2 focuses on practice and presents case studies in environmental practice. In Chapter 6, *Ben Shepard* presents a case study of his involvement in community gardens, creative community organizing, and environmental activism in New York. He outlines the potential for social workers to be involved in community activism by tracing the history of the *More Gardens Coalition*, a successful campaign to save urban gardens in New York City. Community gardens are located mostly in areas of poor neighbourhoods, highest asthma levels, high density housing, and lowest income. The community gardeners have brought safety, food, beauty, fresh air, and sense of community back to their streets and people. Given their orientation to civic rather than commercial purposes, these public spaces have faced myriad threats from corporate globalizers, real estate, and social pressures against unregulated open public space, especially in the last ten years. Shepard describes the More Gardens Coalition and its fight to preserve public space for those at the margins. Through creative community organizing, it builds a diverse coalition to defend community gardens and represents a best practice case study in organizing against urban gentrification. This case study offers images of how regular people can stake a claim and successfully build the components necessary to create healthy communities.

Daniela Stehlik (Chapter 7) discusses social work practice with drought-affected families in Australia, where there has been renewed interest in the impact of longstanding drought and its longer-term consequences. However, the social impacts of drought have been underexplored. This chapter outlines the importance of varied, accessible, and appropriate services and information to improve the quality of life for women and their families in regional, rural, and remote areas of Australia during periods of climatic variability or drought. Building social capital in such times requires trust-based partnerships between individuals, community stakeholders, and the public sector. How might social workers become involved in seeking solutions to this issue? The potential for micro and macro practice interventions is discussed.

In Chapter 8, *Thomas Ryan* shows animals, too, are part of the family in his discussion of an extended moral framework for social work practice. Given the focus on environmental social work, this chapter makes the overall argument that respect and concern for the environment cannot be conceptualized as being circumscribed by the interests and well-being of human beings. The natural world is not here to environ merely the human animal. The increasing recognition that the human species is deeply embedded within the natural world is a most gratifying development, serving to redress the anthropocentrism that has characterized social work's worldview. Remaining largely unacknowledged is the moral claims of our fellow creatures – the non-human animals with which the world is shared. An abiding concern for habitats and ecosystems should obviously include the interests of non-domestic animals, and the fact that domesticated animals are part and parcel of the social environment, the world within which social workers practise, should, of necessity, serve to widen the scope of social work's moral compass. Indeed, animals are routinely regarded as family members by many of those people with whom social workers work, and by social workers themselves in their private lives. Practice scenarios are presented to tease out the moral obligations owed by social workers to both the people and animals involved.

Christine Lynn Norton, Barbara Holguin, and *Jarid Manos* (Chapter 9) examine how social workers engage in environmental initiatives as part of a holistic eco-social work program for young offenders – 'Restoration Not Incarceration' – offered by the Great Plains Restoration Council in Houston, Texas. Its dual focus is the 'restoration' of the prairies, bayous, wetlands, and Gulf Coast shore and 'rehabilitation' of juveniles in the Harris County Corrections System. The program promotes environmentally friendly values as part of productive work: Restoring the land restores human well-being. It uses nature as a vehicle to reintegrate young people into society, prevent recidivism, and achieve improved life outcomes. The chapter describes this multidisciplinary program focusing in particular on social workers' contribution to the program.

In Chapter 10, *Dyann Ross* explores social work and the struggle for corporate social responsibility, noting social work has a valuable knowledge and skills set to inform debates and practice in the area of corporate social responsibility. How might social workers engage in the struggle between multinational corporate mining companies and impacted neighbouring communities? Drawing on research from the small town of Yarloop in Western Australia in the conflict over social, health, and environmental concerns associated with mining, this chapter explores the need for social justice for people and sustainability for the local environment. Profit unhinged from the parallel considerations of people and place threatens sustainability as well as social justice. A key insight is the creative potential of building stakeholder relationships in collaboratively dialoguing about the conflict to find common ground and ways forward.

Part 3 examines how social work education challenges social work students and the local community to respond to environmental issues beginning with *Peter Jones'* (Chapter 11) discussion of preparing social work students for ecosocial 'just' practice. As a profession, social work has been relatively slow, some would say reluctant, to begin exploring the ways in which it might contribute to the challenges presented by the current and looming ecological crisis. However, there are clear signs issues of the natural environment are finally beginning to push themselves into the consciousness of the profession, as both the causes and consequences of issues – such as climate change – emerge with greater clarity. As a result of this growing awareness, there is also recognition social work practitioners need to be better equipped with specific knowledge, skills, and values on the 'natural' environment if the profession is to play a role in addressing the ecological crisis. This presents a clear challenge for social work education. Jones explores social work education and how it might prepare students for practice founded in principles of ecosocial justice and an environmental orientation. The author reviews the environmental, ecological, and sustainability content of key social work education journals, as well as the availability of social work degree programs that include content with a specific focus on the 'natural' environment. Through describing an example of environmentally oriented social work education, the author attempts to capture a sense of where social work education stands in terms of environmental concerns and where it might need to go in the future.

Mishka Lysack (Chapter 12) examines ways to engage the local community with environmental issues and explores linkages between environmental community-based education and the creation of conditions for environmental citizenship and advocacy. How might social workers engage or deepen community members' sense of motivation and commitment to acting on climate change? Drawing on examples from the Alberta Acts program in Canada, whose mandate is to increase 'environmental citizenship' from community members, the author outlines the community engagement processes whereby residents are encouraged to identify the climate change solutions they believe are appropriate for their own communities. Opportunities and potential strategies for social work practitioner involvement and social work education are discussed.

Anna Hayward, Shari Miller, and *Terry Shaw* (Chapter 13) explore social workers' beliefs about environmental issues and argue much more needs to be done to infuse social work with an understanding of the interplay between human society and the natural environment. Social workers need to continue to examine issues surrounding environmental justice and develop methods to address racial and socio-economic inequities. By becoming more aware of the effects of environmental issues, the social work profession might be able to increasingly instigate positive personal and systemic changes.

Cathryne Schmitz, Tom Matyók, Channelle James, and *Lacey Sloan* (Chapter 14) examine responses to the complexity of environmental transformation through educating social workers to work in multidisciplinary response teams. The interconnection between environmental concerns and issues of peace, war, and natural disasters are explored, focusing on the role of multidisciplinary education and transformative learning environment where students experience the dilemmas and the strengths of engagement in team projects and are thus enriched through envisioning, creating, and designing solutions to address the complex factors involved in meaningful and sustainable change. In this chapter, the role of the university and the place of social work are the focus as multidisciplinary courses, curriculum development, and integration across the curriculum are highlighted, models are presented, dilemmas encountered are shared, resultant changes are described, strengths outlined, and student projects highlighted – one at the local level and another with global implications – as exemplars of potential value.

Lena Dominelli (Chapter 15) explores social work education for disaster relief work, arguing communities need to be prepared for natural and human-made disasters because these can strike anywhere, regardless of location, culture or history. The literature on disaster management reveals vulnerable populations tend to be the ones suffering most. How can social workers play important roles in disaster management response? How might disaster relief be incorporated into social work education? Drawing on examples from the Chilean earthquake and tsunami disaster, this chapter outlines how the social work profession can be involved in responding to and rebuilding communities affected by natural disasters.

These chapters mirror the diversity of environmental activity and the methodology involved, and reveal partnerships with other professionals, churches, businesses, and community service organizations. The significant level of collaboration appears more common than not. In the conclusion, we build from the chapters and draw from this and additional literature to identify new directions for social theory development, and social work educational practices. Environmental social work expands practice into new areas and pushes the boundaries of traditional practice paradigms and acceptable educational content. While relationship remains fundamental, environmental social work emphasizes interdependence and links between ecological and social justice, and encourages the profession to reconsider its adherence to positivism and dualistic assumptions, as well as the traditional valuing of individualism, and materialistic definitions of progress. Such reconsiderations may open new directions for more effective ways to understand and address individual and social problems.

References

Albrecht, G., Sartore, G-M., Connor, L., Higginbotham, N., Freeman, S., Kelly, B., Stain, H., Tonna, A., and Pollard, G. (2007). Solastalgia: The distress caused by environmental change. *Australasian Psychiatry, 15*(1), S95–98.

Bardi, U. (2009). Peak oil: The four stages of a new idea. *Energy, 34*(3), 323–326.

Baskin, C. (2002). Circles of resistance: Spirituality in social work practice, education and transformative change. *Currents: New Scholarship in the Human Services, 1*(1). Retrieved July 2, 2011 from http://wcmprod2.ucalgary.ca/currents/files/currents/v1n1_baskin.pdf.

Baskin, C. (2011). *Strong helpers' teachings: The value of Indigenous knowledges in the helping professions.* Toronto: Canadian Scholars Press.

Berger, R., and Kelly, J. (1993). Social work in the ecological crisis. *Social Work, 38,* 521–526.

Berry, T. (1999) *The great work: Our way into the future.* New York: Bell Tower.

Berry, W. (1999). *A timbered choir.* Washington, DC: Counterpoint.

Besthorn, F.H. (1997). *Reconceptualizing social work's person-in-environment perspective: Explorations in radical environmental thought.* Unpublished doctoral dissertation, University of Kansas, Lawrence.

Besthorn, F.H. (2000). Toward a deep-ecological social work: Its environmental, spiritual and political dimensions. *The Spirituality and Social Work Forum, 7*(2), 2–7.

Besthorn, F.H. (2001). Transpersonal psychology and deep ecological philosophy: Exploring linkages and applications for social work. *Social Thought: Journal of Religion in the Social Services, 22*(1/2), 23–44.

Besthorn, F.H. (2002). Expanding spiritual diversity in social work: Perspectives on the greening of spirituality. *Currents: New Scholarship in the Human Services, 1*(1). Retrieved January 27, 2012 from http://fsw.ucalgary.ca/currents/fred_besthorn/besthorn.htm.

Besthorn, F.H. (2003). Radical ecologisms: Insights for educating social workers in ecological activism and social justice. *Critical Social Work: An Interdisciplinary Journal Dedicated to Social Justice, 4*(1), unpaginated. Retrieved November 7, 2011 from http://www.uwindsor.ca/criticalsocialwork/2003-volume-4-no-1.

Besthorn, F.H. (2004). Globalized consumer culture: Its implications for social justice and practice teaching in social work. *Journal of Practice Teaching in Health and Social Work, 5*(3), 20–39.

Besthorn, F. (2011). Deep Ecology's contributions to social work: A ten-year retrospective. *International Journal of Social Welfare, 21.* Article first published online: 9 DEC 2011 | DOI: 10.1111/j.1468-2397.2011.00850.x.

Besthorn, F., and Canda, E. (2002). Deep ecology for education and teaching in social work. *Journal of Teaching in Social Work, 22*(1), 79–101.

Besthorn, F.H., and McMillen, D.P. (2002). The oppression of women and nature: Ecofeminism as a framework for a social justice oriented social work. *Families in Society: The Journal of Contemporary Human Services, 83*(3), 221–232.

Besthorn, F.H., and Saleebey, D. (2003). Nature, genetics, and the biophilia connection: Exploring linkages with social work values and practice. *Advances in Social Work, 4*(1), 1–18.

Bibby, R.W. (1987). *Fragmented Gods: The poverty and potential of religion in Canada.* Toronto, ON: Irwin Publishing.

Brundtland Commission (1987). *Report of the World Commission on Environment and Development: Our Common Future.* New York: Oxford.

Bullard, R.D. (1990). *Dumping in Dixie: Race, class, and environmental quality.* Boulder, CO: Westview.

Bullard, R.D. (1993). *Confronting environmental racism: Voices from the grassroots.* Boston: South End Press.

Capra, F. (1982). *The turning point.* New York: Simon and Schuster.

Catton, W., Jr., and Dunlap, R. (1980). A new ecological paradigm for post-exuberant sociology. *American Behavioural Scientist, 24*(1), 15–47.

Chavis, B., and Lee, C. (1987). *Toxic wastes and race in the United States: A national report on the racial and socio-economic characteristics of communities with hazardous waste sites.* New York: United Church of Christ Commission for Racial Justice.

Clinebell, H. (1996). *Ecotherapy: Healing ourselves, healing the Earth.* Minneapolis: Fortress Press.

Coates, J. (2003). *Ecology and social work: Toward a new paradigm.* Halifax, NS: Fernwood Books.

Coates, J., and Besthorn, F. (Eds). (2010). Building bridges and crossing boundaries: Dialogues in professional helping. Special Issue, *Critical Social Work, 11*(3). Retrieved January 27, 2012 from http://www.uwindsor.ca/criticalsocialwork/building-bridges-and-crossing-boundaries-dialogues-in-professional-helping.

Coates, J., and Gray, M. (2011). The environment and social work: An overview and introduction. *International Journal of Social Welfare, 21.* Article first published online: 13 DEC 2011 | DOI: 10.1111/j.1468-2397.2011.00851.x.

Coates, J., Gray, M., and Hetherington, T. (2006). Ecology and spirituality: Finally, a place for Indigenous social work. *British Journal of Social Work, 36,* 381–399.

Demetriades, J., and Esplen, E. (2010). The gender dimensions of poverty and climate change adaptation. In R. Mearns and Norton, A. (Eds). *Social dimensions of climate change: Equity and vulnerability in a warming world.* Washington, DC: The World Bank. 133–144.

Diamond, J. (2005). *Collapse: How societies choose to fail or succeed.* New York: Viking Press.

Diamond, J. (2007). *Guns, germs, and steel: The fates of human societies.* New York: Random House.

Dryzek, J. (2005). *The politics of the earth: Environmental discourses* (2nd ed.). Oxford, England: Oxford University Press.

Durkin, M. (2007). *The great global warming swindle.* Documentary. Original Broadcast, UK Channel 4, 8 March.

Dylan, A., and Coates, J. (2012). The spirituality of justice: Bringing together the eco and the social. *Journal of Religion and Spirituality in Social Work: Social Thought, 31*(1–2), 128–149.

Freeman, C., Fenner, N., Ostle, N. J., Kang, H., Dowrick, D. J., Reynolds, B., Lock, M.A., Sleep, D., Hughes, S., and Hudson, J. (2004). Export of dissolved organic carbon from peatlands underelevated carbon dioxide levels. *Nature, 430*(6996), 195–198.

Fuller, R.J. (2010). Beyond cliché: Reclaiming the concept of sustainability. *Australian Journal of Environmental Education, 26,* 7–18.

Germain, C.B. (1973). An ecological perspective in casework practice. *Social Casework, 54*(6), 323–330.

Giddens, A. (2009). *The politics of climate change.* Cambridge: Polity Press.

Giroux, H. (2001). *The mouse that roared: Disney and the end of innocence.* Oxford: Rowman and Littlefield.

Gleick, P.H. (2011). *2010 Hottest Year on Record: The graph that should be on the front page of every newspaper.* Posted: January 13, 2011 05:11 PM. Retrieved January 18, 2012 from http://www.huffingtonpost.com/peter-h-gleick/the-graph-that-should-be-_b_808747.html.

Godrej, D. (2001). *The no-nonsense guide to climate change.* London: Verso.

Gray, M. (2008). Viewing spirituality in social work through the lens of contemporary social theory. *British Journal of Social Work, 38*(1), 175–196.

Gray, M., and Coates, J. (2011). Environmental ethics for social work: Social work's responsibility to the non-human world. *International Journal of Social Welfare, 21.* Article first published online: 13DEC2011 | DOI: 10.1111/j.1468-2397.2011.00852.x.

Gray, M., Coates, J., and Hetherington, T. (2007). Hearing Indigenous voices in mainstream social work. *Families in Society, 88*(1), 53–64.

Grinnell, R.M. (1973). Environmental modification: Casework's concern or casework's neglect. *Social Service Review, 47*(2), 208–220.

Hamilton, C. (2003). *Growth fetish.* Sydney: Allen and Unwin.

Harper, C. (2008). *Environment and society: Human perspectives on environmental issues* (4th ed.). Upper Saddle River, NJ: Pearson.

Heinsch, M. (2011). Getting down to earth: Finding a place for nature in social work practice. *International Journal of Social Welfare, 21.* Article first published online: 9DEC2011 | DOI: 10.1111/j.1468-2397.2011.00860.x.

Hirsch, R.L. (2008). Mitigation of maximum world oil production: Shortage scenarios. *Energy Policy, 36*(2), 881–889.

Hoff, M.D., and McNutt, J.G. (Eds). (1994). *The global environmental crisis: Implications for social welfare and social work.* Brookfield, VT: Ashgate.

Hoff, M.D., and Polack, R. (1993). Social dimensions of the environmental crisis: Challenges for social work. *Social Work, 38*(2), 204–211.

Hofrichter, R. (1993). *Toxic struggles: The theory and practice of environmental justice.* Philadelphia, PA: New Society.

Holthaus, G. (2008). *Learning Native wisdom: What traditional cultures teach us about subsistence, sustainability and spirituality.* Lexington, KY: University Press of Kentucky.

Intergovernmental Panel on Climate Change (IPCC). (2001). *Climate Change 2001: Synthesis Report.* A Contribution of Working Groups I, II, and III to the Third Assessment Report of the Intergovernmental Panel on Climate Change. R.T. Watson and the Core Writing Team (Eds). Cambridge: Cambridge University Press.

Intergovernmental Panel on Climate Change (IPCC). (2007). *Climate change 2007: Synthesis Report. A contribution of working groups I, II, and III to the fourth assessment report of the Intergovernmental Panel on Climate Change.* [Core Writing Team, Pachauri, R.K. & Reisinger, A. (Eds).] Geneva: IPCC. Retrieved August 5, 2011 from http://www.ipcc.ch/publications_and_data/ar4/syr/en/contents.html.

Jarman, M. (2007). *Climate change.* London: Palgrave.

Korten, D. (2009). *Agenda for a new economy: From phantom wealth to real wealth.* San Francisco, CA: Berrett-Koehler.

Laurie, D., Bender, L., Burns, S.Z. (Producer) and Guggenheim, D. (Director) (2006). *An inconvenient truth* (documentary featuring Al Gore). Hollywood, Paramount. http://www.climatecrisis.net/.

Lomborg, B. (2001). *The skeptical environmentalist.* Cambridge, MA: Cambridge University Press.

Lysack, M. (2010). Environmental decline, loss, and biophilia: Fostering commitment in environmental citizenship. *Critical Social Work, 11*(3). Retrieved January 27, 2012 from http://www.uwindsor.ca/criticalsocialwork/environmental-decline-loss-and-biophilia-fostering-commitment-in-environmental-citizenship.

Lysack, M. (2011). Building capacity for environmental engagement and leadership: An ecosocial work perspective. *International Journal of Social Welfare, 21.* Article first published online: 13 DEC 2011 | DOI: 10.1111/j.1468-2397.2011.00854.x.

Marlow, C., and van Rooyen, C. (2001). How green is the environment in social work? *International Social Work, 44*(2), 241–254.

Mary, N. (2008). *Social work in a sustainable world.* Chicago, IL: Lyceum Books.

McNeill, J. (2001). *Something new under the sun: An environmental history of the twentieth century.* New York: Norton.

Merchant, C. (1990). Ecofeminism and feminist theory. In I. Diamond and Orenstein, G.F. (Eds). *Reweaving the world: The emergence of ecofeminism.* San Francisco: Sierra Club Books. 100–105.

Meyer, C. (1970). *Social work practice: A response to the urban crisis.* New York: The Free Press.

Meyer, C. (1983). *Clinical social work in the eco-systems perspective.* New York: Columbia University Press.

Molyneux, R. (2010). The practical realities of eco-social work: A review of the literature. *Critical Social Work, 11*(2), 61–69.

Morrissette, V., McKenzie, B., and Morrissette, L. (1993). Towards an Aboriginal model of social work practice: Cultural knowledge and traditional practices. *Canadian Social Work Review, 10*(1), 91–108.

Morton, T. (2007). *Ecology without nature.* Cambridge, MA: Harvard University Press.

Muldoon, A. (2006). Environmental efforts: The next challenge for social work. *Critical Social Work, 7*(2). Retrieved January 27, 2012 from http://www.uwindsor.ca/criticalsocialwork/environmental-efforts-the-next-challenge-for-social-work.

Närhi, K., and Matthies, A-L. (2001). What is the ecological (self-)consciousness of social work? Perspectives on the relationship between social work and ecology. In A.-L. Matthies, Nähri, K., and Ward. D. (Eds). *The eco-social approach in social work.* Jyväskylä: Sophi. 16–53.

Norton, C.L. (2009). Ecopsychology and social work: Creating an interdisciplinary framework for redefining person-in-environment. *Ecopsychology, 1*(3), 138–145.

Norton, C.L. (2011). Social work and the environment: An ecosocial approach. *International Journal of Social Welfare, 21.* Article first published online: 9DEC2011|DOI: 10.1111/j.1468-2397.2011.00853.x.

One World. (2012). *Environmental Activism Guide.* Retrieved January 18, 2012 from http://uk.oneworld.net/guides/environmentalactivism.

Park, K. (1996). The personal is ecological: Environmentalism of social work. *Social Work, 41,* 320–323.

Patel, R. (2009). *The value of nothing: How to reshape market society and redefine democracy.* Melbourne: Black Inc.

Peeters, J. (2011). The place of social work in sustainable development: Towards ecosocial practice. *International Journal of Social Welfare, 21,* 1–12. Article first published online: 13 DEC 2011 DOI: 10.1111/j.1468-2397.2011.00856..

Pincus, A., and Minahan, A. (1973). *Social work practice: Model and method.* Itasca, IL: F.E. Peacock Publishers.

Plant, J. (Ed.). (1989). *Healing the wounds: The promise of ecofeminism.* Philadelphia, PA: New Society Publishers.

Polack, R., Wood, S., and Smith, K. (2010). An analysis of fossil-fuel dependence in the United States with implications for community social work. *Critical Social Work, 11*(3). Retrieved January 27, 2012 from http://www.uwindsor.ca/criticalsocialwork/an-analysis-of-fossil-fuel-dependence-in-the-united-states-with-implications-for-community-social-wo.

Princen, T. (2010). *Treading softly: Paths to ecological order.* Cambridge, MA: MIT Press.

Pulido, L. (1996). *Environmentalism and economic justice: Two Chicano struggles in the Southwest.* Tucson, AZ: University of Arizona Press.

Rifkin, J. (2009). *The empathic civilization: The race to global consciousness in a world in crisis.* New York: Tarcher/Penguin.

Rogge, M.E. (1994a). Environmental justice: Social welfare and toxic waste. In M.D. Hoff and McNutt, J.G. (Eds). *The global environmental crisis: Implications for social welfare and social work.* Brooklyn, VT: Ashgate. 53–74.

Rogge, M.E. (1994b). Field education for environmental hazards: Expanding the person-in-environment perspective. In M.D. Hoff and McNutt, J.G. (Eds). *The global environmental crisis: Implications for social welfare and social work.* Brooklyn, VT: Ashgate. 258–276.

Roof, W.C. (1999). *Spiritual marketplace: Baby boomers and the remaking of American religion.* Ewing, NJ: Princeton University Press.

Ross, D. (2009). Emphasizing the 'social' in corporate social responsibility: A social work perspective. *Professionals' Perspectives of Corporate Social Responsibility, 4,* 301–318.

Ruether, R. (1992). *Gaia and god: An ecofeminist theology of Earth healing.* New York: HarperCollins.

Sachs, W. (1995). The Sustainability Debate in the Security Age. *Development, 4,* 26–31.

Schmitz, C.L., Stinson, C.H., and James, C.D. (2010). Reclaiming community: Multidisciplinary approaches to environmental sustainability. *Critical Social Work, 11*(3), 83–95. http://www.uwindsor.ca/criticalsocialwork/2010-volume-11-no-3.

Schmitz, C.L., Matyók, T., Sloan, L., and James, C.D. (2011). The relationship between social work and environmental sustainability: Implications for interdisciplinary practice. *International Journal of Social Welfare, 21.* Article first published online: 13 DEC 2011 DOI: 10.1111/j.1468-2397.2011.00855.

Schor, J.B. (2010). *Plentitude: The new economics of wealth.* New York: Penguin Press.

Shabecoff, P. (1993). *A fierce green fire: The American Environmental Movement.* New York: Hill and Wang.

Shiva, V. (1989). *Staying alive: Women, ecology, and development.* London: Zed Books.

Shiva, V. (2003). *Earth democracy: Justice, sustainability, and peace.* London: Zed Books.

Singer, S.F., and Avery, D.T. (2007). *Unstoppable global warming.* New York: Rowman & Littlefield.

Soine, L. (1987). Expanding the environment in social work: The case for including environmental hazards content. *Journal of Social Work Education, 23*(2), 40–46.

Solomon, L. (2008). The climate change deniers. *The Washington Times.* Retrieved July 15, 2008 from http://washingtontimes.com/news/2008/may/06/the-climate-change-deniers/.

Spretnak, C. (1990). Ecofeminism: Our roots and flowering. In I. Diamond and Orenstein, G.F. (Eds). *Reweaving the world: The emergence of ecofeminism.* San Francisco: Sierra Club Books. 3–14.

Swimme, B., and Berry, T. (1992). *The Universe story: From the primordial flaring forth to the ecozoic era – a celebration of the unfolding of the cosmos.* New York: Harper One.

Tester, F. (1983). *No weka, whale or kauri: Environmentalism, praxis and the human image.* Ocean Monograph No. 9, for the Waikato Workers Educational Association. Hamilton, New Zealand: Outrigger Publishers.

United Nations. (1998). *Kyoto Protocol to the United Nations Framework Convention on Climate Change.* Retrieved January 18, 2012 from http://unfccc.int/resource/docs/convkp/kpeng.pdf.

Urry, J. (2010). Consuming the planet to excess. *Theory, Culture and Society, 27*(2–3), 191–212.

Van Wormer, K., and Besthorn, F.H. (2011). *Human behavior and the social environment: Groups, communities and organizations* (2nd ed.). New York: Oxford University Press.

Wilson, E.O. (1984). *Biophilia.* Cambridge, MA: Harvard University Press.

World Commission on Environment and Development (WCED). (1987). Brundtland Commission. *Report of the World Commission on Environment and Development: Our Common Future.* New York: Oxford.

World Wide Fund (WWF). (2010). *Living planet report 2010: Biodiversity, biocapacity and development.* Gland, Switzerland: World Wide Fund for Nature. Retrieved January 27, 2012 from http://awsassets.panda.org/downloads/lpr2010.pdf.

Zapf, M.K. (2005a). The spiritual dimension of person and environment: Perspectives from social work and traditional knowledge. *International Social Work, 48*(5), 633–642.

Zapf, M.K. (2005b). Profound connections between person and place: Exploring location, spirituality and social work. *Critical Social Work, 6*(2). Retrieved January 19, 2012 from http://www.criticalsocialwork.com/#.

Zapf, M.K. (2009). *Social work and the environment: Understanding people and place.* Toronto, Ontario: Canadian Scholars Press.

Part 1

Theory

Mapping the terrain of environmental social work

1 Radical equalitarian ecological justice

A social work call to action

Fred H. Besthorn

> Social work must eventually change the central philosophical ground of its conceptualization of justice. In a practical sense, no matter how social work languages its idea of justice, in the end all justice is ecological (Fred Besthorn)

In September 2008, the small South American country of Ecuador became the first nation in the world to ratify a radical new constitution recognizing the inalienable rights of nature and natural systems (Revkin, 2008). Article one of the constitution states:

> Nature or Pachamama, where life is reproduced and exists, has the right to exist, persist, maintain and regenerate its vital cycles, structure, functions and its processes in evolution. Every person, people, community or nationality, will be able to demand the recognitions of rights for nature before the bodies.
>
> (Margil, 2008: 1)

Similarly, in April 2011, the Bolivian National Congress passed historic legislation entitled the *Law of Mother Nature*. This regulatory decree insures that nature and all of its natural systems have the right to life, the right to their normal regenerative processes, and the right to maintain their naturally occurring biodiversity. It emphasizes that all human activities *must align* with the natural world in achieving 'dynamic balance with the cycles and processes inherent in Mother Earth' (Environmental News Services (ENS), 2011: 1). Introductions to the Bolivian statute affirm nature as 'a living dynamic system made up of the undivided community of all living beings, who are all interconnected, interdependent and complementary, sharing a common destiny' (Buxton, 2011).

The Ecuadorian constitution and Bolivian legislation presages a radical reorientation in the way institutions, communities, and societies understand conventional notions of justice in the context of environmental concerns. They highlight the emergence in many countries around the world of initiatives to reconceptualize conventional notions of justice which are historically anthropocentric, emphasizing the human side of justice questions to the minimization of the interests of nature (Besthorn, 2011; Cullinan, 2010; Dryzek and Schlosberg, 2005; Margil, 2011). They force attention to the fact that 'human societies can only be viable and flourish if they regulate themselves as part of the wider Earth community and do so in a way that is consistent with the fundamental laws and principles that govern how the universe functions' (Cullinan, 2010: 144–145).

Social work's emerging concern for environmental justice, particularly the impact of deteriorating ecological conditions on marginalized human populations, has grown precipitously in recent years (Besthorn, 2011; Miller, Hayward, and Shaw, 2011). Clearly, many in the profession are critically reflective with respect to social work's environmental responsibilities. This has yielded a robust scholarly agenda seeking to sensitize the profession to its role in the context of increasingly deteriorating environmental conditions (Coates, 2005; Hawkins, 2010; Jones, 2010; Lysack, 2010; Shaw, 2006). The profession's commitment to social justice provides a conceptual launch-point underpinning this new awareness. Unfortunately, social work's notion of social justice is lodged within broader contexts of modernity and liberal democratic theories defining what constitutes 'just action' and who or what deserves 'just treatment' (Besthorn, 2011; McLaughlin, 2006; Solas, 2008).

This chapter reviews social work's historic commitment to social justice and the profession's evolving interest in environmental justice. It traces the philosophical linkage between social and environmental justice and suggests that both are deeply embedded in utilitarian and anthropocentric worldviews. It examines ecological justice and its critique of modern systems of environmental justice which, according to proponents, have accomplished very little to actually protect the environment or to sustain ecological systems for future generations. Finally, it offers a call to action for social work to reevaluate and radically reconceptualize its notions of social and environmental justice to make them more consistent with core principles of a radical equalitarian ecological justice.

Social justice in social work: An organizing framework

Advocating for social justice is a longstanding tradition of Western social work (Healy, 2008; Ife, 2008a; Lundy and Van Wormer, 2007; Reichert, 2003; Schriver, 2010). The International Federation of Social Workers (IFSW) (2004) declared that 'principles of ... social justice are fundamental to social work' (p. 3). Social work has variously defined social justice as 'an ideal condition in which all members of a society have the same basic rights, protections, opportunities, obligations, and social benefits ... social justice entails advocacy to confront discrimination, oppression, and institutional inequities' (Barker, 2003: 404). Concomitantly, human rights dovetail with social justice with respect to 'the struggle for dignity and fundamental freedoms which allow the full development of human potential' (IFSW, 1996).

Social justice is so intricately interwoven with social work that several have suggested the future of the profession depends upon the degree to which it is able to integrate social justice into an overarching conceptual framework unifying all social work theory and practice (Mohan, 1999; Wakefield, 1988, 1998). Undoubtedly, the combined focus on social justice and human rights is one of the profession's most important conceptual orientations, even surpassing one of its most cherished orientations: the person-in-environment perspective (McLaughlin, 2006; Swenson, 1998).

Environmental justice and social work: An emerging synthesis

In recent years, a new generation of social workers, many from North America, Europe, and Australia, has spoken forcefully concerning the importance of incorporating environmental awareness into the profession's theoretical formulations and practice modalities (Besthorn, 2008, 2011; Coates, 2003; Coates, Gray, and Hetherington, 2006; Hoff, 1998; Hoff and McNutt, 1994; Mary, 2008; McKinnon, 2008; Muldoon, 2006; Van Wormer and Besthorn, 2011; Zapf, 2009). This is a welcome development for a profession for too long unengaged in the emerging international consensus that Earth's carrying capacity and its ability to support life are in deep trouble.

During this same period, social work has expanded its traditional emphasis on social justice to include a more dedicated focus to issues of environmental justice (Coates, 2004; Keefe, 2003; Hawkins, 2010; Jones, 2006; Miller *et al.*, 2011; Rogge, 2008; Shaw, 2006). A spontaneous reading of social work's national and international policy statements and ethical codes clearly illustrates the profession's growing interest in linking social and environmental justice (Australian Association of Social Workers (AASW), 2010; British Association of Social Workers (BASW), 2002; Canadian Association of Social Workers (CASW), 2005; International Federation of Social Workers (IFSW), 2005; US National Association of Social Workers (NASW), 2008). Discerning this trend, Coates (2004) observes that 'issues of well-being, participation and equality – longstanding concerns of radical and structural social work – rise in importance as social justice incorporates environmental justice' (p. 6). Keefe (2003), in his review of the bio-psycho-social-spiritual dimension of social justice, notes that social work's conventional notion of social justice is not complete 'unless environmental justice and its temporal perspective and sustainability criteria are added' (p. 6). Similarly, Hawkins (2010) submits that 'social work must extend its mission to include environmental justice' (p. 68).

While commendable, efforts to integrate environmental justice into social work's core mission raise several important questions. First, what does environmental justice mean, both historically and philosophically, and how is it related to social work's commitment to social justice? Second, does environmental justice provide a sound basis for social work action in the context of deteriorating environmental threats?

Environmental justice: Environment in service to humanity

The environmental justice movement, particularly in the United States, gathered momentum in the early 1980s (Agyeman, 2005; Bullard, 2005; Melosi, 2004; Page, 2006). Several studies, such as the 1983 United States General Accounting Office (USGAO, 1983) report on the state of hazardous waste landfills and the 1987 United Church of Christ Commission on Racial Justice (Chavis and Lee, 1987) report entitled *Toxic Wastes and Race*, demonstrated that poor communities and communities of colour were saddled with highly inequitable shares of environmental harms. Thereafter, racism and the distribution of environmental ills became inextricably connected (Bullard, 2005). Chavis (1993) compellingly outlined the issue with the assertion that 'People of color bear the brunt of the nation's pollution problem' (p. 3). From a broader frame, Dowie (1995) points out that while all Americans were ostensibly created equal 'all Americans were not, as things turned out, being poisoned equally' (p. 141). Over time, environmental justice became increasingly linked with and often an extension of social justice (Taylor, 2000). The environmental justice discourse offered promise in bridging a number of complicated social, ethical, political, and environmental issues into one overarching framework.

The logic of environmental justice is comparatively simple. The central interrogative is: how do societies do justice within the human species and among human communities in the context of environmental issues? Shaw (2006) suggests that nested within this core concern is the notion of 'the inherent right of humanity to a clean and safe environment' (p. 19). Every human being and human community is entitled to a life unencumbered by deleterious environmental conditions. For environmental justice advocates, the natural environment is presumed a relatively stable resource upon which humans depend for survival. The task of individuals, societies, institutions, and governmental entities is to ensure this standing reserve is rationally managed and protected for the benefit of human populations. When environmental risks or, in some cases, environmental calamities do impact human populations, the mission of environmental justice is to ensure that these environmental harms are not disproportionally distributed to any specific person or group.

Environmental justice, although relatively new to the justice discourse, shares important likenesses with liberal notions of social justice. Solas (2008) suggests that several philosophical frameworks have tended to inform modern, Western thinking on social justice ranging 'from traditions that stress the concept of desert or merit, through those based on rights, to others for which the notion of a social contract is central' (p. 814). Each of these traditions has a central concern with how members of a society share and ultimately distribute the benefits and harms of living. As Dobson (1998) points out, 'at its broadest sense, social justice is about the distribution of benefits and burdens' (p. 73). Benefits and burdens are endemic to human existence. They are in one sense – intermittently transitory and abundant – resources which, by virtue of merit, right, or contract, must be distributed in such a manner so as to ensure the viability and right-ordering of human affairs (Dobson, 1998; Gudorf and Huchingson, 2010).

Solas (2008) asserts additionally that the most prominent philosophical basis of social justice is rooted in the Enlightenment idea of utilitarianism. Utilitarianism is a moral philosophy which, at its most basic, is a form of consequentialism. That is, the rightness or wrongness of an action is assessed based on the consequences of such action. Actions which bring more harm than benefit are judged wrong while those bringing greater net or aggregate benefit than harm are right. Social justice, based on utilitarian principles, emphasizes an equitable, although not necessarily equal, distribution of primary benefits or goods, such as property, opportunities, and wealth in such a manner that tends to bring about the most good for the greatest number of people.

Environmental justice is an extension of the distributional and utilitarian aspects of modern Western ideas of social justice (Dobson, 1998; Drengson and Devall, 2010; Dryzek and Schlosberg, 2005; Naess, 2008; Schlosberg, 2009). It emphasizes the minimization of environmental harms and an equitable distribution of environmental benefits or goods, such as protecting clean water, maintaining species integrity, ensuring climate stability, and guarding wilderness areas in such a manner as to bring about the most good for the greatest number of people. In a significant way, *environment* is the common denominator for both social and environmental justice, but is understood in different ways. Environmental justice's first task is to preserve the integrity of the natural environment and its resource potential for the benefit of human welfare. In other words, the environment exists in service to humanity. Social justice is concerned with the negative consequences primary benefits, including Earth's natural capital, are inequitably distributed among human populations (Schlosberg, 2009). Thus, social justice and environmental justice have historically always pulled in the same direction.

Ecological justice: Humanity in service to environment

Social and environmental justice share a common interest in human beings and the natural world. But, much like social work's struggle to clearly balance its commitment to both person-and-environment, the pre-ponderance of energy, activity, and rhetoric of environmental justice falls squarely on the person side of the justice equation. When environmental justice speaks of justice, as Schlosberg (2009) points out, 'their concern is most often (though not exclusively) for *people and communities* facing environmental risks, rather than on doing justice to an external, nonhuman *nature*' (p. 130 original emphasis).

In recent years, the justice discourse has gradually expanded to include an articulation of *ecological justice* and the difference between it and environmental justice (Baxter, 2004; Gudorf and Huchingson, 2010; Schlosberg, 2009). To be sure, ecological justice shares similar conceptualizations with its ethical cousin environmental justice. There is talk of rights, responsibilities, fairness, recognition, and distributive standards in the context of environmental concerns. But, at another level, ecological justice is radically different from environmental justice.

This difference may best be summarized in the central maxim of Aldo Leopold's (1949) *land ethic*. Leopold, North American naturalist and environmental advocate, is considered by many the progenitor of the modern ecological justice movement (Callicott, 1989, 1999; Naess, 1989; Sessions, 1995; Westra, 2001). Leopold asserted, with respect to ethical decision making, 'a thing is right when it tends to preserve the integrity, stability, and beauty of the biotic community. It is wrong when it tends otherwise' (Leopold, 1949: 224). The key is Leopold's understanding of right action as grounded in the *biotic community* or natural world. Callicott (1997) points out that this grounding of ethical decision making in nature is not a novel idea. North American Indigenous tribes and many non-Western cultures have held for centuries that ethical decision making must be grounded in and subordinate to the interests of the natural world. They recognized their deep interconnectedness with and dependency upon the natural world in all human activities. To pretend otherwise would not only be wrong but suicidal.

Ecological justice asserts that modern Western culture, with its obsession with material consumption, continuous economic growth, and ever higher standards of living, has become suicidal. Despite the best and, at times, heroic efforts of environmental justice to protect vulnerable and underrepresented peoples, the movement has largely failed with respect to the natural environment. This failure is not a result of a lack of effort but largely because its metaphysics is misplaced (Besthorn, 2004, 2011; Gudorf and Huchingson, 2010; Rolston, 2001). That is, the philosophical foundation of its ethical activity is firmly situated, first and foremost, in human welfare and the human experience (Eckersley, 1996; Matthews, 2003; Taylor, 2000). It is consistently anthropocentric. Despite environmental justice's respect for and duty to the interests of the natural world, human interests, except under extraordinary circumstances, frequently, if not always, trump the interests of the natural world. For environmental justice, it is not that nature has no value but simply that nature has no *intrinsic* or *objective* value apart from that which the human species ascribes to it. Philosopher Holmes Rolston (2001) explains this idea:

> Nature simply *is* without objective value; the preferences of human subjects establish value; and these human values, appropriately considered, generate human duties. Only humans are ethical subjects

and only humans are ethical objects. Nature is amoral; the moral community is interhuman ... with the resulting paradox that the sole moral species acts only in its collective self-interest toward all the rest.

(p. 126, original emphasis)

Ecological justice proponents are not anti-environmental justice nor, for that matter, anti-social justice. They support efforts to protect vulnerable human populations and to equitably distribute the positive goods of the natural world for benefit of human beings. They also support the eradication of social injustice. They do, however, advocate for a deeper, ecocentrically informed conceptualization of justice, a *deep justice* (Besthorn, 2011; Dryzek, 2005; Naess, 2008). Indeed, they support a comprehensive reordering of conventional conceptualization of environmental justice toward a *radical egalitarian ecological* justice where non-sentient beings and natural systems are given equal moral standing. Their *raison d'être* begins and ends with the natural world. Theirs is a justice of humanity in service of environment. For a detailed review and comparative analysis of ecological and environmental justice see, for instance, the works of Armstrong and Botzler (2003), Baxter (2004), Dobson (1998, 2007), Dryzek (2005), Dryzek and Schlosberg (2005), Light and de-Shalit (2003), Light and Rolston (2003), Regan (2003), Rolston (1989, 2011), Sandler and Pezzullo (2007), Schlosberg (2009), Singer (2009), Stone (2010), Wenz (2001), Westra, Westra, and Bosselman (2008), Zimmerman, Callicott, Sessions, and Clark (2001).

Radical equalitarian ecological justice: A social work call to action

The previous discussion suggests social work has gradually integrated concerns for environmental justice alongside its historic commitment to social justice. Unfortunately, social work's conventional ideas of social and environmental justice are still construed within the context of the human enterprise. In their review of social work's history of environmental concern, Miller *et al.* (2011) note, 'As is the case with social work's notion of social justice, theories of *environmental* justice tend to offer a rights based framework focusing on justice as it relates to human rights and needs' (p. 4), reflecting a 'decisive human-centered orientation grounded in the longstanding humanistic values of the profession' (p. 2). Responsibilities to and inalienable rights of non-human entities in the natural world, except to the extent these impinge upon human well-being, are often ignored.

The current environmental crisis is clearly, on one level, a concern of environmental and social justice. There are disastrous potentials in the ways pollution, climate change, overpopulation, and excessive consumption impact human well-being and social cohesiveness. But the environmental crisis is also a moral issue of a different order. Its long-term negative impact extends to all non-sentient beings and to every sphere of the ecological order. It is not simply an anthropocentric issue.

The broader context of the environmental crisis is intensely philosophical. It is an issue of how and in what way human beings think about or consider the biotic community (Leopold, 1949). Considering the biotic community means respecting the diversity and otherness of nature for its own sake and suggests non-human entities are ends in themselves rather than instruments of human need or wealth creation. It means all species, human and non-human alike, are entitled to a just and equal claim to existence that ensures their well-being and enduring ability to thrive. Considering the biotic community recognizes that any system of justice must have its philosophical grounding in the natural world. Without this as a starting point there can be no meaningful human existence, in fact, no human existence at all.

In his critique of social work's conceptualization of social justice, Australian scholar John Solas (2008) notes that social work has historically held to a minimalist scheme of social justice. This restrictive perspective does not necessarily require that everyone has 'fair and equal access to rights and opportunities as well as resources' (p. 818). Solas (2008) advocates a *radical equalitarianism* which expands the boundaries of social justice. This is both a pressing and practical concern for 'the establishment of a more comprehensive and generous system of social justice is not an abstract matter, but rather a matter of life or death' (p. 19).

Similarly, it is this author's contention that an ecocentrically situated theory of justice, as explicated in this chapter, is *radically equalitarian*. It expands the boundaries of justice to include, fully and completely, the entire natural world, imaging the natural world as the centre and ground informing all our consideration of just action. As Besthorn (2011) concluded, this kind of deeper justice is 'the proper and necessary framework for social work as it moves into the troubled waters of a world on the edge of environmental and economic collapse' (p. 21). A radically equalitarian ecological justice of the kind envisioned here is a fundamentally different orientation and portends nothing short of sweeping change in social work's conventional ideas of justice. It establishes the foundation of a new social work understanding of and mandate for justice. It is not simply a reordering of professional commitments and tasks applied to environmental concerns, neither can it be subsumed under social work's conventional notion of social justice as a subdivision or additional focus of attention.

In a practical sense, no matter how social work languages its idea of justice, in the end all justice is ecological. That is, to be philosophically and metaphysically consistent, any theory of justice, including the conclusions it draws and actions it contemplates, must be grounded in the natural world. Philosopher Mick Smith (2001) points out that in the final analysis the defining measure of any system of justice is the degree to which it considers 'the emergence into significance of the other' (p. 219). This other is the *otherness of the natural world*. Indeed, without this ecocentric grounding social and environmental justice, as conventionally conceived in social work, becomes superfluous: 'The long heritage of severing justice from biological embodiment helps make clear why "environmental justice" seems a latter day indulgence, entirely dispensable' (Hamlin, 2008: 146). The depth and range of environmental catastrophe suggest that Western, liberal democratic notions of justice are not sufficient to address the crushing scope of the problems. Social and environmental injustices are not simply problems that may be 'tinkered with at the margins' (Ife, 2008b: 139) or that can be resolved by refined technical solutions.

A radical equalitarian ecological justice stresses that humans are systemically embedded and biologically embodied beings whose ethical responsibilities *emerge from* and *extend to* all non-human beings and entities. The fact that humans are also social beings with ethical responsibilities to other human beings ultimately flounders without this reorientation. This is precisely why the Ecuadorian constitution and Bolivian statutes have worked so judiciously to redefine the foundational basis of justice and to inculcate into law recognition of the inalienable right of nature (Cullinan, 2010; Margil, 2011). Many in the developing world, particularly Indigenous groups, have long recognized and will not soon forget they have often been the unwitting and unfortunate inheritors of the legacy of Western-style social and environmental justice. The promise of equal social opportunity and environmental protection were encouraging but the outcomes have been dismal. However well-meaning the rhetoric to the contrary, in the end, developing nations and many tribal cultures continue to experience the disastrous and often escalating effects of unrestrained environmental and human exploitation. What they have learned through hard experience is that Western notions of justice do not necessarily guarantee either social or environmental justice. They simply determine how much, how often, and to what degree nature, and by extension human beings, may be exploited.

Conclusion

In 1993, psychologist James Hillman, with colleague Michael Ventura, wrote a provocative book entitled *We've had a hundred years of psychotherapy – And the world is getting worse*. Their theme was that the psychotherapeutic community, notwithstanding best intentions, has done little to meaningfully address human problems of living and in most cases has actually made things worse for individuals and society. Whether one agrees with the conclusion or not, the point is that proponents of ecological justice share a similar sort of lament: *we've had forty years of environmental justice and the world is getting worse*. For them, the environmental justice movement is profoundly anthropocentric and is, at best, a *shallow* form of justice. It is shallow not because its rationale for just action is not sufficiently complex and detailed, but precisely because it uncritically accepts the humanistic predilection to reify the preeminence of human beings in the cosmic order while leaving out or significantly minimizing non-sentient beings and ecosystems as legitimate objects of moral concern (Callicott, 1991; Eckersley, 1996; Naess, 1973, 1989; Rodman, 1995; Rolston, 2011). The deeply embedded humanistic bias creates a situation where attempts to slow the ravages of environmental dis-ease go on at pace but, in the process, the patient – Earth – dies.

Social work must eventually change the central philosophical ground of its conceptualization of justice. This, of course, will be no easy task considering the profession's historic alignment with the anthropocentric and utilitarian principles underlying current notions of social and environmental justice (Miller et al., 2011). It also may be unlikely that social work is ready to engage fully in a critically reflective process of change even in light of the urgency presented by escalated environmental crises (Ife, 2008b). But, it is this author's contention this must begin and it must begin with the profession redefining and operationalizing justice from an ecocentric perspective.

It is not immediately obvious what a new social work orientation to justice might be called. A radically equalitarian, ecocentrically informed, ecological justice is not likely to marshal a ground swell of support. Indeed, it might only inspire confusion and, perhaps, even derision. Social work is trapped by the limitations of its linguistic conventions. But, as this discussion makes clear, we are not alone. Philosophers and environmental ethicists have struggled for decades attempting to articulate a vibrant and comprehensive reorientation to conventional notions of justice. Part of that struggle has involved how to language a revised justice perspective that most can agree to. This task is arduous partly because the prevailing social, cultural, economic, and political order (whether liberal or conservative) has become so profoundly and unconsciously tied to their preferred paradigmatic language. Language is always, at least for a time, inadequate in keeping pace with significant paradigmatic shifts. There is often great misunderstanding, muddle, and no small degree of linguistic overlay. So, whether the profession jettisons the language of social and environmental justice in preference to, for instance, ecological justice, eco-social justice, ecocentric justice, eco-environmental justice is not for me the central concern. The core issue is: can the profession be a meaningful part of the evolving discourse seeking to define an expanded and comprehensive vision of justice for the *whole world*, however that may eventually be languaged. We may not have long to decide, but I am hopeful the profession has the requisite commitment to join the debate. Social work has much to offer the discussion.

References

Agyeman, J. (2005). *Sustainable communities and the challenge of environmental justice.* New York: New York University Press.

Armstrong, S., and Botzler, R. (Eds). (2003). *Environmental ethics: Divergence and convergence.* Columbus, OH: McGraw-Hill.

Australian Association of Social Workers [AASW]. (2010). *Code of ethics.* Retrieved July 29, 2011 from http://www/aasw.asn.au/document/item/740.

Barker, R.L. (2003). *Social work dictionary* (5th ed.). Washington, DC: NASW Press. http://www.amazon.com/Social-Work-Dictionary-Robert-Barker/dp/087101355X

Baxter, B. (2004). *A theory of ecological justice.* New York: Routledge.

Besthorn, F.H. (2004). Restorative justice and environmental restoration – Twin pillars of a just global environmental policy: Hearing the voice of the victim. *Journal of Societal and Social Policy, 3*(2), 33–48.

Besthorn, F.H. (2008). Environment and social work practice. *Encyclopedia of Social Work (vol. 2)* (20th ed.). New York: Oxford University Press. 132–136.

Besthorn, F. (2011). Deep Ecology's contributions to social work: A ten-year retrospective. *International Journal of Social Welfare, 21,* 1–12. Article first published online: 9 DEC 2011 | DOI: 10.1111/j.1468-2397.2011.00850..

British Association of Social Workers [BASW]. (2002). *Code of ethics.* Retrieved July 26, 2011 from the British Association of Social Workers website http://www/basw/co.uk/about/code-of-ethics/.

Bullard, R. (Ed.). (2005). *The quest for environmental justice: Human rights and the politics of pollution.* San Francisco: Sierra Club Books.

Buxton, N. (2011). The law of mother earth: Behind Bolivia's historic bill. The Rights of Nature website. Retrieved July 29, 2011 from http://therightsofnature.org/bolivia-law-of-mother-earth/.

Callicott, J.B. (1989). *In defense of the land ethic.* Albany, NY. State University of New York Press.

Callicott, J.B. (1991). The case against moral pluralism. *Environmental Ethics, 12*(1), 99–124.

Callicott. J.B. (1997). *Earth's insights: A multicultural survey of ecological ethics from the Mediterranean basin to the Australian outback.* Berkeley, CA: University of California Press.

Callicott, J.B. (1999). *The land ethic revisited.* Albany, NY: State University of New York Press.

Canadian Association of Social Workers [CASW]. (2005). *Code of ethics.* Retrieved July 20, 2011 from http://www.casw-acts.ca/practice/codeofethics_e.pdf.

Chavis, B.F. (1993). Foreword. In R. Bullard (Ed.). *Confronting environmental racism: Voices from the grassroots.* Boston, MA: South End Press. 3–6.

Chavis, B., and Lee, C. (1987). *Toxic wastes and race in the United States: A national report on the racial and socio-economic characteristics of communities with hazardous waste sites.* Report of the United Church of Christ Commission on Racial Justice. Retrieved February 9, 2012 from http://www.ucc.org/about-us/archives/pdfs/toxwrace87.pdf.

Coates, J. (2003). *Ecology and social work: Toward a new paradigm.* Halifax: Fernwood.

Coates, J. (2004). From ecology to spirituality and social justice. *Currents: New Scholarship in the Human Services, 3*(1), 1–10. Retrieved February 9, 2012 from http://wcmprod2.ucalgary.ca/currents/files/currents/v3n1_coates.pdf.

Coates, J. (2005). The environmental crisis: Implications for social work. *Journal of Progressive Human Services, 16*(1), 25–49.

Coates, J., Gray, M., and Hetherington, T. (2006). An 'ecospiritual' perspective: Finally, a place for indigenous approaches. *The British Journal of Social Work, 36*(3), 381–399.

Cullinan, C. (2010). Earth jurisprudence: From colonization to participation. In E. Assadourian & World Watch Institute (Eds). *State of the world 2010: Transforming cultures from consumerism to sustainability.* New York: W.W. Norton & Company. 143–148.

Dobson, A. (1998). *Justice and the environment: Conceptions of environmental sustainability and dimensions of social justice.* New York: Oxford University Press.

Dobson, A. (2007). *Green political thought* (4th ed.). New York: Routledge.

Dowie, M. (1995). *Losing ground: American environmentalism at the close of the twentieth century.* Cambridge, MA: MIT Press.

Drengson, A., and Devall, B. (2010). The deep ecology movement: Origins, development and future prospects. *The Trumpeter: Journal of Ecosophy, 26*(2), 48–69.

Dryzek, J. (2005). *The politics of the earth: Environmental discourses.* New York: Oxford University Press.

Dryzek, J., and Schlosberg, D. (Eds). (2005). *Debating the earth: The environmental politics reader* (2nd ed.). New York: Oxford University Press.

Eckersley, R. (1996). Greening liberal democracy: The rights discourse revisited. In B. Doherty and de Geus. M. (Eds). *Democracy and green political thought.* London: Routledge. 213–225.

Environmental News Service (ENS). (2011). Bolivia celebrates law granting rights to mother earth. Retrieved July 27, 2011 from http://www.ens-newswire.com/ens/apr2011/2011-04-20-01.html.

Gudorf, C., and Huchingson, J. (2010). *Boundaries: A casebook in environmental ethics.* Washington, DC: Georgetown University Press.

Hamlin, C. (2008). Is all justice environmental? *Environmental Justice, 1*(3), 145–147.

Hawkins, C. (2010). Sustainability, human rights, and environmental justice: Critical connections for contemporary social work. *Critical Social Work, 11*(3), 68–81.

Healy, E. (2008). Exploring the history of social work as a human rights profession. *International Social Work, 51,*745–746.

Hillman, J., and Ventura, M. (1993). *We've had a hundred years of psychotherapy – And the world's getting worse.* New York: Harper One.

Hoff, M. (Ed.). (1998). *Sustainable community development: Studies in economic, environmental, and cultural revitalization.* Boston, MA: Lewis.

Hoff, M.D., and McNutt, J.G. (Eds). (1994). *The global environmental crisis: Implications for social welfare and social work.* Brookfield, VT: Ashgate Publishing.

Ife, J. (2008a). *Human rights and social work: Towards rights-based practice.* New York: Cambridge University Press.

Ife, J. (2008b). Invited commentary – Comment on John Solas: 'What are we fighting for?' *Australian Social Work, 61*(2), 137–140.

International Federation of Social Workers [IFSW]. (1996). *International policy on human rights.* Retrieved from International Federation of Social Workers website: http://www.ifsw.org/p38000212.html.

International Federation of Social Workers [IFSW]. (2004). *Ethics in social work, statement of principles.* Retrieved from International Federation of Social Workers website: http://www.ifsw.org/p38000324.html.

International Federation of Social Workers [IFSW]. (2005). *International policy statement on globalization and the environment.* Retrieved from International Federation of Social Workers website: http://www.ifsw.org/p38000222.html.

Jones, P. (2006). Considering the environment in social work education: Trans-formations for eco-social justice. *Australian Journal of Adult Learning, 46*(3), 364–382.

Jones, P. (2010). Responding to the ecological crisis: Transformative pathways for social work. *Journal of Social Work Education, 46*(1), 67–84.

Keefe, T. (2003). The bio-psycho-social-spiritual origins of environmental justice. *Critical Social Work, 3*(1), 1–17.

Leopold, A. (1949). *The sand county almanac and sketches here and there.* New York: Oxford University Press.

Light, A., and Rolston, H. (Eds). (2003). *Environmental ethics: An anthology.* Malden, MA: Blackwell Publishing.

Light, A., and de-Shalit, A. (Eds). (2003). *Moral and political reasoning in environmental practice.* Cambridge, MA: MIT Press.

Lundy, C., and Van Wormer, K. (2007). Social and economic justice, human rights and peace: The challenge for social work in Canada and the USA. *International Social Work, 50,* 727–739.

Lysack, M. (2010). Environmental decline, loss, and biophilia: Fostering commitment in environmental citizenship. *Critical Social Work, 11*(3), 48–66.

Margil, M. (2008). Ecuador approves new constitution: Voters approve rights of nature. Community Environmental Defense Fund. Retrieved July 28, 2011 from http://celdf.org/article.php?id=302.

Margil, M. (2011). *Los derechos de la naturaleza: Rights based protection for puchamama.* Retrieved July 26, 2011 from The Rights of Nature website http://www.therightsofnature.org/wp-content/uploades/pdfs.

Mary, N. (2008). *Social work in a sustainable world.* Chicago: Lyceum Books.

Matthews, F. (2003). *For love of mater: A contemporary panpsychism.* Albany, NY: State University of New York Press.

McKinnon, J. (2008). Exploring the nexus between social work and the environment. *Australian Social Work, 61*(3), 256–268.

McLaughlin, A.M. (2006). Liberal interpretations of social justice for social work. *Currents: New Scholarship in the Human Services, 5*(1), 1–18.

Melosi, M. (2004). *Garbage in the cities: Refuse, reform, and the environment.* Pittsburgh, PA: University of Pittsburgh Press.

Miller, S.E., Hayward, R.A., and Shaw, T.V. (2011). Environmental shifts for social work: A principles approach. *International Journal of Social Welfare, 21,* 1–8. Article first published online: 13 DEC 2011 | DOI: 10.1111/j.1468-2397.2011.00848.

Mohan, B. (1999). *Unification of social work: Rethinking social transformation.* Westport, CT: Praeger.

Muldoon, A. (2006). Environmental efforts: The next challenge for social work. *Critical Social Work, 7*(2), 84–93.

Naess, A. (1973). The shallow and the deep, long-range ecology movement: A summary. *Inquiry, 16*(2), 95–100.

Naess, A. (1989). *Ecology, community and lifestyle: Outline of an ecosophy.* New York: Cambridge University Press.

Naess, A. (2008). The basics of the deep ecology movement. In A. Drengson and Devall, B. (Eds). *The ecology of wisdom.* Emeryville, CA: Counterpoint Press. 105–119.

National Association of Social Workers (2003). *Environmental Policy. Social Work Speaks.* Washington, DC: NASW Press.

National Association of Social Workers [NASW]. (2008). *Code of ethics.* Retrieved July 28, 2011 from http://www.naswdc.org/pubs/code/code.asp

Page, E. (2006). *Climate change, justice and future generations.* Cheltenham, UK: Edward Elgar

Regan, T. (2003). *Animal rights, human wrongs: An introduction of moral philosophy.* Lanham, MD: Rowman and Littlefield.

Reichert, E. (2003). *Social work and human rights: A foundation for policy and practice.* New York: Columbia University Press.

Revkin, A. (2008). Ecuador constitution grants rights to nature. *New York Times,* 29 September. Retrieved July 29, 2011 from http://dotearth.blogs.nytimes.com/2008/09/29/ecuador-constitution-grants-nature-rights/.

Rodman, J. (1995). Four forms of ecological consciousness reconsidered. In A. Drengson and Inoue, Y. (Eds). *The deep ecology movement: An introductory anthology.* Berkeley, CA: North Atlantic Books. 242–256.

Rogge, M. (2008). Environmental justice. In National Association of Social Workers (NASW), *Encyclopedia of social work.* New York: Oxford University Press. 136–139.

Rolston, H. (1989). *Environmental ethics: Duties to and values in the natural world.* Philadelphia: Temple University Press.

Rolston, H. (2001). Challenges in environmental ethics. In M. Zimmerman, Callicott, J.B., Sessions, G., Warren, K., and Clark, J. (Eds). *Environmental philosophy: From animal rights to radical ecology* (3rd ed.). Upper Saddle River, NJ: Prentice Hall. 82–101.

Rolston, H. (2011). *A new environmental ethics: The next millennium for life on earth.* New York: Routledge.

Sandler, R., and Pezzullo, P. (Eds). (2007). *Environmental justice and environmentalism: The social justice challenge to the environmental movement.* Cambridge, MA: MIT Press.

Schlosberg, D. (2009). *Defining environmental justice: Theories, movements, and nature.* New York: Oxford University Press.

Schriver, J. (2010). *Human behavior and the social environment: Shifting paradigms in essential knowledge for social work practice* (5th ed.). Boston, MA: Allyn and Bacon.

Sessions, G. (1995). Ecocentrism and the anthropocentric detour. In G. Sessions (Ed.). *Deep ecology for the 21st century: Readings on the philosophy and practice of the new environmentalism.* Boston, MA: Shambhala. 156–183.

Shaw, T.V. (2006). Environmental equity and environmental racism. *Perspectives on Social Work – Doctoral Journal, 4*(2), 17–22. Retrieved October 23, 2011 from http://www.sw.uh.edu/documents/phdprogram/perspectives/fall2006.pdf

Singer, P. (2009). *Animal liberation: The definitive classic of the animal movement.* New York: Harper Perennial.

Smith, M. (2001). *The ethics of place: Radical ecology, postmodernity, and social theory.* Albany, NY: State University of New York Press.

Solas, J. (2008). What kind of social justice does social work seek? *International Social Work, 51*(6), 813–822.

Stone, C. (2010). *Should trees have standing: Law, morality and the environment* (3rd ed.). New York: Oxford University Press.

Swenson, C. (1998). Clinical social work's contribution to a social justice perspective. *Social Work, 43*(6), 527–537.

Taylor, D. (2000). The rise of the environmental justice paradigm: Injustice framing and social construction of environmental discourses. *American Behavioral Scientist, 43*(4), 508–580.

United States General Accounting Office. (1983). *Siting of hazardous waste landfills and their correlation with racial and economic status of surrounding communities.* Washington, DC: Government Printing Office.

Van Wormer, K., and Besthorn, F.H. (2011). *Human behavior and the social environment: Groups, communities, and organizations* (2nd ed.). New York: Oxford University Press.

Wakefield, J. (1988). Psychotherapy, distributive justice, and social work part 1: Distributive justice as a conceptual framework for social work. *Social Service Review, 62*(2), 187–211.

Wakefield, J. (1998). Psychotherapy, distributive justice and social work revisited. *Smith College Studies in Social Work, 69*(1), 25–57.

Wenz, P. (2001). *Environmental ethics today.* New York: Oxford University Press.

Westra, L. (2001). From Aldo Leopold to the wildlands project: The ethics of integrity. *Environmental Ethics, 23*(3), 261–274.

Westra, L., Westra, R., and Bosselman, K. (Eds). (2008). *Reconciling human existence with ecological integrity: Science, ethics, economics and law.* Oxford, UK: Earthscan.

Zapf, M. (2009). *Social work and the environment: Understanding people and place.* Toronto: Canadian Scholars Press.

Zimmerman, M., Callicott, J.B., Sessions, G., Warren, K., and Clark, J. (Eds). (2001). *Environmental philosophy: From animal right to radical ecology* (3rd ed.). Upper Saddle River, NJ: Prentice Hall.

2 Ecosocial work with marginalized populations

Time for action on climate change

Tiani Hetherington and Jennifer Boddy

> It is not enough for people [social workers] to know about climate change in order to be engaged; they also need to care about it, be motivated and able to take action (Lorenzoni, Nicholson-Cole, and Whitmarsh, 2007: 446).

While there is an emerging social work literature on climate change (Alston and Whittenbury, 2011, forthcoming; Dominelli, 2011, forthcoming; Lysack, 2007, 2008), there has been little engagement with its effects on marginalized communities. Consequently, this chapter explores the potential effects of climate change on marginalized communities, as well as the science of climate change, in the belief that social workers need to understand these issues in order to respond appropriately for the welfare of current and future generations. Despite repeated calls for social work's unique person-in-environment construct to be reconceptualized to incorporate not only the built and social environments, but also the natural environment, mainstream social work has yet to take up this challenge. Yet, there are tremendous social, economic, and political consequences of climate change that will adversely affect many of the people with whom social workers practise. This chapter documents the inequalities resulting from environmentally unsustainable policies in an effort to inform social work practitioners and provide foundational knowledge for environmental social work scholarship, critique, education, and activism.

Social work and climate change

While there has been a push for social work to engage with environmental issues since the 1970s, the social work profession has been slow to respond to climate change and environmental degradation (Coates, 2005; Coates and Gray, 2011). However, social work's focus on the 'person-in-environment' or ecosystems perspective places the profession in a strong position to address environmental issues (Norton, 2011; Schmitz, Matyók, Sloan, and James, 2011). For example, Matthies, Närhi, and Ward (2001) believe social workers' 'person-in-environment' approach predisposes them to 'a new multidimensional and holistic way of working [which] can re-build connections between service users, decisions and politics in a given living area' (p. 141). Yet, social work has tended to focus solely on the social rather than the physical or natural environment, despite repeated calls for a reconceptualization of the person-in-environment perspective (see, for example, Besthorn, 2000; Coates, 2003; Norton, 2009, 2011; Rogge and Cox, 2001; Zapf, 2009). Besthorn (2003) argues that social workers must incorporate environmental justice into mainstream practice as 'concern for any oppression necessitates concern for all oppression' (p. 14) (see Chapter 1).

Much of the literature to date on ecosocial work and climate change is highly theoretical and normative in nature (Molyneux, 2010). Several social work writers have highlighted the impact of environmental issues on economically disadvantaged populations in industrial and developing nations (see, for example, Coates, 2005; Hoff, 1996; Kaufman and Slonim-Nevo, 2004; Rogge, 2000; Stehlik, 2003). A number of social work conferences and special journal issues have been devoted to the environment and climate change (see *Critical Social Work 11*(3); Coates and Besthorn, 2010; and the Global Alliance for a Deep Ecological Social Work, 2011).

Additionally, social work codes of ethics espouse a social justice value base, with an increasing number recognizing the importance of ecological justice principles. For example, the Australian Code of Ethics (2010) claims that the social work profession 'promotes the protection of the natural environment as inherent to social wellbeing' (p. 13), while the Canadian Code of Ethics (2005) says that 'social workers promote social development and environmental management in the interests of all people' (p. 5). Similarly, the International Federation of Social Workers (2004) claims that 'social workers should be concerned with the whole person, within the family, community, societal and natural environments, and should seek to recognise all aspects of a person's life' (p. 2). Despite these policy statements, a clear role for social workers in relation to climate change has yet to be determined and some might question whether working with marginalized groups to deal with the fallout from climate change is the 'core' business of social work.

However, ecological questions are also social questions and there is a connection between social and ecological problems (and between social and ecological justice). As well, climate change and environmental degradation are political issues (Giddens, 2009). Several writers adopt a rights-based approach to ecological justice and climate change. For example, Lysack (2011) sees climate change as a human rights issue while others emphasize people's right to live in a safe, clean, and healthy environment (Molyneux, 2010). Närhi and Matthies (2001) claim that 'social workers should act as political actors, and ... have a political agenda ... to guide society in the direction of sustainable development' (p. 33).

The science of climate change: A contested discourse

The science of climate change is contested with political and media discourses primarily revolving around two opposing groups: the climate change 'skeptics' (or deniers) and the 'greens' (Giddens, 2009). This is a highly contentious area based on the extent of belief about whether or not climate change is human induced or part of nature's natural cycles (with skeptics pointing to prior ice and heat ages). However, the full weight of scientific evidence suggests that the climate is changing and that human activities are exacerbating environmental change (see the Intergovernmental Panel on Climate Change [IPCC], 2007).

Through dominant 'promethean' views (Dryzek, 2005), humans have interfered, and continue to interfere, in the natural environment, and thus have contributed to climate change (see Pielke, 2005). Predictions link future changes to the physical environment and ecosystems to human actions, particularly around greenhouse gas emissions (Giddens, 2009). According to scientist David King (2004), 'Climate change is real, and the causal link to increased greenhouse emissions is now well established' (p. 176; see also Oreskes, 2004).

Climate change is likely to manifest in four ways: slow changes in mean climate conditions, increased interannual and seasonal variability, increased frequency of extreme events, and rapid climate changes causing catastrophic shifts in ecosystems (IPCC, 2001, 2007). On all continents and in most oceans, changes in natural systems have been observed. These include, but are not limited to, changes in marine and freshwater biological systems, earlier timing of spring events, reduced ice cover, and warmer lakes and rivers. Over the past century, temperatures have risen between 0.6°C and 0.8°C, with much of the increase over recent decades (Folland *et al.*, 2001; Mishra, Singh, and Jain, 2010). Additionally, global sea levels have risen by 20 cm, and ice caps on mountain peaks are melting (Rignot, Rivera, and Casassa, 2003; Thompson *et al.*, 2002). These are all phenomena that represent the impact of a changing climate, but are, at the same time, only early signs of what might come to pass. From a review of the literature, Tubiello and Rosenzweig (2008) concluded that in the short term moderate warming might benefit crops and pastures in temperate regions, while reducing yields in semi-arid and tropical regions, but further warming would have adverse effects on yields in all regions.

Climate change would be compounded by anticipated water shortages, with 80 per cent of the world's population facing extreme problems in relation to water security as a result of population and economic growth, particularly those in less wealthy nations who are unable to offset high stressor levels (Vörösmarty, Green, Salisbury, and Lammers, 2000; Vörösmarty *et al.*, 2010). Additionally, Hsiang, Meng, and Cane (2011) revealed that weather patterns, such as El Niño, with its higher temperatures and higher drought rates, have a direct impact on civil unrest. Hsiang *et al.* (2011) claim El Niño has contributed to 21 per cent of civil conflicts internationally since 1950 (see also Scheffran and Battaglini, 2011). As the climate changes, it is anticipated that the El Niño cycle will worsen and have significant implications for all people (see Adger, Huq, Brown, Conway, and Hulme, 2003; Trenberth and Hoar, 1997). Barnett and Adger (2007) argue:

> … change increasingly undermines human security in the present day, and will increasingly do so in the future, by reducing access to, and the quality of, natural resources that are important to sustain livelihoods. Climate change is also likely to undermine the capacity of states to provide the opportunities and services that help people to sustain their livelihoods. We argue that in certain circumstances these direct and indirect impacts of climate change on human security may in turn increase the risk of violent conflict.
>
> (p. 639)

In a world of increasing complexity and insecurity, the impacts of the planet's natural changes, together with human interference and alterations to the environment, are difficult to grasp, let alone contain. It is unclear what the likely speed of impacts and the probabilities of particular future scenarios might be (Schneider, 2001). There is also debate about whether change will mean irreversible global heating with catastrophic outcomes or whether changes will be relatively slow, allowing nations time to adjust (Szerszynski and Urry, 2010). However, what is clear is that some regions will be more vulnerable to the risks associated with climate change (Adger *et al.*, 2003); for example, it is predicted that those living in Africa, South Asia, the Arctic, and Small Island Developing States will fare particularly poorly (Crowley, 2011; Hare, Cramer, Schaeffer, Battaglini, and Jaeger, 2011). Thus, within societies, it is likely that different types of climate change will bring opportunities to some and increased vulnerability to others, based on economics and geography (Giddens, 2009). As the Stern Review (2007) argues:

> No two countries will face exactly the same situation in terms of impacts of the costs and benefits of action, and no country can take effective action to control the risk that they face alone. International collective action to tackle the problem is required because climate change is a global public good – countries can free-ride on each others' efforts – and because co-operative action will greatly reduce the costs of both mitigation and adaptation. The international collective response to the climate change problem is therefore unique, both in terms of complexity and depth.
>
> (p. 450)

Effects on marginalized populations

Almost two decades of research on vulnerability to climate change shows that, although all people will be affected, inevitably it is marginalized and disadvantaged people who suffer and will continue to suffer the greatest impacts of changing environmental conditions (see, for example, Adger *et al.*, 2003; Adger, Kelly, and Ninh, 2001; Bullard, 1993, 2000; Downing, 2003; Ribot, Magalhães, and Panagides. 1996; Smit and Pilifosova, 2001). This includes, but is not limited to, women, people living in poverty and in rural areas, Indigenous Peoples, and older people, all of whom experience varying inequities in mobility and access to wealth, food, water, and safe places in which to live. While in some areas, child poverty and HIV and AIDS appear to be more significant concerns, it is expected that there will be some 150–200 million displaced persons from climate change by 2050 as a result of rising seas, famine, and disease, making it a major issue for current and future generations (Stern, 2007). Climate change is thus not only an environmental phenomenon but also a social, economic, and political issue.

Poverty and climate change

Poverty is inextricably linked to climate change, as well as the capacity to adapt to, and mitigate the impact of, emergencies and durable changes of living conditions (Adger, 2003; Adger *et al.*, 2003). Although it is antici-pated that the degree to which people living in poverty will be affected by climate change will vary (Adger *et al.*, 2003; Hertel and Rosch, 2010), the poor, particularly those in developing countries, are expected to be disproportionately affected (Mendelsohn, Dinar, and Williams, 2006). According to Tol, Fankhauser, Richels, and Smith (2000):

> Although our knowledge of the impact of climate change is incomplete and uncertain, economic valuation is difficult and controversial, and the effect of other developments on the impacts of climate change is largely speculative, we find that poorer countries and people are more vulnerable than are richer countries and people.
>
> (p. 1)

People living in poverty not only lack material goods, but also the means by which to cope with impending environmental changes, as they have less access to key economic and social capital, such as education, private savings, and mobility, and to water, food, livelihoods, infrastructure, health, housing, and services (Hope, 2009; Meza, 2010). Thus, the projected impacts of climate change mean there will be a disruption or decrease in access to such commodities.

In rural areas, small-scale agriculture and fisheries are threatened by projected changes in precipitation, dry and wet seasons, and temperature, particularly in regions that are more severely affected by climate change (Hertel and Rosch, 2010; Hope, 2009; Meza, 2010). For example, in the Himalayan region of Nepal, the number of water sources near villages has decreased and there have been increased rates of water contamination resulting in disease. Agricultural production decreased by 50 per cent in 2008 due to a lack of rainfall, and there have been more displaced peoples as a result of floods and landslides over the last decade (Charmakar and Mijar, 2009). Further, 'de-peasantisation' (Davis, 2007), whereby poor rural people displaced by war and climate change impacts are forced to move to urban areas, leads to difficulties in finding work as these people are unlikely to have the education and job skills and experience required for urban labour markets (Hardoy and Pandiella, 2009; Hope, 2009; Meza, 2010).

Poor people in cities are more likely to build their homes in the least desirable areas and become disproportionately affected by floods, droughts, mudslides, and tsunamis (Hardoy and Pandiella, 2009). For example, in New Orleans, African-American and poor people were most adversely affected by Hurricane Katrina, with multiple negative life events linked to poverty. They were often unable to access transport to evacuate and they lived largely in low-lying, flood-prone areas (Hawkins, 2009). Additionally, all else being equal, African-American workers were four times more likely to lose their job in the month following the disaster than others. In reality, seven times as many African-American people lost their jobs during this time (Elliott and Pais, 2006). Consequently, poor people are more vulnerable to health problems induced by increased heatwaves and reduced urban air quality, as well as transmissible diseases, including malaria, dengue, and cholera, and rodent-borne infections following floods or droughts (Hardoy and Pandiella, 2009). Poor people also suffer from health problems from living near environmentally toxic locations more so than wealthy people (see, for example, Bullard, 2000; Hofrichter, 1993; Rogge, 1993, 2000).

Women and climate change

The effects of environmental climate change and environmental degradation are not gender neutral. Women continue to be the most vulnerable to climate change (Crate and Nuttall, 2009; Denton, 2002), and the highly gendered impacts of climate change have only recently been recognized. Women worldwide have less access than men to land, decision making, technology, and education (Aguilar, 2008). Although largely overlooked, women contribute significantly to the survival of agriculture and farming families, including work on the farm, income generation away from the farm, and in caring for children and the household (Alston, 2000). In many parts of the world, women and girls are the prime agriculturalists and carers of children, while men generally work outside the home. Women grow, gather, and cook much of the family's food, yet in many cultures they must eat only after the men and older male children have eaten. Thus, women bear the brunt of the fight to secure food, and are often solely responsible for the production of food for their families (Phillips, 2009).

As access to food is threatened due to droughts and floods associated with climate change, women suffer disproportionately more due to predefined gender roles, tighter cultural constraints regarding roles and mobility, and unequal power relations between men and women (Ahsan and Khatun, 2004; Demetriades and Esplen, 2008; Juran, 2012; Meza, 2010; Neumayer and Pluemper, 2007; Phillips, 2009; Röhr, Hemmati, and Lambrou, 2009; Sultana, 2010; Tol *et al.*, 2000). For example, during floods in Bangladesh many women do not leave their homes due to cultural constraints. They can be unaware of the impending danger as announcements are made in public places which women do not frequent, and if they do leave their homes they are often unable to swim (Röhr, in Demetriades and Esplen, 2008; see also Sultana, 2010). Additionally, women are more likely than men to experience reduced nutritional health (often ensuring the family is fed first) and increased workloads (such as greater distances to collect water, food, and fuel, and increasing work demands to generate income) as a result of climate changes (Alston, 2007; Denton, 2002). Food shortages and increasing food insecurity associated with climate change mean women face greater risks to their health when pregnant, particularly anaemia, and further risks due to limited resources in pre- and ante-natal care (Denton, 2002). In adapting to the impacts of climate change, women generally prioritize the emotional health and well-being of their family and community at the expense of their own (Alston, 2010).

Whether they live in developed or developing countries, poor and disadvantaged women are unequally affected by natural disasters and overrepresented in death tolls (Alston, 2010). For example, the majority of the people who died in the 2004 Indonesian tsunami were women (Oxfam, 2005; see also, Pittaway, Bartolomei, and Rees, 2007; Rees, Pittaway, and Bartolomei, 2005). During times of conflict over competition for scarce resources, women also face greater risks of violence, rape, anxiety, and human trafficking (Osei-Agyemang, 2007). The increasing risks to women caused by climate change inequalities point to the urgent need for a feminist approach to the issue of women and food insecurity, and the need for enhanced support and protection of women in marginalized and impoverished communities (Shiva, 2008).

Indigenous Peoples and minority race groups

The effects of climate change on Indigenous populations as well as other minority race groups are expected to be early and severe (Bullard, 1993, 1994, 2000; Chavis and Lee, 1987). Many Indigenous communities are situated in vulnerable areas with fragile ecosystems, including small islands, high altitude regions, deserts, and the Arctic. This is compounded in areas where local Indigenous Peoples rely upon natural resources for their livelihoods (Salick and Byg, 2007) and there are inadequate health services and infrastructure (Hennessy *et al.*, 2007). In some areas, Indigenous Peoples are no longer able to rely on traditional methods of farming and knowledge of weather patterns, ocean currents, and tides (Kalanda-Joshua, Ngongondo, Chipeta, and Mpembeka, 2011; Turner and Clifton, 2009). Top-down institutional processes, lack of recognition of Indigenous cultures, marginalization of Indigenous Peoples in debates about climate change, dismissal of Indigenous Peoples' rights to live in a safe and clean environment, and poor communication and engagement, have all reinforced oppressive practices that disempower Indigenous Peoples in their attempt to counteract the effects of climate change in their communities (Crowley, 2011; Petheram, Zander, Campbell, High, and Stacey, 2010). According to Lakhani, Oliver, Yee, Jackson, and Flicker (2010), 'climate change associated with industrialisation has continued the colonial legacy disrupting Indigenous connections to the land and has fuelled migration to urban centres' (p. 206).

Indigenous Peoples, however, are not only victims of climate change, but their knowledge and experience will provide insights and understanding into the phenomena, as well as potential adaptation measures (McLean, Ramos-Castillo, and Rubis, 2011; Schlosberg and Carruthers, 2010). More recently, scientific research has begun to draw from the experiences and observations of local Indigenous people (see for example, Alexander *et al.*, 2011; Green, Billy, and Tapim, 2010; Herman-Mercer, Schuster, and Maracle, 2011; Krupnik and Jolly, 2002; Kalanda-Joshua *et al.*, 2011; Laidler, 2006; Martello, 2008; Nyong, Adesina, and Elasha, 2007; Petheram, Zander, *et al.*, 2010; Turner and Clifton, 2009). Luseno *et al.* (2003) suggest that, since Indigenous climate prediction is needs-driven, focused on timing of rains and on locality, and is provided by '"experts" known and trusted by pastoralists' (p. 1,484), it may complement and improve other seasonal forecasts. Additionally, Indigenous Peoples' belief in their role as caretakers of the Earth, embracing 'all life forms as well as sustainability for the planet' (Gray, 2008: 192), provides insightful understandings of ways to respond to climate change (Coates, Gray, and Hetherington, 2006; Morrissette, McKenzie, and Morrissette, 1993). Thus, not only to ensure the effectiveness of climate change strategies, but also as a matter of equity and justice, Indigenous Peoples and minority race groups should be included in discussions about climate change (Sakona and Denton, 2001; Patt and Schröter, 2008; World People's Conference on Climate Change and the Rights of Mother Earth, 2010).

Older people and climate change

Although the effects of climate change for older people vary according to health and socioeconomic status, social connections, geographical location, and psychological well-being, older people more generally are particularly vulnerable to the adverse effects of climate change as a result of decreased mobility, poor physiology, and diminished access to resources (Filiberto *et al.*, 2009; Horton, Hanna, and Kelly, 2010). During extreme weather events, older people have increased susceptibility to disease, greater vulnerability to the effects of shortages or contamination of food and water supplies, and higher mortality rates (Filiberto *et al.*, 2009). The European heatwave in 2003, for example, killed approximately 30,000 people through heatstroke, and cardiovascular, cerebrovascular, and respiratory diseases, most of whom were elderly (Haines, Kovats, Campbell-Lendrum, and Corvalan, 2006; Argaud *et al.*, 2007). In heat waves older people are also more likely to experience heat exhaustion, cramps, strokes, renal failure, and heart attacks (Horton *et al.*, 2010). At the other extreme, the cold snap in 2009–2010 in the UK killed approximately 26,000 people, the majority of whom were over 75 (Hajat, Kovats, and Lachowycz, 2007). Additionally, during bushfires – which are exacerbated by heatwaves – older people are often dependent on others to evacuate and, if they have a respiratory disease, this will be aggravated due to exposure to smoke and air pollution (Horton *et al.*, 2010). Thus, the implications of climate change for older people are significant.

Conclusion: Ecosocial work, climate change, and marginalized populations

What then might we glean about an ecosocial work model to promote ecological justice? Social workers are already proactively engaged in working with those most disadvantaged and at the margins of society. However, they need to educate themselves and others about climate change and the opportunities for micro and macro practice interventions (see typology in introduction). For example, social workers can focus their energies on a range of issues from resource depletion, to global warming, air and water pollution, and species extinction to name a few. They can redirect policy toward green energy solutions, work in communities in the aftermath of natural disasters, bringing their crisis intervention and community engagement skills to the fore, and work with others to provide emergency health services (see Chapter 15).

The adverse effects of climate change on marginalized people and communities mean that social workers need to respond appropriately for the welfare of current and future generations. Social workers, with their focus on social justice, are uniquely positioned to respond to the effects of climate change on marginalized populations. Based on the belief that climate change and environmental degradation are already occurring, and that those most marginalized will be most directly affected, social workers should be at the forefront of debates about rights and ecological justice and move towards a more informed stance if the profession is to manage the fallout from climate change. Social workers have an important role to play in informing themselves and others about the science of climate change, the effects on marginalized populations, and the interconnected nature of human well-being and the natural environment, while also mobilizing people to take action and overtly challenge practices, beliefs, policies, and laws that are environmentally unsustainable. Social work has a role to play in ensuring that social and ecological justice shapes society's responses to climate change and a sustainable future will be available to all.

References

Adger, W.N. (2003). Social capital, collective action and adaptation to climate change. *Economic Geography, 79*(4), 387–404.

Adger, W.N., Huq, S., Brown, K., Conway, D., and Hulme, M. (2003). Adaption to climate change in the developing world. *Progress in Development Studies, 3*(3), 179–195.

Adger, W.N., Kelly, P.M., and Ninh, N.H. (Eds). (2001). *Living with environmental change: Social resilience, adaptation and vulnerability in Vietnam.* London: Routledge.

Aguilar, L. (2008). *Is there a connection between gender and climate change?* International Union for the Conservation of Nature (IUCN): Office of the Senior Gender Advisor.

Ahsan, R., and Khatun, H. (2004). *Disaster and the silent gender.* In R. Ahsan and Khatun, H. (Eds). *Disaster and the silent gender: Contemporary studies in geography.* Dhaka: The Bangladesh Geographical Society. 1–8.

Alexander, C., Bynum, N., Johnson, E., King, U., Mustonen, T., Neofotis, P., Oettle, N., Sakakibara, C., Shadrin, V., Vicarelli, M., Waterhouse, J., and Weeks, B. (2011). Linking Indigenous scientific knowledge of climate change. *BioScience, 61*(6), 477–484.

Alston, M. (2000). *Breaking through the grass ceiling: Women, power and leadership in rural Australia.* Churr, Switzerland: Harwood Publishers.

Alston, M. (2007). Gender and climate change: Variable adaptations of men and women. *Just Policy, 46,* 29–35.

Alston, M. (2010). Gender and climate change in Australia. *Journal of Sociology, 47*(1), 53–70.

Alston, M., and Whittenbury, K. (Eds). (forthcoming). *Research, action and policy: Addressing the gendered impacts of climate change.* New York: Springer.

Alston, M., and Whittenbury, K. (2011). Climate change and water policy in Australia's irrigation areas: A lost opportunity for a partnership model of governance. *Environmental Politics, 20*(6), 899–917.

Argaud, L., Ferry, T., Le, Q.H., Marfist, A., Ctorba, D., Achache, P., and Robert, D. (2007). Short- and long-term outcomes of heatstroke following the 2003 heat wave in Lyon, France. *Archives of Internal Medicine, 167,* 2177–2183.

Barnett, J., and Adger, W.N. (2007). Climate change, human security and violent crime. *Political Geography, 26,* 639–655.

Besthorn, F.H. (2000). Toward a deep-ecological social work: Its environmental, spiritual and political dimensions. *The Spirituality and Social Work Forum, 7*(2), 2–7.

Besthorn, F.H. (2003). Radical ecologisms: Insights for educating social workers in ecological activism and social justice. *Critical Social Work: An Interdisciplinary Journal Dedicated to Social Justice, 3*(1), 66–106. Retrieved February 9, 2012 from http://www.criticalsocialwork.com/CSW_2003_1.html.

Bullard, R. (1993). Anatomy of environmental racism and the environmental justice movement. In R.D. Bullard (Ed.). *Confronting environmental racism: Voices from the grassroots.* Boston: South End Press. 15–39.

Bullard, R. (Ed.). (1994). *Unequal protection.* San Francisco: Sierra Club Books.

Bullard, R. (2000). *Dumping in Dixie: Race, class, and environmental quality* (3rd ed.). Boulder, CO: Westview Press.

Charmakar, S., and Mijar, D. (2009). Impact of climate change on poor and marginalised people in high mountain region, Nepal. *IOP Conference Series: Earth and Environmental Science, Climate Change: Global Risks, Challenges and Decisions, 6.* Retrieved December 31, 2011 from http://iopscience.iop.org/1755-1315/6/14/142017.

Chavis, B., and Lee, C. (1987). *Toxic wastes and race in the United States: A national report on the racial and socio-economic characteristics of communities with hazardous waste sites.* New York: United Church of Christ Commission for Racial Justice.

Coates, J. (2003). *Ecology and social work: Toward a new paradigm.* Halifax, NS: Fernwood Books.

Coates, J. (2005). Environmental crisis: Implications for social work. *Journal of Progressive Human Services, 16*(1), 25–49.

Coates, J., and Besthorn, F. (Eds). (2010). Building bridges and crossing boundaries: Dialogues on professional helping. Special Issue. *Critical Social Work, 11*(3). Downloaded from http://www.uwindsor.ca/criticalsocialwork/2010-volume-11-no-3.

Coates, J., and Gray, M. (2011). The environment and social work: An overview and introduction. *International Journal of Social Welfare, 21,* 1–9. Article first published online: 13 DEC 2011 | DOI: 10.1111/j.1468-2397.2011.00851.x.

Coates, J., Gray, M., and Hetherington, T. (2006). An 'ecospiritual' perspective: Finally, a place for Indigenous approaches. *British Journal of Social Work, 36*(3), 381–399.

Crate, S., and Nuttall, M. (2009). *Anthropology and climate change: From encounters to actions.* Walnut Creek, CA: Left Coast Press.

Crowley, P. (2011). Interpreting 'dangerous' in the United Nations framework convention on climate change and the human rights of Inuit. *Global Environmental Change, 11*(S1), 265–274.

Davis, M. (2007). *Planet of slums.* London, England: Verso.

Demetriades, J., and Esplen, E. (2008). The gender dimensions of poverty and climate change adaptation. *IDS Bulletin, 39*(4), 24–31.

Denton, F. (2002). Climate change vulnerability, impacts, and adaptation: Why does gender matter? *Gender & Development, 10*(2), 10–20.

Dominelli, L. (2011). Climate change: Social workers' roles and contributions to policy debates and practice interventions. *International Journal of Social Welfare, 20*(4), 430–438.

Dominelli, L. (forthcoming). Gendering climate change: Implications for debates, policies and practice. In M. Alston and Whittenbury, K. (Eds). *Women and climate change.* Melbourne: Monash University.

Downing, T. (2003). Toward a vulnerability/adaptation science: Lessons from famine early warning and food security. In J. Smith, Klein, R., Huq, S. (Eds). *Climate change adaptive capacity and development*. London: Imperial College Press. 77–100.

Dryzek, J. (2005). *The politics of the earth: Environmental discourses* (2nd ed.). Oxford: Oxford University Press.

Elliott, J.R., and Pais, J. (2006). Race, class, and Hurricane Katrina: Social differences in human responses to disaster. *Social Science Research, 35,* 295–321.

Filiberto, D., Wethington, E., Pillemer, K., Wells, N.M., Wysocki, M., and Parise, J.T. (2009). Older people and climate change: Vulnerability and health effects. *Generations, 33*(4), 19–25.

Folland, C.K., Karl, T.R., Christy, J.R., Clarke, R.A., Gruza, G.V., Jouzel, J., Mann, M.E., Oerlemans, J., Salinger, M.J., and Wang, S.W. (2001). Observed climate variability and change. In J.T.,Houghton, Ding, Y., Griggs, D.J., Noguer, M., van der Linden, P.J., Dai, X., Maskell, K., and Johnson, C.A. (Eds). *Climate Change 2001: The Scientific Basis. Contribution of Working Group I to the Third Assessment Report of the Intergovernmental Panel on Climate Change.* Cambridge: Cambridge University Press. 99–182.

Giddens, A. (2009). *The politics of climate change.* Cambridge: Polity Press.

Global Alliance for a Deep Ecological Social Work. (2011). Downloaded from http://ecosocialwork.org/.

Gray, M. (2008). Viewing spirituality in social work through the lens of contemporary social theory. *British Journal of Social Work, 38*(1), 175–196.

Green, D., Billy, J., and Tapim, A. (2010). Indigenous Australians' knowledge of weather and climate. *Climatic Change, 100,* 337–354.

Haines, A., Kovats, R.S., Campbell-Lendrum, D., and Corvalan, C. (2006). Climate change and human health: Impacts, vulnerability and public health. *Public Health, 120,* 585–596.

Hajat, S., Kovats, R.S., and Lachowycz, K. (2007). Heat-related and cold-related deaths in England and Wales: Who is at risk? *Journal of Occupational and Environmental Medicine, 64,* 93–100.

Hardoy, J., and Pandiella, G. (2009). Urban poverty and vulnerability to climate change in Latin America. *Environment and Urbanization, 21*(1), 203–224.

Hare, W.L., Cramer, W., Schaeffer, M., Battaglini, A., and Jaeger, C.C. (2011). Climate hotspots: Key vulnerable regions, climate change and limits to warming. *Regional Environmental Change, 11*(S1), 1–13.

Hawkins, R.L. (2009). Same as it ever was, only worse: Negative life events and poverty among New Orleans Katrina survivors. *Families in Society, 90*(4), 375–381.

Hennessy, K., Fitzharris, B., Bates, B.C., Harvey, N., Howden, S.M., Hughes, L., Salinger, J., and Warrick, R. (2007). Australia and New Zealand. Climate change 2007: Impacts, adaptation and vulnerability. In M.L. Parry, Canziani, O.F., Palutikof, J.P., van der Linden, P.J., and Hanson, C.E. (Eds). *Contribution of Working Group II to the Fourth Assessment Report of the Intergovernmental Panel on Climate Change.* Cambridge, UK: Cambridge University Press. 507–540.

Herman-Mercer, N., Schuster, P.F., and Maracle, K.B. (2011). Indigenous observations of climate change in the lower Yukon River Basin, Alaska. *Human Organization, 70*(3), 244–252.

Hertel, T.W., and Rosch, S.D. (2010). Climate change, agriculture, and poverty. *Applied Economic Perspectives and Policy, 32*(3), 355–385.

Hoff, M.D. (1996). Poverty, environmental decline and intergroup violence: An exploration of the linkages. In J.S. Ismael (Ed.). *International social welfare in a changing world*. Calgary: Detseling Enterprise, Ltd. Press. 167–183.

Hofrichter, R. (1993). *Toxic struggles: The theory and practice of environmental justice*. Philadelphia, PA: New Society.

Hope, K.R. (2009). Climate change and poverty in Africa. *International Journal of Sustainable Development and World Ecology, 16*(6), 451–461.

Horton, G., Hanna, L., and Kelly, B. (2010). Drought, drying and climate change: Emerging health issues for ageing Australians in rural areas. *Australasian Journal on Ageing, 29*(1), 2–7.

Hsiang, S.M., Meng, K.C., and Cane, M.A. (2011). Civil conflicts are associated with the global climate. *Nature, 476,* 438–441. Retrieved February 9, 2012 from http://ochaonline.un.org/NewsInFocus/ClimateChangeHumanitarianImpact/Cli... http://www.circleofblue.org/waternews/2010/world/peter-gleick-climate-change-deniers-versus-the-scientific-societies-of-the-world-who-should-we-listen-to/.

Intergovernmental Panel on Climate Change (IPCC). (2001). *The Third Assessment Report: Climate Change 2001*. New York: Cambridge University Press.

Intergovernmental Panel on Climate Change (IPCC). (2007). *The Fourth Assessment Report: Climate Change 2007*. New York: Cambridge University Press.

Juran, L. (2012). The gendered nature of disasters: Women survivors in post-tsunami Tamil Nadu. *Indian Journal of Gender Studies, 19*(1), 1–29.

Kalanda-Joshua, M., Ngongondo, C., Chipeta, L., and Mpembeka, F. (2011). Integrating indigenous knowledge with convention science: Enhancing localised climate and weather forecasts in Nessa, Mulanje, Malawi. *Physics and Chemistry of the Earth, 36,* 996–1003.

Kaufman, R., and Slonim-Nevo, V. (2004). Food insecurity and hunger among disadvantaged populations in the Negev: Findings from an exploratory research. *Social Security, 65* (Hebrew), 33–54.

King, D.A. (2004). Climate change science: Adapt, mitigate, or ignore? *Science, 303,* 176–177.

Krupnik, I., and Jolly, D. (Eds). (2002). *The Earth is faster now: Indigenous observations of Arctic environmental change*. Fairbanks, AK: Arctic Research Consortium of the United States.

Laidler, G.J. (2006). Inuit and scientific perspectives on the relationship between sea ice and climate change: The ideal complement? *Climatic Change, 78,* 407–444.

Lakhani, A., Oliver, V., Yee, J., Jackson, R., and Flicker, S. (2010). Keep the fire burning brightly: Aboriginal youth using hip-hop to decolonize in a chilly climate. In L.A. Sandberg and Sandberg, T. (Eds). *Climate change: Who's carrying the burden?* Toronto, CA: Canadian Centre for Policy Alternatives. 205–215.

Lorenzoni, I., Nicholson-Cole, S., and Whitmarsh, L. (2007). Barriers perceived to engaging with climate change among the UK public and their policy implications. *Global Environmental Change, 17,* 445–459.

Luseno, W.K., McPeak, J.G., Barrett, C.B., Little, P.D., and Gebru, G. (2003). Assessing the value of climate forecast information for pastoralists: Evidence from southern Ethiopia and northern Kenya. *World Development, 31*(9), 1477–1494.

Lysack, M. (2007). Family therapy, the ecological self, and global warming. *Context, 91*, 9–11.

Lysack, M. (2008). Global warming as a moral issue: Ethics and economics of reducing carbon emissions. *Interdisciplinary Environmental Review, 10*(1/2), 95–109.

Lysack, M. (2011). Building capacity for environmental engagement and leadership: An ecosocial work perspective. *International Journal of Social Welfare, 21.* Article first published online: 13 DEC 2011 | DOI: 10.1111/j.1468-2397.2011.00854.x.

Martello, M.A. (2008). Arctic Indigenous Peoples as representations and representatives of climate change. *Social Studies of Science, 38*(3), 351–376.

Matthies, A.-L., Närhi, K., and Ward, D. (Eds). (2001). *The eco-social approach in social work.* Jyväskylä, Finland: Sophi Publishers.

McLean, K.G., Ramos-Castillo, A., and Rubis, J. (2011). Indigenous Peoples, Marginalized Populations and Climate Change: Vulnerability, Adaptation and Traditional Knowledge. *IPMPCC Workshop Report. *Retried February 2, 2012 from http://www.unutki.org/downloads/File/2011_IPMPCC_Mexico_Workshop _Summary_Report_web.pdf.

Mendelsohn, R., Dinar, A., and Williams, L. (2006). The distributional impact of climate change on rich and poor countries. *Environment and Development Economics, 11*, 159–178.

Meza, L.E.R. (2010). Climate change, poverty and migration processes in Chiapas, Mexico. *International Journal of Labour Research, 2*(2), 187–210.

Mishra, A.K., Singh, V.P., and Jain, S.K. (2010). Impact of global warming and climate change on social development. *Journal of Comparative Social Welfare, 26*(2–3), 239–260.

Molyneux, R. (2010). The practical realities of ecosocial work: A review of the literature. *Critical Social Work, 11*(2), 61–69. Retrieved February 2, 2011 from www.uwindsor.ca/criticalsocialwork.

Morrissette, V., McKenzie, B., and Morrissette, L. (1993). Towards an Aboriginal model of social work practice: Cultural knowledge and traditional practices. *Canadian Social Work Review, 10*(1), 91–108.

Närhi, K., and Matthies, A.-L. (2001). What is the ecological (self-)consciousness of social work? Perspectives on the relationship between social work and ecology. In A.-L. Matthies, Nähri, K., and Ward, D. (Eds). *The eco-social approach in social work.* Jyväskylä: Sophi. 16–53.

Neumayer, E., and Pluemper, T. (2007). *The gendered nature of natural disasters: The impact of catastrophic events on the gender gap in life expectancy, 1981–2002.* Retrieved November 10, 2009 from http://papers.ssrn.com/sol3/papers.cfm?abstract_ id=874965.

Norton, C.L. (2009). Ecopsychology and social work: Creating an interdisciplinary framework for redefining person-in-environment. *Ecopsychology, 1*(3), 138–145.

Norton, C.L. (2011). Social work and the environment: An ecosocial approach. *International Journal of Social Welfare, 21.* Article first published online: 9DEC2011|DOI: 10.1111/j.1468-2397.2011.00853.x.

Nyong, A., Adesina, F., and Elasha, B.O. (2007). The value of indigenous knowledge in climate change mitigation and adaption strategies in the African Sahel. *Mitigation Adaption Strategies for Global Change, 12*(5), 787–797.

Oreskes, N. (2004). The scientific consensus on climate change. *Science, 306*, 1686.

Osei-Agyemang, M. (2007). Temperatures rising: Understanding the relationship between climate change, conflict and women. *Women & Environments International Magazine, 74/75*, 25–27.

Oxfam (2005). *The tsunami's impact on women.* Oxfam International. Retrieved February 9, 2012 from www.oxfam.org/en/policy/bn050326-tsunami-women.

Patt, A.G., and Schröter, D. (2008). Perceptions of climate risk in Mozambique: Implications for the success of adaptation strategies. *Global Environmental Change, 18*, 458–467.

Petheram, L., Zander, K.K., Campbell, B.M., High, C., and Stacey, N. (2010). 'Strange changes': Indigenous perspectives of climate change and adaption in NE Arnhem Land (Australia). *Global Environmental Change, 20*(4), 681–692.

Phillips, R. (2009). Food security and women's health: A feminist perspective for international social work. *International Social Work, 52*(4), 485–498.

Pielke, R.A. (2005). Land use and climate change. *Science, 310*, 1625–1626.

Pittaway, E., Bartolomei, L., and Rees, S. (2007). Gendered dimensions of the 2004 tsunami and a potential social work response in post-disaster situations. *International Social Work, 50*(3), 307–319.

Rees, S., Pittaway, E., and Bartolomei, L. (2005). Waves of violence: Women in post-tsunami Sri Lanka. *Australasian Journal of Disaster and Trauma Studies, 2.* Retrieved February 2, 2012 from http://www.massey.ac.nz/~trauma/issues/2005-2/rees. htm.

Ribot, J.C., Magalhães, A.R., and Panagides, S.S. (Eds). (1996). *Climate variability, climate change and social vulnerability in the semi-arid tropics.* Cambridge, England: Cambridge University Press.

Rignot, E., Rivera, A., and Casassa, G. (2003). Contribution of the Patagonia Icefields of South America to sea level rise. *Science, 302*, 434–437.

Rogge M.E. (1993). Social work, disenfranchised communities, and the natural environment: Field education opportunities. *Journal of Social Work Education, 29*, 111–120.

Rogge, M.E. (2000). Children, poverty, and environmental degradation: Protecting current and future generations. *Social Development Issues, 22*(2/3), 46–53.

Rogge, M.E., and Cox, M.E. (2001). The person-in-environment perspective in social work journals: A computer assisted content analysis. *Journal of Social Services Research, 28*(2), 47–68.

Röhr, U., Hemmati, M., and Lambrou, Y. (2009). Towards gender equality in climate change policy: Challenges and perspectives for the future. In E. Enarson and Dar Chakrabarti, P.G. (Eds). *Women, Gender and Disaster.* London: Sage. 289–303.

Sakona, Y., and Denton, F. (2001). Climate change impacts: Can Africa cope with the challenges? *Climate Policy, 1*(1), 117–123.

Salick, J., and Byg, A. (2007). *Indigenous Peoples and climate change.* Oxford: Tyndall Centre for Climate Change Research.

Scheffran, J., and Battaglini, A. (2011). Climate and conflicts: The security risks of global warming. *Regional Environmental Change, 11*(S1), 27–39.

Schlosberg, D., and Carruthers, D. (2010) Indigenous struggles, environmental justice and community capabilities. *Global Environmental Politics, 12*(4), 12–35.

Schmitz, C.L., Matyók, T., Sloan, L., and James, C.D. (2011). The relationship between social work and environmental sustainability: Implications for interdisciplinary practice. *International Journal of Social Welfare, 21.* Article first published online: 13 DEC 2011 DOI: 10.1111/j.1468-2397.2011.00855.x.

Schneider, S.H. (2001). What is 'dangerous' climate change? *Nature, 411,* 17–19.

Shiva, V. (2008). *Soil, not oil: Climate change, peak oil and food insecurity.* London, England: Zed Books.

Smit, B., and Pilifosova, O. (2001). Adaptation to climate change in the context of sustainable development and equity. In J.J. McCarthy, Canziani, O., Leary, N.A., Dokken, D.J., and White, K.S. (Eds). *Climate change 2001: Impacts, adaptation and vulnerability.* Cambridge: Cambridge University Press. 877–912.

Stehlik, D. (2003) Australian drought as lived experience: Social and community impacts. In L. Botterill and Fisher, M. (Eds). *Beyond drought in Australia: People, policy and place.* Canberra: CSIRO Press.

Stern, N. (2007). *Stern review of the economics of climate change.* Cambridge, England: Cambridge University Press. Part VI: International Collective Action. 450–467. Retrieved February 9, 2012 from http://webarchive.nationalarchives.gov. uk/20100407174731/http://www.hm-treasury.gov.uk/stern_review_report.htm.

Sultana, F. (2010). Living in hazardous waterscapes: Gendered vulnerabilities and experiences of floods and disasters. *Environmental Hazards, 9*(1), 43–53.

Szerszynski, B., and Urry, J. (2010). Changing climates: Introduction. *Theory Culture Society, 27*(2–3), 1–8.

Thompson, L.G., Mosley-Thompson, E., Davies, M.E., Henderson, K.A., Brecher, H.H., Zagorodnov, V.S., Mashiotta, T.A., Lin, P.N., Mikhalenko, V.N., Hardy, D.R., and Beer, J. (2002). Kilimanjaro ice core records: Evidence of Holocene climate change in tropic Africa. *Science, 298,* 589–593.

Tol, R.S.J., Fankhauser, S., Richels, R.G., and Smith, J.B. (2000). *How much damage will climate change do? Recent estimates.* Working Paper SCG-2, Research Unit Sustainability and Global Change.

Trenberth, K.E., and Hoar, T.J. (1997). El Niño and climate change. *Geophysical Research Letters, 24*(3), 3057–3060.

Tubiello, F.N., and Rosenzweig, C. (2008). Developing climate change impact metrics for agriculture. *Integrated Assessment Journal, 8*(1), 165–184.

Turner, N.J., and Clifton, H. (2009). 'It's so different today': Climate change and indigenous lifeways in British Columbia, Canada. *Global Environmental Change, 19,* 180–190.

Vörösmarty, C.J., Green, P., Salisbury, J., and Lammers, R.B. (2000). Global water resources: Vulnerability from climate change and population growth. *Science, 289,* 284–288.

Vörösmarty, C.J., McIntrye, P.B., Gessner, M.O., Dudgeon, D., Prusevich, A., Green, P.A., Glidden, S., Bunn, S.E., Sullivan, C.A., Reidy, C.A., and Davies, P.M. (2010). Global threats to human water security and river biodiversity. *Nature, 467,* 555–561.

World People's Conference on Climate Change and the Rights of Mother Earth (2010). Peoples Agreement. Retrieved on October 12, 2011 from http://pwccc. wordpress.com/support /.

Zapf, M.K. (2009). *Social work and the environment: Understanding people and place.* Toronto, ON: Canadian Scholars' Press.

3 Environmental sustainability, sustainable development, and social work

Arielle Dylan

> In the long run, sustainable living demands a fundamental shift in values.
> But action invariably precedes a profound shift in values, so actually doing
> something is important. In the process, one learns and becomes committed
> (Suzuki, McConnell, and Mason, 2007: 302).

The twenty-first century has brought into focus the cumulative concerns
and warnings heralded by environmental thinkers, scholars, and activists
since the time of industrialization (see, for example, Carson, 1962; Leopold,
1949; Marsh, 1864; Muir, 1914; Pinchot, 1947). Indeed the post-industrial
era is marked by such extensive human-generated environmental damage
that the term *anthropocene* has been used to describe this epoch (Crutzen
and Stoermer, 2000). A review of the environmental challenges commonly
inventoried forecasts a precarious future: irrefutable climate change,
persistent chemical toxins polluting air and water, toxic loads bio-
accumulated in human beings and other species, diminishing potable water
supply, deforestation, desertification and soil degradation, coral reef
dieback around the world, species loss, and new disease vectors and
infestations (Barlow, 2007; Korten, 2009; Monbiot, 2006; Speth, 2008). This
context of diminished environmental quality and uncertain futurity,
together with the growing attention to climate change, garnered in public
discourse, has underscored the interdependence of social and environmental
well-being. Increasing awareness of the human–environment relationship
has mobilized concerned citizens to defend inhabited and life-supporting
places and protect and enshrine rights of access to natural necessities, such
as water and air.

Many have recognized the fit between social work and environmental
considerations given the central metaphor of 'person-in-environment'
and the profession's historical and continued commitment to addressing
social, political, material, and structural realities and injustices (Besthorn,
1997; Rogge, 1994a; Rogge and Cox, 2001; Zapf, 2009). As early as the
beginning of the twentieth century, Jane Addams, during her Settlement
House experiences, observed the challenges of urban overcrowding and

sanitation, and documented the profound relationship between environmental and public health: 'nothing was more painfully clear than the fact that pliable human nature is relentlessly pressed upon by its physical environment' (Addams, 1990: 111). In their most recent articulation of the life model for social work practice, Gitterman and Germain (2008) have given greater attention to the 'natural world, our life-sustaining environment' (p. 249). For more than two decades now, social work, in its professional and scholarly purview, has increasingly called attention to the importance of the human–nature relationship. Soine (1987), in many ways picking up the mantle from Addams, argued for the need to include the physical environment, especially 'environmental hazards content', more amply in social work curricula. Rogge (1994b), building on the Chavis and Lee's (1987) US Racial Justice report (1987) and Bullard's (1990) sociological examination of environmental racism, was among the first to suggest the need for social work to concentrate on environmental injustice issues. This concern has been further developed to include a strong international perspective encompassing poverty, social justice, and the environment (Rogge and Darkwa, 1996; Rogge, 2000). Some have argued for the value of expanding and reworking the foundational person-in-environment metaphor into a more ecocentric, accurate representation of the human–nature relationship (Besthorn, 1997; Hoff and Polack, 1993; Rogge, 1994a; Zapf, 2009), while others have stressed the significance of theoretical frameworks new to social work, such as Deep Ecology and ecofeminism (Besthorn, 2003; Besthorn and McMillen, 2002; Ungar, 2002). Hoff and Polack (1993) traced environmental issues, and related social, political, and economic concerns, to neoclassical economics and scientific rationalism. Coates (2003), similarly seeking to uncover causes for contemporary sociopolitical and environmental ills, holds modernity culpable and identifies how social work, forged in modernity and shaped by its tenets, potentially perpetuates the human–nature divide. One prominent concept in the environmental social work literature, perhaps because of the shared humanistic underpinnings, is that of sustainability (Estes, 1993; Gamble and Hoff, 2005; Hoff, 1994, 1998; Lusk and Hoff, 1994; Mary, 2008).

According to the World Wildlife Fund (2008), humankind is consuming resources 'faster than they can be replenished' (p. 1), is responsible for an ecological footprint that 'exceeds the planet's regenerative capacity by about 30%' (p. 3), and will require two planets by the early 2030s should business as usual persist. In this context, the appeal of sustainability, with its potentiality for inherent solution-focused, multisectoral, and multiscalar pragmatism, is understandable. This chapter investigates the relevance of sustainability and sustainable development to environmental social work, examining its fit, strengths, roles, and applications.

Historical development of sustainability and sustainable development

Definitions and influences

Sustainability and sustainable development (hereafter, SD) are different but related concepts, though often used interchangeably. The term sustainability has been conceived as having weak and strong forms: weak sustainability being more consistent with market imperatives and faith in technological interventions while strong sustainability has an ecosystemic focus, that is, a desire to preserve natural capital and the ability to substitute human-made for ecologically-derived resources (Agyeman, Bullard, and Evans, 2003; Sneddon, Howarth, and Norgaard, 2006). The word 'development' in the phrase SD ties the construct to development theory, which often, in its conventional formulations, is associated with economic growth. For the purposes of this chapter, and in keeping with the majority of literature on the subject, sustainability and SD are used as approximate synonyms.

Sustainability is not a static construct but rather an evolving notion that advocates a particular method of investigation that varies in accordance with context, goals, and newly emerging ecosystemic understandings (Bagheri and Hjorth, 2007). A blueprint approach to SD is impracticable because the contingency of sustainability forecloses unequivocal, universal, and decontextualized forms of planning (Leach, Scoones, and Stirling, 2010; Voss and Kemp, 2005). Despite the fluid status of SD, it is the preferred and leading development paradigm at multiscalar levels in countries of the Global North and South (Castro, 2004). Yet handily defining SD remains elusive as there are myriad definitions reflecting sociopolitical differences. For example, a Marxist understanding of SD would involve an idea of an ecological commons and a communitarian-based ecological democracy (Burkett, 2005); a poststructuralist SD approach would analyse and expose power relations determining socioenvironmental needs, capacities, and courses of action (Murdoch, 2006); and a less radical form of SD would likely give primacy to economic considerations.

Given the definitional challenges, a useful way to obtain an understanding of sustainability and SD is through their historical development, the surfacing of the terms in the context of decades-long international discourse, commissions, conferences, summits, and other fora. The concepts are an extension of development theory which theorizes broadly how best to achieve desired alterations to societies, conventionally through mimicking processes used by 'developed' countries (Bilbao-Ubillos, 2011; Escobar, 1996). The inability of economic development models to provide useful responses to conditions of environmental degradation, world poverty, and international economic inequities, especially between North and South, called for a new paradigm (Estes, 1993). Sometimes understood as developing in response to radical environmentalism and the limits-to-growth argument, SD is often

Table 3.1 Chronology of sustainable development

Date	Organization or event	Key developments
1972	UN Conference on the Human Environment, also called the Stockholm conference	United Nations Environment Program created Stockholm Declaration developed 109 recommendations produced to guide international environmental action
1980	International Union for Conservation of Nature and Natural Resources (IUCN)	Produced a document titled the World Conservation Strategy First significant use of the term sustainable development
1987	World Commission on Environment and Development (WCED)	Produced a report titled *Our Common Future*, often referred to as the Brundtland Report Integrated environmental, economic, and social strategies into development work Expanded compass of development practice by including rich and poor countries in sustainability policies Advanced the focus on poverty alleviation Helped foster emergence of international environmental community
1992	UN Conference on Environment and Development (UNCED), also known as the Rio conference or Earth Summit	Adopted Rio Declaration on Environment and Development, Agenda 21, and Non-legally Binding Authoritative Statement of Principles for a Global Consensus on the Management, Conservation and Sustainable Development of All Types of Forests Agenda 21 promotes community participation, grassroots developments, respect for local knowledge, and multisectoral collaborations Agenda 21 argues for global partnership dedicated to sustainable development while underscoring the need for a localist approach
1994	Green Cross International and the Earth Council	Induction of the Earth Charter Initiative
2000	UN Education, Scientific and Cultural Organization	Consensus reached by more than 40 Earth Charter committees on the final version of the Charter Earth Charter seeks to develop a global partnership dedicated to the well-being of all Earth's life forms and a present and long-term responsibility to Earth security Sustainability as articulated by the Earth Charter was to be achieved by 16 guiding principles
2000	UN Millennium Summit	Millennium Declaration produced emphasizing respect for nature and a rededication to sustainable development Development of eight Millennium Development Goals

Date	Organization or event	Key developments
2002	World Summit on Sustainable Development, sometimes called Rio+10	Johannesburg Declaration on Sustainable Development produced, a document that reasserts international commitment to SD as described in Rio Declaration
		Summit attempted to respond to unsatisfactory progress in sustainable development following Rio
		Failed attempt to have the Earth Charter document formally accepted
		Earth Charter nonetheless recognized as a global consensus statement on sustainability
2012	UN Conference on Sustainable Development, also termed Rio+20	Will seek to renew political commitment to sustainable development, evaluate progress, identify gaps, and address new issues

positioned in the 'wise use' tradition, a kind of stewardship of the natural environment, as first articulated by Gifford Pinchot in 1910 (Colgan, 1997; Martinez-Alier, 2002).

The beginnings of sustainability have been traced to environmental scholarship that detailed the devastation humanity was inflicting on the Earth through population pressures, technological advances, and economic practices. Two works in particular are cited as helping to foster the emergence of sustainability in the USA: Carson's (1962) *Silent Spring*, which chronicled environmental impacts of chemical toxins, and Meadows, Meadows, Randers, and Behrens (1972) *Limits to Growth*, which stressed the consequences of fast-growing populations in a world with finite resources and questioned the continued value of the growth paradigm (see, for example, Agyeman, Bullard, and Evans, 2003; Castro, 2004; Cuthill, 2010). These works underscored the need for greater attention to human–nature relations and precipitated a sudden increase in concerns about human well-being vis-à-vis the natural world.

Stockholm Conference 1972

Awareness of environment and development challenges globally is often attributed to the United Nations Conference on the Human Environment (UNCHE) held in Stockholm in 1972, the first international meeting with environmental considerations central to the agenda. This conference is responsible for the creation of the United Nations Environment Programme (UNEP) and produced the Stockholm Declaration comprising 26 principles 'to inspire and guide the peoples of the world in the preservation and enhancement of the human environment' (UNEP, 1972). The language of the Declaration is highly anthropocentric and androcentric and nowhere is the term sustainability or SD used. However, the seeds of sustainable thought are present and articulated in the language of wise use. Principle 1 states,

> Man [sic] has the fundamental right to freedom, equality and adequate conditions of life, in an environment of a quality that permits a life of dignity and well-being, and he bears a solemn responsibility to protect and improve the environment for present and future generations. In this respect, policies promoting or perpetuating apartheid, racial segregation, discrimination, colonial and other forms of oppression and foreign domination stand condemned and must be eliminated.
>
> (UNEP, 1972: 2)

The success of the Stockholm conference consists in the development of an international structure, the UNEP, to advocate environmental issues. The 26 principles of the Stockholm Declaration comprise the first effort toward creating non-binding international environmental policy, and an action plan of 109 recommendations to guide international environmental action (Meinhard and Tollefson, 2009; Quental, Lourenço, and da Silva, 2011). Since 1972, the UNEP has played a considerable role in foregrounding environmental issues for the international community and engendering multilateral environmental agreements (Meinhard and Tollefson, 2009).

World Conservation Strategy 1980

The first significant use of the term SD is found in the *World Conservation Strategy* (WCS), a 1980 publication of the International Union for Conservation of Nature and Natural Resources (IUCN). The IUCN, founded in 1948, is an international organization, involving governments and various stakeholders. Collaborative development strategies are a keystone of the IUCN and the WCS exemplifies this principle while concurrently making links among escalating environmental issues and equity-related socioeconomic concerns, and securing a safe, healthy future for humankind. Development is defined in the WCS as:

> the modification of the biosphere and the application of human, financial, living and nonliving resources to satisfy human needs and improve the quality of human life. For development to be sustainable it must take account of social and ecological factors, as well as economic ones; of the living and the non-living resource base; and of the long term as well as the short term advantages and disadvantages of alternative actions.
>
> (IUCN, 1980: 18)

Attending to social, ecological, and economic factors requires adapted conservation strategies to respond appropriately to dire survival conditions.

SD, therefore, has a strong commitment to poverty alleviation where applications of conservation are coupled with measures designed to accommodate short- and long-term economic needs through grassroots participation and the creation of 'lasting and secure livelihoods that minimize resource depletion, environmental degradation, cultural disruption, and social instability' (Barbier, 1987: 109).

Brundtland Report

Various economic reforms promoted by the International Monetary Fund (IMF) and the World Bank (WB), during the economic downturn in the 1980s, increased international socioeconomic inequalities. These prescriptions were designed to achieve macroeconomic stabilization and ultimately ushered in trade liberalization, extensive resource use and concomitant plunder, and the market approach now known as neoliberalism. It was in this context that SD was catapulted to the world stage. Though central to the *World Conservation Strategy*, the concept of SD was not common in public discourse prior to the 1987 report of the World Commission on Environment and Development (WCED), *Our Common Future*, often called the Brundtland Report after its Chairperson, then Prime Minister of Norway, Gro Harlem Brundtland. The General Assembly of the United Nations asked the WCED to devise a 'global agenda for change' (WCED, 1987: 5). The concept of SD, as defined in the Brundtland Report, not only integrates environmental, economic, and social strategies into development work but also expands the compass of development practice beyond the 'Third World', requiring countries of the North and South, rich and poor, to participate in international sustainability policies.

The most oft-cited definition of SD is articulated in the Brundtland Report: 'Sustainable development is development that meets the needs of the present without compromising the ability of future generations to meet their own needs' (WCED, 1987: 41). The concept of SD here implies limits but not 'absolute limits', only those associated with current technologies and social formations and the restricted biospheric ability to handle human activities. The report argues at once for conservation and a 'new era of economic growth', adopting a kind of middle ground or third way where the two goals are not only desirable but eminently compatible. Building on the Stockholm Declaration in which humankind is stated to have a 'fundamental right to ... [the] adequate conditions of life' (Principle 1), the Brundtland Report advances the focus on poverty alleviation maintaining that 'sustainable development requires meeting the basic needs of all and extending to all the opportunity to fulfil their aspirations for a better life' (WCED, 1987: 16).

This definition altered the conservation orientation prominent in the IUCN's 1980 articulation of SD, promoting instead a tripartite environmental, socioeconomic, and political framework (Agyeman *et al.*, 2003). Significant sustainable development policy objectives include 'reviving growth; changing the quality of growth; meeting essential needs for jobs, food, energy, water, and sanitation; ensuring a sustainable level of population; conserving and enhancing resource base; reorienting technology and managing risk; and merging environment and economics in decision making' (WCED, 1987: 41). In many respects, the preparation and presence of the Brundtland Report, the ideas contained therein, helped to foster the emergence of an international environmental community.

Key post-Brundtland developments

Following the Brundtland Report, the 1992 United Nations Conference on Environment and Development (UNCED) held in Rio de Janeiro, also known as the Earth Summit, made a critical contribution to SD. At this conference, the United Nations Framework Conventions on Climate Change and on Biological Diversity were signed by more than 150 states. The UNCED adopted the 'Rio Declaration on Environment and Development, Agenda 21 and the Non-legally Binding Authoritative Statement of Principles for a Global Consensus on the Management, Conservation and Sustainable Development of All Types of Forests' (UN, 1993: 2). Agenda 21 is a 40-chapter guide to SD, and contained within these chapters is a strong argument for community participation, grassroots developments, deference to local knowledge, and the need for multisectoral collaborations. Moreover, Agenda 21 calls for a global partnership dedicated to SD because its objective to realize 'integration of environment and development concerns [which] ... will lead to the fulfillment of basic needs, improved living standards for all, better protected and managed ecosystems, and a safer, more prosperous future' (p. 3) cannot be achieved by a single nation alone. Reinforcing key themes in the Stockholm Declaration, the Rio Declaration's first principle asserts 'Human beings are at the centre of concerns for sustainable development [and] ... are entitled to a healthy and productive life in harmony with nature' (p. 3). However, the main strength of Agenda 21 is countering the 'globalist thrust of orthodox approaches to sustainable development' through endorsing a 'localist' turn and strategies to develop 'local programmes for realising community sustainability' (Yanarella and Bartilow, 2000: 126).

In 1994, the Earth Charter Initiative was inaugurated by Green Cross International and the Earth Council. At a March 2000 meeting convened at the United Nations Education, Scientific and Cultural Organization head office in Paris, the Earth Charter Commission, after numerous drafts and revisions by more than 40 Earth Charter committees, arrived at a consensus on the Charter. Although efforts to have the Earth Charter formally adopted at the 2002 World Summit on Sustainable Development (WSSD) in Johannesburg failed, the document is understood to be a global consensus statement on sustainability, SD, and principles central to their achievement.

The Earth Charter (2000) was an attempt to develop a global partnership that would 'recognize the common destiny of all creatures and life forms on Earth and ... foster a sense of responsibility for the present and future well-being of the living world' (Agyeman *et al.*, 2003: 11). The aim of the initiative is to promote sustainability through 16 principles guided by 'a shared ethical framework that includes respect and care for the community of life, ecological integrity, universal human rights, respect for diversity, economic justice, democracy, and a culture of peace' (Earth Charter, 2000: 1). However, the Earth Charter, irrespective of international signatories and multilateral agreement, did not have the weight or means to steer the shift to SD (Quental, Lourenço, and da Silva, 2011).

During the same year that the Earth Charter was launched, the United Nations convened a Millennium Summit with environmental and development concerns as its primary focus. From this meeting, the Millennium Declaration was produced emphasizing the values of 'freedom, equality, solidarity, tolerance, respect for nature, and shared responsibility' as 'essential to international relations in the twenty-first century' (UN, 2000: 2). Respect for nature as articulated in this document is a rededication to the principles of SD, a pledge to alter unsustainable human production and consumption patterns for the sake of humankind's collective future. The Millennium Summit also resulted in the creation of eight Millennium Development Goals (eradicate extreme poverty and hunger; achieve universal primary education; promote gender equality and empower women; reduce child mortality; improve maternal health; combat HIV and AIDS, malaria, and other diseases; ensure environmental sustainability; and develop a global partnership for development) which clearly indicate a commitment to all three components – equity, economy, and environment – of SD.

In 2002, Johannesburg hosted the World Summit on Sustainable Development (WSSD), attended by 104 heads of state and government and more than 20,000 other participants, including delegates, nongovernmental organization representatives, and members of the press. The Summit resulted in the Johannesburg Declaration on Sustainable Development which reasserted the international commitment to SD as expressed ten years earlier in the Rio Declaration:

> We reaffirm our pledge to place particular focus on, and give priority attention to, the fight against the worldwide conditions that pose severe threats to the sustainable development of our people, which include: chronic hunger; malnutrition; foreign occupation; armed conflict; illicit drug problems; organized crime; corruption; natural disasters; illicit arms trafficking; trafficking in persons; terrorism; intolerance and incitement to racial, ethnic, religious and other hatreds; xenophobia; and endemic, communicable and chronic diseases, in particular HIV/AIDS, malaria and tuberculosis.
>
> (UN, 2002: 5)

This 2002 Summit, sometimes called Rio+10, was a response to the unsatisfactory SD progress during the ten-year period following the UNCED conference in Rio and represents a global effort to safeguard the destiny of world cultures, peoples, and species, and to promote collective responsibility for the continued well-being of Earth systems through a commitment to the Plan of Implementation of the World Summit on Sustainable Development. This Plan intended to advance further the 1992 UNCED accomplishments while accelerating progress on the remaining goals. The main thrust of the plan is to work concertedly at multiple levels (local, regional, grassroots, governmental, and NGO) to develop and execute concrete measures to foster international cooperation in the pursuit of SD: 'These efforts will also promote the integration of the three components of sustainable development – economic development, social development and environmental protection – as interdependent and mutually reinforcing pillars' (UN, 2002: 8). Central to this document is a continued commitment to eradicating poverty, transforming unsustainable production and consumption models, and managing the natural resource base essential to economic and social security.

A United Nations Conference on Sustainable Development (UNCSD), also termed Rio+20, in Brazil in 2012 on the twentieth anniversary of the UNCED Rio conference has as its objectives: renewing political commitment to SD, gauging implementation progress to date, identifying persistent gaps, and addressing emerging issues. Given that poverty eradication remains pivotal, once again conference participants aim to collaborate to develop a practicable framework for SD.

Sustainability and sustainable development: A critical analysis

As this brief historical overview attests, SD has developed iteratively through a number of summits, declarations, implementations, reaffirmations, and revisions, but it has remained a lasting and prominent feature in environment and development discourse. Part of SD's longevity resides in its pragmatism, its coalescence of social, environmental, and economic concerns into a single framework. While this has facilitated the easy adoption of sustainability into mainstream public and political discourse (Cuthill, 2010), SD has both proponents and detractors. This section examines the arguments of each.

Critique of SD

Sustainability is a contested construct for a variety of reasons, some of which are explored here. A recurring critique of SD is the problematic manner in which it is defined. The widely cited Brundtland definition is faulted for its lack of clarity, failure to explicate what is meant by needs, vulnerability to a variety of interpretations, and 'intellectual emptiness' (Luke, 2005: 228, see also Castro, 2004). SD and sustainability are concepts that are adopted and used by people with differing, sometimes conflicting, values, goals, and political interests, making it difficult to know the meaning or shape (i.e., conventionalism (incremental development) or radicalism (profound structural change)) SD might take for them (Hopwood, Mellor, and O'Brien, 2005). The 'polysemic' nature of sustainable development leaves it open to diverse sociocultural, economic, philosophical, and political interpretations (Hopwood *et al.*, 2005). Its appeal to all sides of politics leads to its cooptation and misuse. While most would agree with its goals, there are widely divergent views as to the best way these might be achieved (Sneddon *et al.*, 2006). It is unlikely then that an unambiguous definition of SD would assist in its implementation given the resource implications it entails. Definitions, in any way, cannot resolve the inherent contradictions of those who privilege environmental sustainability over economic growth (Daly, 1996; Redclift, 1987). Contradictions in SD might be strategic manoeuvres for 'political compromise' to win over critics and increase its acceptability (Castro, 2004; Giddings, Hopwood, and O'Brien, 2002; Keirstead and Leach, 2008) or deliberate attempts to commodify nature under the pretext of an ethic of care (Escobar, 1996). This might account for the disappointing sustainability outcomes since the 1992 Earth Summit (Castro, 2004).

Given its lofty and conflicting goals, critics believe SD is not only unattainable, but also undesirable if economic growth, despite negative environmental influences, continues to be its dominant driver (Castro, 2004; Jacob, 1997; Yanarella and Bartilow, 2000). The Brundtland Report states:

> [I]t is essential that global economic growth be revitalized. In practical terms, this means more rapid economic growth in both industrial and developing countries, freer market access for the products of developing countries, lower interest rates, greater technology transfer, and significantly larger capital flows, both concessional and commercial.
>
> (UN, 1987: 72)

The Rio Report also seeks to promote 'information exchange and appropriate technology transfer among all countries, with particular attention to developing countries, for resource management in construction, particularly for non-renewable resources' (UN, 1992: 91). Hence SD might be seen as part of the neoliberal agenda to enforce trade liberalization, economic growth, environmental colonialism, and the free market as the means to promote social and environmental justice (Castro, 2004; Daly, 1996; Goldsmith, 1996; McLaren, 2003; Sneddon *et al.*, 2006; Venn, 2010). The costs, source, and direction of technology transfer are a major consideration. Technology is expensive and 'most countries of the periphery will have to export natural resources, thereby creating more environmental destruction, to be able to purchase the technology [needed for SD]' (Castro, 2004: 200; see also Goldsmith, 1996). Multinational corporations stand to benefit the most since they control the research agenda, and nation states in the Global South lack the power and competitive edge to produce the technologies needed to meet contemporary development objectives (Glasmeier and Farrigan, 2003).

While SD aims to eliminate absolute poverty in developing countries, it ignores the escalation of poverty in developed countries and the increasing gap between the rich and poor globally. Capitalism thrives on inequalities as profits essentially depend on supplies of cheap labour and natural resources. As a neoliberal economic framework, SD is unlikely to upset the market logic which benefits the Global North at the expense of the Global South (Castro, 2004; Glasmeier and Farrigan, 2003). It is unlikely, then, that SD will yield transformative policies to address global inequities (Jacob, 1997; Sneddon *et al.*, 2006). Existing international structures constrain social and environmental justice efforts, as the International Monetary Fund and the World Bank function largely in the service of wealthy elites in the Global North, providing loans to the South as a means to control development processes (Goldsmith, 1996; Venn, 2010). While the language of sustainability might be used, the practices of SD are expansionist and growth-oriented (i.e., GDP focused), rendering a weak form of sustainability (Castro, 2004; Glasmeier and Farrigan, 2003; Hay, 2010).

Although most SD documents stress the importance of grassroots organisations and citizen participation in decision making (UN, 1987, 1992), an absence of multilateral agreement on how to accomplish this objective and the indifference of corporate and executive leaders to such practices makes participation largely a nominal rather than meaningful practice. As Escobar (1995) notes, 'Development was – and continues to be for the most part – a top-down, ethnocentric, and technocratic approach, which treated people and cultures as abstract concepts, statistical figures to be moved up and down in the charts of "progress"' (p. 44). SD is seen by some as a new form of colonialism – an environmental colonialism – where resources move from the periphery to the centre, hegemonic benefits accrue to the North, and neoclassical economic practices and neoliberal institutions are strengthened (Goldsmith, 1996; McLaren, 2003; Sneddon *et al.*, 2006). Its colonizing thrust is justified by claims that poverty in developing nations 'reduces people's capacity to use resources in a sustainable manner [and] ... intensifies pressure on the environment' (UN, 1987, p. 29) when, ironically, the Global North has the worst track record for unsustainable resource use, environmental degradation, and overconsumption but these are not seen as explicit targets of change.

Support for SD

For all its drawbacks, SD has brought disparate disciplinary perspectives and political interests together in a cohesive development model. It has led to a greater focus on world health, food security, and child poverty through linking social and environmental justice with economic growth (Poland and Dooris, 2010; Plummer, 2006). In the aftermath of the Brundtland Report, it ignited the international development imagination, motivating nations, peoples, and multinational and national corporations to work toward a sustainability agenda and seek multilevel approaches to social, environmental, and economic challenges (Rixecker and Tipene-Matua, 2003). Sustainability as a catch cry has galvanized diverse stakeholders – governments, international agencies, researchers, scholars, specialists, and citizens – around development issues in a manner heretofore unseen (Estes, 1993; Haberl *et al.*, 2011; Plummer, 2006). Its project is ambitious given the competing interests of economic growth, environmental protection, and international development (Jacob, 1997). SD points to the inseparability of social, economic, and environmental objectives. Nevertheless, ways have yet to be found to move beyond 'ideological and epistemological straightjackets that deter more cohesive and politically effective interpretations of SD' (Sneddon *et al.*, 2006: 261). But supporters like Sneddon *et al.* (2006) call for radical change to 'ecological economics, political ecology, freedom-oriented development, deliberative democracy, [and] ... universal notions of justice and equity' (p. 264). Others seeking transformative change in society argue for a rethinking of 'growth' (Daly, 1996), a valuing of qualitative rather than economic growth (Jackson, 2005), and an advancement toward the 'fullest possible human development' (Estes, 1993: 12).

Social work, sustainability, and sustainable development

Environmental circumstances today are grave. The ecological footprint of humankind is so large that the Earth's carrying capacity is overshot. Global heating, climate change, cultural and biodiversity loss, environmental refugees, contaminated waters, polluted air, and depleted soils, are reminders of the failed relationship between humankind and the natural world in the Anthropocene. Sustainability and SD, despite the many critiques, offer a valuable direction forward given their ability to bring together divergent groups with manifold interests in the service of environmental protection and human rights.

Writing from a public health perspective, Poland and Dooris (2010) advanced six principles to help build health, equity, and sustainability. Of interest is the commensurability of these principles with social work and the extent to which they illustrate social work's professional aptitude for responding to environmental challenges, a point acknowledged by Rifkin (2004). The six principles are:

1   adopt an ecological 'whole system' perspective;
2   start where people are;
3   root practice in place;
4   deepen sociopolitical analysis;
5   capitalize on strengths and successes; and
6   build resilience.

These principles are compatible with social work's worldview but call for a new environmental paradigm (Mary, 2008), an ecological, community-based, holistic model (Coates, 2003) eschewing the person-in-environment metaphor and asserting instead the importance of place (Zapf, 2009).

Place

While the Brundtland definition has a temporal focus on future generations, SD also has important spatial dimensions tied to locality and *place*. Juxtaposing the competing interests of global and local concerns necessitates an understanding of international, national, and local policy as it impacts on SD (Morse, Vogiatzakis, and Griffiths, 2011). Social workers engaged with SD need to be operating at both local and global levels and drawing from a variety of knowledge sources (Hoff, 1994) to work holistically with the complexities of social, cultural, economic, political, and environmental relations. Since social work is largely urban-based, it is well placed to engage in SD with the more than 50 per cent of the global population now residing in cities to reduce the biosphere burden by creating sustainable consumption patterns, energy generation, and waste management (Keierstead and Leach, 2008). With its acute focus on poor and marginalized communities it is well placed to attend to the 'hypersusceptibility' of low-income and racialized communities, as well as poor children, to environmental hazards (Rogge, 1994b, 2000).

Community practice and policy

Hall (1996) suggests community social workers adopt a 'combative role' to work with communities to militate against social, economic, and environmental threats; assume an 'educational role' to help foster a collectivity; and act as networkers forging alliances with funders, agencies, sympathetic government workers, and other allies. Community participation requires that community members be invested and engaged meaningfully in project design, goals, implementation, administration, outcomes, and evaluation (Pandey, 1998). Community participation is central to sustainable development for it provides accurate information on community needs while simultaneously being a methodologically equitable, non-hierarchical approach. Moreover, community participation is an invaluable tool for helping citizens feel empowered and unified (Kauffman, 1994), which is critical because more powerless communities are typically at greatest risk (Lovell and Johnson, 1994). Citizen organizing that attends robustly to issues of power together with social action planning can help surmount thoughts of powerlessness (Kauffman, 1994; Shubert, 1994). Social workers engaged with sustainability work must be mediators between communities and the state, transforming policies into practicable programmes for community members and bringing community needs to the attention of the state. Subscribing to an irreconcilable schism between community and state is counterproductive and hampers the lasting success of SD (Pandey, 2010). Unfortunately, seeking citizen input in development initiatives, though discussed repeatedly in SD agendas, is not legally required (Kauffman, 1994). Social workers could raise awareness about the negative effects of non-participatory models, seeking to instigate SD policy and implementation changes making community participation mandatory.

SD also necessitates considerable attention to poverty and justice issues. While much of the SD literature and policy work focuses on poverty alleviation and oppression in the Global South, there are peoples living in abject poverty and contending with disproportionate environmental burdens in the urban centres of industrialized nations where most social workers are found (Cuthill, 2010). Consistent with SD principles, social workers can endeavour to ensure that all people have adequate and accessible housing, sustenance, education, and opportunities to participate meaningfully in civic life. Masuda, Poland, and Baxter (2010) recommend a 'three-fold process' based on tenets of equity, access, and respect, that restructure the three sustainability pillars in specific community contexts in a manner that rectifies historical and persistent discrimination. This redressing of discriminatory practices needs to focus not only on environmental 'bads' but also 'goods', meaning ensuring access to amenities as well as healthy, secure social and physical environments (Masuda et al., 2010; Roberts, 2003). The continued failure of the dominant political-economic models to foster socially just and sustainable communities, locally and internationally, invites critical community practice work and a more active policy role for social workers in dismantling and redefining unsustainable political-economic institutions (Tester, 1994).

Globally, many SD projects have not succeeded because a blueprint approach was used and community members were not adequately involved (Hall, 1996; Leach et al., 2010). Community-based participatory research (CBPR) is invaluable to learning community perspectives; building buy-in to multilevel social, economic, environmental, and political analyses; and promoting community cohesion and project ownership (Masuda et al., 2010; St. Martin and Hall-Arber, 2007). CBPR findings and processes can then be applied to grassroots SD which involves localized, small-scale community-based initiatives designed to work on equity, economic, and environmental challenges (Stevens and Morris, 2001). Environmental social workers with well-honed community practice skills are highly suited to ensure issues of equity, rights, access, participation, and relevant structural concerns are attended to in this process (Cuthill, 2010; Kauffman, 1994; Shubert, 1994).

Education

A key component of SD and sustainability work is education (Hall, 1996; Kauffman, Walter, Nissly, and Walker, 1994; Mary, 2008; Rogge, 1994a). In part, this involves educating about the scope of environmental challenges and burdens; the differential exposure to those burdens based on marginalization; the institutional, structural, and global economic systems that support environmental degradation and discriminatory effects; and the sustainable approaches to addressing these challenges. Sustainability education and solutions necessitate transdisciplinary understandings, drawing on a range of knowledge bases, which is a historical practice of social work. Mary (2008) deems interdisciplinary understandings crucial to achieving a shift toward a non-hierarchical sociopolitical model which is essential to sustainability. Sustainable education looks not only at global forces and their impact on locality, place and communities but also at the force of centralized policy decisions and the paternalism of distant, disconnected government and other regulative authorities. As sustainability requires consideration of both space and time scales, education surrounding immediate and long-term planning at community, international, and policy levels is critical (Jepson, 2004; Morse *et al.*, 2011). This involves replacing the expansionist perspective which dominates much international policy discourse, including mainstream SD, with an appreciation of collectivity and ecological time scales (Diamond, 2005; Jepson, 2004; Lake, 2010).

Rogge's (1994a) suggestion that the person-in-environment perspective be expanded to suit environmental social work objectives has been neatly answered by Zapf's (2009) person as place response. In Zapf's (2009) construction, the new metaphor of 'people as place' elicits a stewardship ethos, a feeling of responsibility toward the natural environment because it is absolutely central to human existence. This 'person as place' construct raises the sustainability quotient. Education that elucidates the connections between SD and rights discourse (a field of knowledge fundamental to social work) helps social workers to realize that championing human rights requires bioregional protection and safeguarding planet Earth (Van Wormer and Besthorn, 2011). Ife (2007) makes the astute observation that human rights must be located in collectivist rights, the rights of a human community, and community development, and, by extension, SD must commence from a position that values these rights. Part of education then is to draw the connections between rights, including environmental and non-human species rights, and SD, providing mentorship, skills training, and advocacy education toward this end (see Hoefer, 2006).

Individual considerations

An examination of individual responsibility and behaviours needs to be included in social work and SD considerations. While critics are right to see the limitations of individual actions (Jensen, 2009), individuals comprise communities, so this unit of analysis should not be ignored. Sustainability involves transforming social, cultural, political, and economic systems, reconceptualizing how to manage individual, community, national, and international practices. Yet there are those in the Global North who believe that greening consumption is enough (Poland and Dooris, 2010). The reluctance many feel toward limiting consumption has been linked to various causes, including centrality to identity formation and preservation (Soron, 2010), addiction to shopping (Wilkinson and Pickett, 2009), denial and feelings of helplessness (Norgaard, 2011), and the decline of social capital (Putnam, 2000). Social capital erosion has negatively impacted on social networks and collective citizen practices. This political and social 'retreatism' stands in opposition to the civic engagement necessary to confront environmental issues. Decreased social capital is best addressed through capacity-building processes and initiatives to stimulate the desire for engagement (Gamble and Hoff, 2012; Peeters, 2011), which again involves working at the group and community level but appealing to the individual desire for meaningful social networking and connection. While SD would benefit from greater social capital, social capital, too, would be enhanced by SD because it has proven to be a rousing concept for peoples of diverse ideological and cultural backgrounds interested in environment and equity issues. Yet SD itself could use reinvigoration.

Toward the future

Haberl *et al.* (2011) have correctly identified the profound differences between the present industrial/post-industrial society and an envisaged sustainable society: 'The challenge of sustainability is, therefore, a fundamental re-orientation of society and the economy, not the implementation of some technical fixes' (p. 1). Social workers, with their well-developed policy understandings, community and strengths-building skills, and transdisciplinary knowledge base, are uniquely situated to be key facilitators in this process. This work would involve myriad practices working in tandem with multidisciplinary groups and organizations, including restructuring the global economy; creating ecological tax reforms; reviving community strengths and networks; combating social and environmental discrimination and redressing associated legacies; responding to environmental health challenges; assisting to mobilize citizen action to support greater response to climate change and coordinated processes to eradicate socio-ecological inequities between North and South; and developing a more concerted, organized approach to health research,

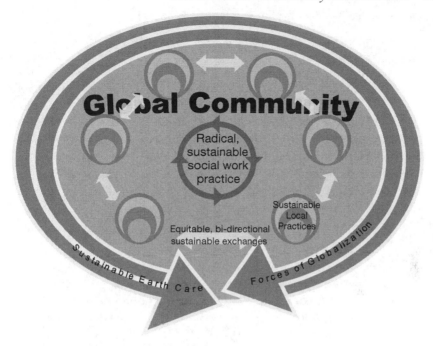

Figure 3.1 Model for environmental social work practice

community action, and policy change (Hoff and McNutt, 1994; Lusk and Hoff, 1994). Central to this sociocultural reorientation are radical sustainability principles, such as the intrinsic worth of all species; democracy of Earth community; centrality of cultural- and biodiversity; economies in service of all peoples; environmental and social injustices redressed; inherent right of all beings to security and sustenance; inherent right of all species to respect; and international economies based on successful local economies (see Shiva's (2005) Principles of Earth Democracy). Figure 3.1 provides a rough schematic of society reoriented to radical sustainability values, where each of the nested circles represents one of innumerable possibilities for sustainable local practices having a sustainable economy situated within a sustainable community, operating within a sustainable environment. The arrows between communities represent equitable bi-directional sustainable exchanges of knowledge, goods, and services. The large circle represents the global community in which all the local sustainable practices occur, with the burgundy arrow signalling the oppressive, inequitable forces of globalization, while the mauve arrow signals liberatory, equitable, radical, sustainable Earth care. The multi-arrowed red circle at the centre represents radical sustainable social work practice operating at the local and global levels, involved in social and environmental justice, collectivist rights discourse, advocacy, restoration, remediation, community work, and multisectoral practices.

Case example

An exciting example of SD in the Canadian context is a Sustainable Community Design (SCD) used to develop a subdivision three kilometres outside the City of Dieppe, New Brunswick. This SCD project developed from an affiliation involving the Province of New Brunswick, the City of Dieppe, and a local developer in a collaboration to create 'Le Village en haut du ruisseau' (the village at the top of the stream). Sustainable community design builds on the idea of conservation design developed by Randall Arendt in the United States (1999, 1996). Conservation design provides an alternative to conventional subdivision zoning by converting no more than half of a buildable land area into homes and streets but building the same number of homes by using a density neutral design that works with the ecosystems of a site and maintains important functions and qualities of the natural environment. This approach allows 'the balance of the property to be permanently protected and added to an interconnected network of green spaces and green corridors crisscrossing one's township or county' (Arendt, 1996: xix). Conservation design adapted and implemented in Canada as SCD creates avenues for multisectoral engagement in subdivision developments by involving communities, developers, local governments, and homeowners in a process that improves neighbourhood quality and protects the environment by developing no more than 50 per cent of the developable land.

SCD represents a shift from conventional to conservation subdivision design by using a flexible model that aims to protect natural landscapes and drainage systems. In a conventional subdivision approach only environmental constraints, such as marshy land, are considered when determining the extent of buildable area. In the SCD model, environmental constraints are considered along with sustainability concerns such as protecting endangered species, and preserving community sites (e.g., picnic areas), cultural sites, mature trees, views, wildflowers and meadows. In the Speech from the Throne 2007, the Government of Canada articulated an environmental action plan that sought to integrate climate change concerns into development planning; promote partnerships; accentuate green building practices; and promote environmental sustainability. SCD incorporates all these considerations. Climate change issues are addressed through the preservation of environmental features which not only enhances quality of life but reduce the carbon footprint. The emphasis is on small lots, limited lawns, environmental design of streets and trails, and tree conservation and landscaping. Built into the SCD model is the goal of reducing the number of vehicular kilometres travelled by prospective community members. The promotion of partnerships is achieved through the necessity of multidisciplinary teams of experts and multisectoral relationships where meaningful input is invited from all members and understanding community needs is essential. Moreover, the goal of creating a sustainable, equitable community is built into the SCD model through ensuring that inexpensive housing is developed having rates consistent with rent levels established by the Canada Mortgage and Housing Corporation. Green construction is addressed through building homes in accordance with the Leadership in Energy and Environmental Design (LEED) Green Building Rating System. This approach emphasizes developing an area sustainably, using water and energy efficiently, and selecting green materials. Through conservation of natural features, maintaining ecosystem integrity, and storm water management environmental sustainability goals are met. Social sustainability is augmented through social equity, community enhancement, and recreational opportunities.

In a meeting with Daniel Savard, Senior Planner, Sustainable Planning Branch, New Brunswick Department of Environment, the author was told 'Le Village' not only meets sustainability goals but also is a more affordable approach than conventional subdivision design models. However, SCD requires complete investment in the theory undergirding SCD and in the model from all stakeholders and partners, which involves understanding the importance of all the basic principles and agreeing on them collectively before implementation. To facilitate reaching this end, the Sustainable Planning Branch of the New Brunswick Department of Environment has created a one-and-a-half-day training module that details the values and principles of the model and provides steps for implementation. Without this training, the probability of realizing a true SCD subdivision design is unlikely. The Canadian housing development community looks to New Brunswick and Dieppe as leaders in SCD implementation.

Conclusion

The contemporary environmental crisis is in many respects at an impasse, marked by incremental changes and responses unequal to the considerable challenges faced today, as evidenced by the weak international response at the United Nations Climate Conference in Copenhagen, 2009. Sustainable Development, conceptualized in its more radical, structurally astute form, holds the promise of transformational change. Social work has a significant role in transitioning to a sustainable future through application of a critical political perspective and a social and environmental justice agenda. Social workers can help facilitate the transition through community action, grassroots initiatives, social capital and capacity building, education, justice initiatives, advocacy, multisectoral and multiscalar planning, and policy change.

References

Addams, J. ([1910], 1990). *Twenty years at Hull House.* Champaign, IL: University of Illinois Press.

Agyeman, J., Bullard, R.D., and Evans, B. (2003). Joined-up thinking: Bringing together sustainability, environmental justice and equity. In J. Agyeman, Bullard, R.D., and Evans, B. (Eds). *Just sustainabilities: Development in an unequal world.* Cambridge, MA: MIT Press. 1–16.

Arendt, R. (1996). *Conservation design for subdivisions: A practical guide to creating open space networks.* Washington, DC: Island Press.

Arendt, R. (1999). *Growing greener: Putting conservation into local plans and ordinances.* Washington, DC: Island Press.

Bagheri, A., and Hjorth, P. (2007). Planning for sustainable development: A paradigm shift towards a process-based approach. *Sustainable Development, 15*(2), 83–96.

Barbier, E. (1987). The concept of sustainable economic development. *Environmental Conservation, 14*(2), 101–110.

Barlow, M. (2007). *Blue Covenant: The global water crisis and the coming battle for the right to water.* Toronto: McClelland and Stewart.

Besthorn, F.H. (1997). *Reconceptualizing social work's person-in-environment perspective: Explorations in radical environmental thought.* Unpublished doctoral dissertation. Lawrence: University of Kansas.

Besthorn, F.H. (2003). Radical ecologisms: Insights for educating social workers in ecological activism and social justice. *Critical Social Work, 4*(1). Retrieved on January 21, 2012 from http://www.uwindsor.ca/criticalsocialwork/radical-ecologisms-insights-for-educating-social-workers-in-ecological-activism-and-social-justice.

Besthorn, F.H., and McMillen, D.P. (2002). The oppression of women and nature: Ecofeminism as a framework for a social justice oriented social work. *Families in Society: The Journal of Contemporary Human Services, 83*(3), 221–232.

Bilbao-Ubillos, J. (2011). The limits of human development index: The complementary role of economic and social cohesion, development strategies and sustainability. *Sustainable Development, 19.* Article first published online: 18 MAY 2011 DOI: 10.1002/sd.525.

Birkin, F. (2001). Steps to natural capitalism. *Sustainable Development, 9,* 47–57.

Bullard, R. (1990). *Dumping in Dixie: Race, class, and environmental quality.* Boulder, CO: Westview Press.

Burkett, P. (2005). Marx's vision of sustainable human development. *Monthly Review, 57*(5), 34–62.

Carson, R. (1962). *Silent spring.* New York: Houghton Mifflin.

Castro, C. (2004). Sustainable development: Mainstream and critical perspectives. *Organization & Environment, 17,* 2, 195–225.

Chavis Jr., B., and Lee, C. (1987). *Toxic wastes and race in the United States: A national report on the racial and socio-economic characteristics of communities with hazardous waste sites.* New York: United Church of Christ: Commission for Racial Justice.

Coates, J. (2003). *Ecology and social work: Toward a new paradigm.* Blackpoint, NS: Fernwood.

Colgan, C.S. (1997). 'Sustainable Development' and economic development policy: Lessons from Canada. *Economic Development Quarterly, 11,* 2, 123–137.

Crutzen, P.J., and Stoermer, E.F. (2000). The 'Anthropocene'. *Global Change Newsletter, 41,* 17–18.

Cuthill, M. (2010). Strengthening the 'social' in sustainable development: Developing a conceptual framework for social sustainability in a rapid urban growth region in Australia. *Sustainable Development, 18,* 362–373.

Daly, H.E. (1996). Sustainable growth? No thank you. In J. Mander and Goldsmith, E. (Eds). *The case against the global economy: And for a turn toward the local.* San Francisco: Sierra Club Books. 192–196.

Diamond, J. (2005). *Collapse: How societies choose to fail or succeed.* New York: Penguin.

Earth Charter. (2000). *Earth Charter.* Retrieved on September 26, 2011 from http://www.earthcharterinaction.org/content/pages/Read-the-Charter.html.

Escobar, A. (1995). *Encountering development: The making and unmaking of the Third World.* Princeton, NJ: Princeton University Press.

Escobar, A. (1996). Constructing nature. In R. Peet and Watts, M. (Eds). *Liberation ecologies: Environment, development, social movements.* New York: Routledge. 46–68.

Estes, R. (1993). Toward sustainable development: From theory to praxis. *Social Development Issues, 15,* 3, 1–30.

Gamble, D.N., and Hoff, M.D. (2005). Sustainable community development. In M. Weil (Ed.). *The handbook of community practice.* Thousand Oaks, CA: Sage.

Gamble, D.N., and Hoff, M.D. (2012). Sustainable community development. In M. Weil (Ed.). *The handbook of community practice* (2nd ed.). Thousand Oaks, CA: Sage Publications. 169–188.

Giddings, B., Hopwood, B., and O'Brien, G. (2002). Environment, economy and society: Fitting them together into sustainable development. *Sustainable Development, 10,* 4, 187–196.

Gitterman, A., and Germain, C. (2008). *The life model of social work practice: Advances in theory and practice* (3rd ed.). New York: Columbia University Press.

Glasmeier, A.K., and Farrigan, T.L. (2003). Poverty, sustainability, and the culture of despair: Can sustainable development strategies support poverty alleviation in America's most environmentally challenged communities? *The ANNALS of the American Academy of Political and Social Science, 590*(1), 131–149.

Goldsmith, E. (1996). Development as colonialism. In J. Mander and Goldsmith, E. (Eds). *The case against the global economy: And for a turn toward the local.* San Francisco: Sierra Club Books. 253–266.

Haberl, H., Fischer-Kowalski, M., Krausmann, F., Martinez-Alier, J., and Winiwarter, V. (2011). A socio-metabolic transition towards sustainability? Challenges for another great transformation. *Sustainable Development, 19,* 1–14.

Hall, A. (1996). Social work or working for change? Action for grassroots sustainable development in Amazonia. *International Social Work, 39,* 27–39.

Hay, R. (2010). The relevance of ecocentrism, personal development and transformational leadership to sustainability and identity. *Sustainable Development, 18,* 163–171.

Hoefer, R. (2006). *Advocacy practice for social justice.* Chicago, IL: Lyceum Books, Inc.

Hoff, M. (1994). Environmental foundations of social welfare: Theoretical resources. In M. Hoff and McNutt, J. (Eds). *The global environmental crisis: Implications for social welfare and social work.* Brookfield, VT: Ashgate. 12–35.

Hoff, M. (1998). *Sustainable community development: Studies in economic, environmental, and cultural revitalization.* Boca Raton, FL: CRC Press.

Hoff, M., and McNutt, J. (Eds). (1994). *The global environmental crisis: Implications for social welfare and social work.* Brookfield, VT: Ashgate Publishing.

Hoff, M., and Polack, R. (1993). Social dimensions of the environmental crisis: Challenges for social work. *Social Work, 38*(2), 204–211.

Hopwood, B., Mellor, M., and O'Brien, G. (2005). Sustainable development: Mapping different approaches. *Sustainable Development, 13,* 38–52.

Ife, J. (2007). Cultural relativism and community activism. In E. Reichert (Ed.). *Challenges in human rights: A social work perspective.* New York: Columbia University Press. 76–96.

International Union for Conservation of Nature and Natural Resources (IUCN). (1980). *World conservation strategy: Living resource conservation for sustainable development.* New York: IUCN-WWF-UNEP.

Jackson, T. (2005). Live better by consuming less? Is there a 'double dividend' in sustainable consumption. *Journal of Industrial Ecology, 9*(1/2), 19–36.

Jacob, M. (1997). Critical theory in political practice: Sustainable development and development theory. *Science Technology & Society, 2*(1), 99–129.

Jensen, D. (2009). Forget shorter showers: Why personal change does not equal political change. *Orion Magazine,* July/August. Retrieved on January 21, 2012 from http://www.orionmagazine.org/index.php/articles/article/4801/.

Jepson, Jr., E.J. (2004). Human nature and sustainable development: A strategic challenge for planners. *Journal of Planning Literature, 19*(1), 3–15.

Kauffman, S.E. (1994). Citizen participation in environmental decisions: Policy, reality, and considerations for community organizing. In M. Hoff and McNutt, J. (Eds). *The global environmental crisis: Implications for social welfare and social work.* Brookfield, VT: Ashgate. 219–239.

Kauffman, S.E., Walter, C.A., Nissly, J., and Walker, J. (1994). Putting the environment into the human behavior and the social environment curriculum. In M. Hoff and McNutt, J. (Eds). *The global environmental crisis: Implications for social welfare and social work.* Brookfield, VT: Ashgate. 277–296.

Keirstead, J., and Leach, M. (2008). Bridging the gaps between theory and practice: A service niche approach to urban sustainability indicators. *Sustainable Development, 16,* 329–340.

Korten, D.C. (2009). *Agenda for a new economy: From phantom wealth to real wealth.* San Francisco, CA: Barrett-Koehler.

Lake, O.O. (2010). *Uprisings for the earth: Reconnecting culture with nature.* Ashland, OR: White Cloud Press.

Leach, M., Scoones, I., and Stirling, A. (2010). *Dynamic sustainabilities: Technology, environment, social justice.* Washington, DC: Earthscan.

Leopold, A. ([1949], 1987). *A sand county almanac.* New York: Oxford.

Lovell, M.L., and Johnson, D.L. (1994). The environmental crisis and direct social work practice. In M. Hoff and McNutt, J. (Eds). *The global environmental crisis: Implications for social welfare and social work.* Brookfield, VT: Ashgate. 199–218.

Luke, T.W. (2005). Neither sustainable nor development: Reconsidering sustainability in development. *Sustainable Development, 13*(4), 228–238.

Lusk, M.W., and Hoff, M. (1994). Sustainable social development. *Social Development Issues, 16*(3), 20–31.

Mander, J., and Goldsmith, E. (Eds). (1996). *The case against the global economy: And for a turn toward the local.* San Francisco: Sierra Club Books.

Marsh, G.P. ([1864], 2003). *Man and nature: Or, physical geography as modified by human action.* Seattle, WA: Washington University Press.

Martinez-Alier, J. (2002). *The environmentalism of the poor: A study of ecological conflicts and valuation.* Northampton, MA: Edward Elgar.

Mary, N.L. (2008). *Social work in a sustainable world.* Chicago, IL: Lyceum Books.

Masuda, J.R., Poland, B., and Baxter, J. (2010). Reaching for environmental health justice: Canadian experiences for a comprehensive research, policy and advocacy agenda in health promotion. *Health Promotion International, 25*(4), 453–456.

McLaren, D. (2003). Environmental space, equity and the ecological debt. In J. Agyeman, Bullard, R.D., and Evans, B. (Eds). *Just sustainabilities: Development in an unequal world.* Cambridge, MA: MIT Press. 19–37.

Meadows, D.H., Meadows, D.L., Randers, J., and Behrens, W.W. (1972). *The limits to growth.* New York: Universe Books.

Meinhard, D., and Tollefson, C. (2009). *Environmental law: Cases and materials.* Toronto, ON: Carswell.

Monbiot, G. (2006). *Heat: How to Stop the Planet from Burning.* Toronto, ON: Anchor Canada.

Morse, S., Vogiatzakis, I., and Griffiths, G. (2011). Space and sustainability: Potential for landscape as a spatial unit for assessing sustainability. *Sustainable Development, 19*(1), 30–48.

Muir, J. ([1914], 1980). *Wilderness essays.* Layton, Utah: Gibbs Smith.

Murdoch, J. (2006). *Post-structuralist geography: A guide to relational space.* Thousand Oaks, CA: Sage.

Norgaard, K.M. (2011). *Living in denial: Climate change, emotions, and everyday life.* Cambridge, MA: MIT Press.

Pandey, A. (2010). Greening Garhwal through stakeholder engagement: The role of ecofeminism, community and the state in sustainable development. *Sustainable Development, 18*(1), 12–19.

Pandey, S. (1998). Women, environment, and sustainable development. *International Social Work, 41,* 339–355.

Peeters, J. (2011). The place of social work in sustainable development: Towards ecosocial practice. *International Journal of Social Welfare, 21,* 1–12. Article first published online: 13 DEC 2011 DOI: 10.1111/j.1468-2397.2011.00856.x.

Pinchot, G. ([1947], 1998). *Breaking new ground.* Washington, DC: Island Press.

Plummer, R. (2006).The evolution of sustainable development strategies in Canada: An assessment of three federal natural resource management agencies. *Sustainable Development, 14,* 16–32.

Poland, B., and Dooris, M. (2010): A green and healthy future: The settings approach to building health, equity and sustainability. *Critical Public Health, 20*(3), 281–298.

Putnam, R. (2000). *Bowling alone: The collapse and revival of American community.* New York: Simon & Schuster.

Quental, N., Lourenço, J.M., and da Silva, F.N. (2011). Sustainable development policy: Goals, targets and political cycles. *Sustainable Development, 19,* 15–29.

Redclift, M. (1987). *Sustainable development: Exploring the contradictions.* London: Methuen.

Rifkin, J. (2004). *The European dream: How Europe's vision of the future is quietly eclipsing the American dream.* New York: Penguin Group.

Rixecker, S.S., and Tipene-Matua, B. (2003). Maori Kaupapa and the inseparability of social and environmental justice: An analysis of bioprospecting and a people's resistance to (bio)cultural assimilation. In J. Agyeman, Bullard, R.D., and Evans,

B. (Eds). *Just sustainabilities: Development in an unequal world.* Cambridge, MA: MIT Press. 252–268.

Roberts, D. (2003). Sustainability and equity: Reflections of a local government practitioner in Southern Africa. In J. Agyeman, Bullard, R.D., and Evans, B. (Eds). *Just sustainabilities: Development in an unequal world.* Cambridge, MA: MIT Press. 187–200.

Rogge, M. (1994a). Field education for environmental hazards: Expanding the person-in-environment perspective. In M. Hoff and McNutt, J. (Eds). *The global environmental crisis: Implications for social welfare and social work.* Brookfield, VT: Ashgate. 258–276.

Rogge, M. (1994b). Environmental injustice: Social welfare and toxic waste. In M. Hoff and McNutt, J. (Eds). *The global environmental crisis: Implications for social welfare and social work.* Brookfield, VT: Ashgate. 53–74.

Rogge, M. (2000). Children, poverty, and environmental degradation: Protecting current and future generations. *Social Development Issues, 22*(2/3), 46–53.

Rogge, M.E., and Cox, M.E. (2001). The person-in-environment perspective in social work journals: A computer-assisted content analysis. *Journal of Social Service Research, 28*(2), 47–68.

Rogge, M., and Darkwa, O. (1996). Poverty and the environment: An international perspective for social work. *International Social Work, 39*(4), 395–409.

Shiva, V. (2005). *Earth democracy: Justice, sustainability, and peace.* Cambridge, MA: South End Press.

Shubert, J.G. (1994). Case studies in community organizing around environmental threats. In M. Hoff and McNutt, J. (Eds). *The global environmental crisis: Implications for social welfare and social work.* Brookfield, VT: Ashgate. 239–257.

Sneddon, C., Howarth, R., and Norgaard, R. (2006). Sustainable development in a post-Brundtland world. *Ecological Economics, 57,* 253– 268.

Soine, L. (1987). Expanding the environment in social work: The case for including environmental hazards content. *Journal of Social Work Education, 23*(2), 40–46.

Soron, D. (2010). Sustainability, self-identity and the sociology of consumption. *Sustainable Development, 18,* 172–181.

Speth, J.G. (2008). *The bridge at the edge of the world: Capitalism, the environment, and crossing from crisis to sustainability.* New Haven, CT: Yale University Press.

Stevens, K., and Morris, J. (2001). Struggling toward sustainability: Considering grassroots development. *Sustainable Development, 9,* 149–164.

St. Martin, K., and Hall-Arber, M. (2007). Environment and development: (Re) connecting community and commons in New England fisheries. In S. Kindon, Pain, R., and Kesby, M. (Eds). *Connecting people, participation and place: Participatory action research approaches and methods.* London and New York: Routledge. 51–59.

Suzuki, D., McConnell, A., and Mason, A. (2007). *The sacred balance: Rediscovering our place in nature.* Vancouver: Greystone Books.

Tester, J.F. (1994). In an age of ecology: Limits to voluntarism and traditional theory in social work practice. In M. Hoff and McNutt, J. (Eds). *The global environmental crisis: Implications for social welfare and social work.* Brookfield, VT: Ashgate. 75–99.

Ungar, M. (2002). A deeper, more social ecological social work practice. *Social Service Review, 76*(3), 480–497.

United Nations. (1992). *United Nations Conference on Environment & Development Rio de Janeiro, Brazil, 3 to 14 June 1992. Agenda 21.* New York: United Nations.

United Nations. (1993). *Report of the United Nations Conference on Environment and Development: Rio de Janeiro, 3–14 June 1992.* New York: United Nations.

United Nations. (2000). *United Nations Millennium Declaration: Resolution adopted by the General Assembly.* New York: United Nations.

United Nations. (2002). *Report of the World Summit on Sustainable Development.* New York: United Nations.

United Nations Environment Programme (UNEP). (1972). Declaration of the United Nations Conference on the Human Environment. Retrieved September 26, 2011 from http://www.unep.org/Documents.Multilingual/Default.Print.asp ?documentid=97&articleid=1503.

United Nations World Commission on Environment and Development. (1987). *Our common future: Report of the World Commission on Environment and Development.* Published as Annex to General Assembly document A/42/427, Development and International Co-operation: Environment August 2, 1987. Retrieved June 7, 2011 from http://www.un-documents.net/wced-ocf.htm.

Van Wormer, K., and Besthorn, F.H. (2007). *Human behavior and the social environment: Groups, communities and organizations* (2nd ed.): New York: Oxford University Press.

Venn, C. (2010). Living individuation, relationality, affect: Rethinking the human in relation to the living. *Body & Society, 16*(1), 129–161.

Voss, J.P., and Kemp, R. (2005). Reflexive governance for sustainable development: Incorporating feedback in social problem-solving. Paper for ESEE Conference, Lisbon, June 14–17.

Wilkinson, R., and Pickett, K. (2009). *The spirit level: Why more equal societies almost always do better.* London: Allen Lane/Penguin.

World Commission on Environment and Development (1987). *Our common future.* Oslo: United Nations.

World Wildlife Fund (WWF). (2008). *Living Planet Report.* Gland, Switzerland: WWF.

Yanarella, E.J., and Bartilow, H. (2000). Beyond environmental moralism and policy incrementalism in the global sustainability debate: Case studies and an alternative framework. *Sustainable Development, 8*(3), 123–134.

Zapf, M.K. (2009). *Social work and the environment: Understanding people and place.* Toronto, ON: Canadian Scholars' Press.

4 Social science research in ocean environments

A social worker's experience

Susan A. Taylor

Over the past 50 years there has been a varied and increasing body of scientific literature on environmental concerns. Within the social sciences, social work has been one of the last disciplines to engage in scientific investigations on the environment. Traditional social work scholarship is nuanced to person-in-environment rather than an environment-including-person focus (Dewane, 2011; McKinnon, 2008), and thereby too narrowly confines investigation. Arguably, the person-in-environment lens limits research to person-centred, anthropogenic, and egocentric explorations that are not useful in ecologically complex investigations (Bay, 2010; Besthorn, 1997, 2008; Besthorn and Canda, 2002; Coates, 2003; Cox 2006). Ironically, if the 'environment' positioning were ecosystem in nature, skillsets that encourage research in the aggregate, with specificity to the individual, make social work valuable as a partner in multidisciplinary research related to environmental concerns. Oceans and public health is one research area where such collaboration is greatly needed.

While a thorough investigation of this topic is beyond the scope of this chapter, the purpose is to: (1) provide a targeted overview of issues connecting humans and marine life; (2) identify areas of research and practice approaches for social scientists in general, and social workers specifically; (3) suggest a framework for future investigation and collaboration; and (4) provide an example of interdisciplinary social work practice. The theoretical lens used in this exploration is an ecocritical approach (Matthies, Närhi, and Ward, 2001), infused with threads of social epidemiology (Krieger, 2001) and an ecosystems perspective (VanLeeuwen, Waltner-Toews, Abernathy, and Smit, 1999). The knowledge base of the author is informed by her three years of university service and participant observation research at the Marine Mammal Center, an internationally recognized rehabilitation, research, and educational facility north of San Francisco, California. As the following discussion shows, this work would not have been possible without a thorough knowledge of the policy and practice context in which scientific research on mammalian marine life is conducted.

An oceans and public health initiative

The United States Oceans and Human Health Act of 2004 provided the impetus for strategic planning related to ocean ecosystem needs and human–environment interactions. The Act established an interagency program and ten-year implementation plan to 'define the goals and priorities for federal research which most effectively advance scientific understanding of the connections between oceans and human health, [and] provide useable information for the prediction of marine-related public health problems' (Interagency Working Group on Harmful Algal Blooms, Hypoxia, and Human Health [IWG-4H], 2008: 1). The Oceans and Human Health Initiative (OHHI), through the National Oceanic and Atmospheric Administration (NOAA), entered into ongoing collaboration with several federal agencies, such as the National Science Foundation (NSF), National Institute of Environmental Health Sciences' (NIEHS) Centers for Oceans and Humans Health, the Centers for Disease Control and Prevention (CDC), Environmental Protection Agency (EPA), Food and Drug Administration (FDA), Marine Mammal Commission (MMC), and National Aeronautics and Space Administration (NASA). The interagency collaboration was designed to better integrate and focus research efforts, including those in the physical and social sciences (Interagency Working Group, 2008, 2009). The initial and concurrent planning efforts opened the door for social science to engage more fully in research in the overlapping areas of ocean environments and public health.

Ocean environments and public health

Ecocritical and *ecosocial* models are congruent with natural science investigations in marine or oceanic environments, which investigate sustainability and human–environmental interaction, and offer a more expansive lens through which to move forward Hoff and McNutt's (1994) early conceptual scholarship. Along with an ecocritical, ecosocial understanding of the interrelatedness of human impacts on the health of the environment, other oft-used social science theories provide a useful lens through which to view ocean research in national and international contexts. For example, *social epidemiology*, often used to explain social inequalities in health, can be used to anchor multidisciplinary social impact investigations. Social epidemiology draws on psychosocial, political-economic, and ecosocial theory and related multilevel frameworks to explain health inequalities (Krieger, 2001). Social epidemiology recognizes 'the impact of social factors on the distribution of health and illness in a population [and] examines the role of social variables on other known and accepted biological and behavioral factors that shape the health status of a community' (Sable, Schild, and Hipp, 2012: 76). Among other things, it uses community assessment methodologies in conducting health and social impact assessments (Ebi and Semenza, 2008; Ebi, Kovats, and Menne, 2006) and geographic information systems to map spatial correlations, both of which are compatible with ocean research which, for example, examines social influences on marine conservation (Jarrett, Gale, and Kontgis, 2010; Reynolds, Marsh, and Ragen, 2009; Wallace, 2003), risk and vulnerability in fishing communities (Clay and Olson, 2008), and social impact assessments as a part of conservation planning strategies (Interorganizational Committee on Principles and Guidelines for Social Impact Assessment, 2003).

VanLeeuwen *et al.* (1999) combine these foci to represent public health as an *ecosystem* which they believe 'provides a more realistic model of the determinants of human health' (p. 205). They explain:

> ecosystem health is a logical extension of the health paradigm (and its accompanying language, values, testing, and procedures) beyond individuals (human or animal health), and populations of the same species in one place (public or herd health), to populations of different species in one place or in many places.
>
> (p. 205)

Multispecies, multispatial research lends itself to a 'one medicine' conceptualization of public health (posited by Calvin Schwade in 1984). Zinsstag, Schelling, Waltner-Toews, and Tanner (2011) built on this work adding that 'sustainable development depends on the mutualism of the health and well being of humans, animals, and the ecosystems in which they coexist' (p. 150). They concluded that 'interactions between human and animal health ... reach far beyond individual clinical issues and includes ecology, public health, and broader societal dimensions' (p. 150). They note two examples of this ecosystems approach: the United States National Institutes of Health, Office of Behavioral and Social Sciences aims to bring 'together in a systematic way behavioural-social-ecological models and molecular, cellular, and ultimately physiological bases of health and disease to improve public health' (p. 153) and Canada was one of the first countries to establish 'a program for integrated surveillance of antibiotic resistance in humans and animals using a systematic approach' (p. 153). Along these lines, other authors have noted interspecies connections. For example, Stewart *et al.* (2008) remind us that 'an estimated 75% of emerging infectious diseases are zoonotic' (p. 10), that is, they are transmitted from animals to humans. The 'one medicine' ecosystem health modelling allows for collaboration among physical and social sciences across research spectrums involving multiple species and multiple spatial interactions.

Economic impact in North America

In 2003 and 2004 respectively, Canada and the United States developed overarching policies specifically related to ocean environments. These reflected the many accords explored in the United Nations Law of the Sea agreement in 1982. However, unsurprisingly, later documents were specific to the interests of each country. In North America, population location and economic activity are dynamically affected by ocean environments and marine life. Over half the US population lives along the 95,000 miles of coastline (Sandifer *et al.*, 2007). In Canada, 'eight of ten provinces and all three territories directly border oceans and marine waterways, and over twenty-five percent of the population live[s] in coastal zones' (Fisheries and Oceans Canada, 2002: 2). Economic activity produced from this concentration of population and wealth is estimated in the United States to represent 'over half of the nation's gross domestic product' (Sandifer *et al.*, 2007: 4) and in Canada, 'over $20 billion in annual economic activity and many billions more in ocean trade through the waterways' (Fisheries and Oceans Canada, 2002: 2). For those who live and work near these ocean environments, the relevance of ocean cycles, as well as the health of ocean ecosystems and marine life, is without question. Although conflicting social, political, economic, and environmental meta-questions arise, the significance of impact is unmitigated.

Why ocean environments?

Seventy-one per cent of Earth's surface is made up of oceans (Bowermaster, 2010), and 'a significant portion of the world's population live within 75 miles of an ocean coast [with] this density of human population increasing daily' (Fleming *et al.*, 2006, p. 2). Oceanographer Sylvia Earle (2010) reminds us that 'even if you have never had the chance to see or touch the ocean, the ocean touches you with every breath you take, every drop of water you drink, every bite you consume' (p. 11). She continues, 'the ocean drives climate and weather, regulates temperature, absorbs much of the carbon dioxide from the atmosphere, holds 97% of the Earth's water, and embraces 95% of the biosphere' (p. 11). Quite simply, variations in the capacity of oceans to maintain biodiversity and ecosystem health affect all life on the planet. Human interdependence with this environment – its biological and chemical properties, along with its non-human inhabitants – is significant to multispecies survivability.

A wealth of research related to the health of ocean environments has developed within the physical sciences over the last fifty years. Concern over the health of the expansive ocean ecosystem is well documented (e.g., Agrawal, 2009; Allsopp, Pambuccian, Johnston, and Santillo 2009; Booth and Zellar, 2006; Danson, 2011; Glover and Earle, 2004; Laws, Fleming, and Stegeman, 2008). Areas of concern include:

- An increase in the degradation of ocean environments – evident in harmful algae blooms, coral bleaching, and marine litter.
- The developing impact of climate change.

- The physiological stresses on the health of marine life from environmental pollution and loss of habitat.
- The increasing ecosystem toxicity of ocean environments and the episodic transmission of disease-causing agents to animals and humans.

In North America, these developments have led to national plans for multidisciplinary research designed to mitigate harm.

Blueprint for policy in the United States

In 2004 the United States Commission of Ocean Policy developed the first comprehensive US plan, *An Ocean Blueprint for the 21st Century*. The 480-page document (plus appendices) was extremely thorough. Divided into 10 distinct sections with 31 subsections, the document provides an overview of historical policy development and a grounded understanding of social, economic, and scientific issues affecting ocean environments. For the purposes of the exploration in this chapter, a brief overview is relevant.

Parts one and two review national policy and federal agency involvement and explore leadership, regional approaches, coordination issues, and federal agency structure. Part three discusses ocean stewardship, education, and public awareness and the promotion of lifelong learning as a key element to successful conservation. Part four emphasizes economic growth and resource conservation in coastal areas. Included is attention to reducing natural hazards to people and property, conserving and restoring natural coastal habitat, managing sediment and shorelines, and supporting marine commerce and transportation. The investigation of coastal and ocean water quality, resource use and protection is developed in Parts five and six. Included is a poignant discussion of water pollution, and efforts aimed at limiting vessel pollution, preventing the spread of invasive species, reducing marine debris, achieving sustainable fisheries, protecting marine mammals and endangered marine species, preserving coral reefs and coral communities, sustainable marine aquaculture, oceans and public health, and managing offshore energy and mineral resources. Parts seven, eight, and nine explore strategies for increasing scientific knowledge, infra-structure and technology development, data and information system needs, international policy participation, funding needs, and recommendations. In North America, this document, combined with previously mentioned provisions from the 1982 UN Convention on the Law of the Sea (Agenda 21), provide a comprehensive assessment of issues facing ocean environments, along with specific recommendations for future research. Combined with Canada's parliamentary efforts, including its Ocean Act of 1996 (Minister of Justice Canada, 1996) and national strategic plans (Fisheries and Oceans Canada, 2002, 2005, 2010), both countries' plans provide a wealth of information designed to enhance research strategies of physical and social scientists within North America and internationally.

An invitation to collaborate in ocean science

In the United States, concurrent with the development of national reports, opportunities for interdisciplinary research in ocean and marine mammal environments continued to develop. The National Oceanic and Atmospheric Administration's (NOAA) ocean research agendas specifically targeted opportunities for the social sciences. Its 2003 report identified potential social science disciplinary partners, and recommended areas of scientific focus that would provide a beneficial intersection of research activities with the physical sciences (NOAA, 2003). Among the social sciences listed in the 2003 report, eight disciplines were highlighted: anthropology, demography, economics, geography, law, political science, psychology (social and cognitive), and sociology. Although social work was not one of the distinct disciplines, the skillsets of the profession are compatible with many of the disciplines mentioned though few social workers are directly involved in environmental research on the health of the oceans and marine life and its impact on human well-being.

The NOAA report (2003) identified social science as a 'process of describing, explaining, and predicting human behaviour and institutional structure in interaction with their environments' and identified data categories as 'economic, demographic, legal/regulatory, political/ institutional, and social/cultural' (p. 10). Specific areas of focus included: the origin of physical, social and cultural development and behaviour; and populations, including size, growth, density, and distribution, as well as statistics regarding birth, marriage, migration, disease, and death. Also noted was study involving 'the allocation of scarce resources among competing ends to understand how individuals, groups, and governments faced limited resources, choose to produce, distribute, and consume goods and services; and, the spatial distribution of human activity and interactions with the environment' (NOAA, 2003: 10). Finally, legal and policy areas were mentioned, specifically, the study of law and law-related subjects and political organizations and institutions, especially governments, along with social and cognitive psychology.

SSWG in their 2009 follow-up report encouraged further work by NOAA to integrate the social sciences into agency work, noting

> a social science research agenda is well articulated within the National Marine Fisheries Service (NMFS) and National Ocean Service (NOS) line offices [and offers] ... rich opportunities for social science research [on] ... climate, coasts and oceans, weather and water, and ecosystems, and commerce and transportation.
>
> (NOAA, 2009: 6)

Against this backdrop of events supporting social scientific research into marine life, I ventured into the Marine Mammal Center (TMMC) located in the Marin Headlands of the Golden Gate National Recreation Area, north of San Francisco.

A social worker ventures into ocean science: The Marine Mammal Center

Over its 38-year history, TMMC has established itself as one of the premiere marine mammal rehabilitation, research, and educational facilities in the world. The Center's primary objective is the rehabilitation of distressed, injured, orphaned, and diseased species of marine mammals which inhabit the California coast, with the ultimate goal of releasing them back into their natural habitat. According to Smalley (1973), its focus is:

- *Marine mammal health*: Acquiring 'knowledge … about diseases, parasites, and the effects of toxic materials discharged into the sea on marine mammal populations' (p. 2).
- *Environmental*: Learning about 'the man-made dangers these animals face [that] are increasing all the time. Oil spills continue to occur; radioactive materials are released into the ocean depths; industrial wastes such as arsenic, lead, and mercury find their way into the sea, contaminating food sources we share with these animals' (p. 2).
- *Animals as sentries*: Exploring how 'animals served by this program might in turn serve as an early warning system alerting us to the buildup of these harmful elements' (p. 2).

TMMC's unique location positions it on the migration path of a great number of Pacific marine mammals and near many birthing rookeries. The facility's development runs parallel to the emergence of scientific protocols related to marine mammal rescue and rehabilitation, marine mammal and ocean science education, and knowledge of marine pathogens and their possible danger to humans. In addition to targeted research, particularly as it relates to California sea lions, northern fur seals, Guadeloupe fur seals, northern elephant seals, Pacific harbour seals, and to a lesser degree other Pacific ocean inhabitants: sea otters, dolphins, and whales, a larger view of the ocean environment these animals inhabit has also emerged.

Beyond the sentimentality present in working with marine mammals, my interest in public health informed my decision to volunteer and research at TMMC. Oceans and public health initiatives benefit from an understanding of the positioning of marine mammals as sentinels of 'environmental stress and potential health threats to humans' (Stewart *et al.*, 2008: 8). Stewart *et al.* (2008) note at least three areas where this recognition is helpful:

1   Wildlife or habitats, 'contaminants, toxins, and/or pathogens from [marine mammal] environment[s] … may provide more biologically

relevant indicators of possible effects than water sampling alone' (p. 9; see also Ragen, 2005).

2 Wildlife diets and physiologies where these factors 'are at least partially similar to those of humans and which therefore demonstrate early indications of potential health effects of environmental levels of contaminants, toxins, and pathogens before they show up in humans (a biological early warning system)' (p. 9; see also O'Hara and O'Shea, 2005).

3 Habitats encompassing 'key ecosystem components and [are] subject to early and often high pollution exposure, thereby indicating potential effects at system or community levels and on people' (p. 9). Examples of such areas are 'sea grass beds, oyster reefs, kelp forests, coral reefs, tidal creeks ... and estuaries' (p. 9, see also Van Dolah, 2005).

Relevance for social work

I ventured into the oceans and public health arena not knowing whether or how my *clinical practice skills* would be useful in this physical science environment. At the first information session, the facilitator asked whether there were any therapists or teachers in the room. Several of us raised our hands. 'We want you' she said. She explained that our unique professional qualities, such as our intuition, ability to nurture change, draw out the best in individuals, maintain a positive attitude, and patience in waiting for progress were transferable to the animal care environment. Also applicable, particularly among therapists, was the ability to handle life and death situations, remain calm and focused during crisis, and collaborate effectively toward positive interventions for individuals and groups. For those who had worked in hospital settings, knowledge of charting, use of medicine, types of public health diseases, and safety protocols were similarly needed in and transferable to the new environment. Once I entered the marine mammal hospital environment, I quickly understood the relevance of my professional skill in an environment that arguably resembled a cross between a health or mental health clinic and a foster care or adoption agency.

I quickly learnt the *seal patients and protocols* in this new clinical environment where particular species of seals are seasonal patients at the hospital. Ages range from those with umbilical cords still attached, to the seal equivalent of toddlers (3–6 months), teenagers (1–3 years), and young adults (4 years plus). Maternal separation, malnutrition, disease, predator wounds, and gunshots are the maladies affecting patients. I started my immersion into veterinary science working with elephant seal pups and California sea lions.

Prior to working with seal patients, I learned the medical universal precautions – gloving, wearing protective clothing, knowing what to do if there was a transfer of bodily fluid (through bites, scrapes, fecal matter on open wounds, exposure to bacteria through splashing of water into one's eyes, mouth, and skin), and other protocols for assuring the team, myself, and the patient remained safe. It felt oddly familiar from my work in AIDS, TB, and other human communicable disease environments. I was also reminded that hospitals of any kind are biohazard environments.

Among the unique attributes of elephant seal pups is that, until instinct kicks in, they are clueless as to how to eat, swim, or manoeuvre 'seal life' for several months after birth in the wild. It is something that they learn in tide pools, among peer groups after the adults have left to re[hy]engage with life at sea. For those who learn slowly or where social learning is stunted by disease or injury, death is imminent. For those who are fortunate enough to be rescued, TMMC becomes their lifeline.

Along with assisting in providing basic medical care, nutritional support, and safe play guidance (i.e., being watchful to house like-tempered animals together so that they feel safe, can relax, heal, and prepare to learn), I also serve as a teacher of *fish school* – the equivalent of psychosocial educational skill development groups. Once seal pups are stabilized, and grouped based on size, disease type, temperament, and 'learning ability', they are 'sent' to fish school to learn basic seal survival skills. The first step is often reducing fear of water, learning how to swim in four to five feet of water (generally by being pushed in by the 'teacher'), and gaining some degree of comfort in a pod of beginning swimmers. Beyond water survival, fish school involves becoming familiar with fish – their touch and taste, how to swallow them, and how to chase them. This process can take weeks. Success produces a confident seal pup who realizes he will not drown in deep water, can actually hold his breath for long periods underwater, can manoeuvre in peer groups, learn from peers, and who becomes excited at the prospect of eating fish. Once these skills have been developed, the patients are released in peer pods near adult colonies so that they can rejoin their species' habitat and recolonize.

Research into and rehabilitation of California sea lions, suffering from malnutrition, disease, and entanglement, is another important aspect of this work. Research with this particular 'seal' species is very unique at TMMC, where scientific and veterinary science protocols developed by veterinary staff and lead scientists at 'the Center' are nationally and internationally recognized as leading contributions in the field. TMMC has one of the largest and oldest repositories of blood, urine, and tissue samples of seal species, particularly pinnepeds (i.e., sea lions). Because the anatomy and physiology of sea lions so closely resembles humans, their vulnerabilities in ocean environments inform similar vulnerabilities in humans. This is particularly true of ocean-borne pathogens (see Loge *et al.*, 2005; National Research Council, 1999) that these animals store in their blubber, brain material, and organs (see Brodie *et al.*, 2006). Domoic acid poisoning among sea lions is one area of staff expertise. While a number of other diseases are prevalent in this population, domoic acid is becoming more present in ocean environments and is an early indicator of harmful algae blooms (HABs) and toxic environments (see O'Hara and O'Shea, 2005; Moore *et al.*, 2008; Reynolds *et al.*, 2005), hazardous to both marine animals and human health.

With this species contributions can be direct, in animal care, and indirect, working with veterinary staff, researchers, and other team members. Observational skills and monitoring patterns of social behaviour within the species are particular areas where social workers are valuable in a multidisciplinary team setting. The interdisciplinary nature of my veterinary science experience requires qualification. The animal care crew to which I am assigned comprises three nurses, three teachers, another social worker, various computer tech professionals, business professionals, and an array of physical science students in various stages of their education. Together, we join our various skillsets and knowledge interests to become a collaborative multidisciplinary medical care team. It is one of the most interesting collaborative experiences of my professional career.

My interest in *macro and policy practice* issues related to oceans and public health grew out of my work with individual patients (a general pattern for social work practitioners). What became apparent after the first full year of volunteering in Veterinary Science was my growing understanding of the interrelatedness of marine mammal and human health, and the increasing degradation of the ocean environment that we shared. During my second year of University service at the Center, in addition to serving in the Veterinary Science area, I decided to also be trained as a member of the Center's Educational department. This training exposed me to science and research related to climate change, ocean debris and plastics, and the chemical alteration of ocean environments, largely influenced by human consumption patterns, industrial innovations, infrastructure vulnerability, and land use. Exposure to national and international scientists studying these patterns, along with interest of the visiting public in many of these issues, prompted me to become a docent at the Center, begin to develop scholarship in the area, guest lecture in social work departments across the United States, and develop curriculum for my own social work graduate and undergraduate students at my home University. While ocean environments and marine mammal content were initially suspect among my social work peers and students, it became apparent after my reframing the macro practice arena in community economic assessment, policy analysis, social impact assessment, and health and wellness projections in this context, how social work research and macro practice could be relevant in this practice arena. Such recognition has led to an increasing interest among some social work students as to how they can become more knowledgeable of the subject area, and collaborate in multidisciplinary practice. Also under consideration from the physical scientists at TMMC is increasing dialogue related to how the social sciences can be included in research and practice contributions of the organization and ocean environmental science research as a whole.

As noted above, social workers have many skills for multidisciplinary research and practice in ocean environments. Given the international focus on climate change, among other related ocean challenges, social workers would be wise to gain and refine practice knowledge in this area. A wealth of literature and policy has developed over the last 15 years that clearly identifies a path for social scientists, and a place where social work researchers and practitioners may look to ocean environments as areas for their professional contributions.

Looking ahead

Without question, the health of oceans and marine mammals impacts directly on human well-being in several key respects. Many coastal communities depend on the oceans for their livelihoods, and the impact of toxic waste, pollution, and marine debris, specifically plastics and fishing gear, can be felt far beyond the immediate cause of the problem. It becomes a public health issue when there is negative impact on humans (see also Chapters 2 and 15). Social workers are often the first responders in such cases through their professional contact with individuals, communities, and the health and welfare issues that confront them. Questions of cross species and environmental sustainability are ones that are equally important to social and physical practitioners and scientists. Environmental research strengthens activism and advocacy practice, suggesting social workers should take advantage of the supportive environment that has been created for social science research in ocean and marine mammal science. As in most areas of environmental activity, this is a multidisciplinary area where social workers can contribute with other social scientists to environmental impact assessments and participatory action research with communities affected by declining ocean health.

References

Agrawal, A. (2009). Local institutions and adaptation to climate change. In R. Mearns and Norton, A. (Eds). *Social dimensions of climate change: Equity and vulnerability in a warming world.* Washington, DC: World Bank. 173–198.

Allsopp, M., Pambuccian, S.E., Johnston, P., and Santillo, D. (2009). *State of the world's oceans.* New York: Springer.

Bay, U. (2010). Social work and the environment: Understanding people and place. *Australian Social Work, 63*(3), 366–367.

Besthorn, F.H. (1997). *Reconceptualizing social work's person in environment perspective: Explorations in radical environmental thought.* Unpublished dissertation. Lawrence, KS: University of Kansas.

Besthorn, F.H. (2008). Environment and social work practice. *Encyclopedia of Social Work* (20th ed.). Oxford: Oxford University Press. 132–136.

Besthorn, F.H., and Canda, E.R. (2002). Revising environment: Deep ecology for education and teaching in social work. *Journal of Teaching in Social Work, 22*(1/2), 79–102.

Booth, S., and Zellar, D. (2006). Mercury, food webs, and marine mammals: Implications of diet and climate change for human health. *Environmental Health Perspectives, 113*(5), 521–526.

Bowermaster, J. (Ed.). (2010). *Oceans: The threats to our seas and what you can do to turn the tide.* New York: Public Affairs (Perseus Books Group).

Brodie, E., Gulland, F.M.D., Grieg, D.J., Hunter, M., Jaakola, J., St.Leger, J., Leighfield, T.A., and Van Dohlah, F.M. (2006). Domoic acid causes reproductive failure in California sea lions (*Zalophus Californianus*). *Marine Mammal Science 22*(3), 700–707.

Clay, P.M., and Olson, J. (2008). Defining 'fishing communities': Vulnerability and Magnuson-Stevens Fishery Conservation and Management Act. *Human Ecology Review, 15*(2), 143–160.

Coates, J. (2003). *Ecology and social work toward a new paradigm.* Nova Scotia, CA: Fernwood Publishing.

Cox, R. (2006). *Environmental communication and the public sphere.* Thousand Oaks, CA: Sage.

Danson, T. (2011). *Oceana: Our endangered oceans and what you can do to save them.* New York: Rodale Books.

Dewane, C.J. (2011). Environmentalism and social work: The ultimate social justice issue. *Social Work Today, 11*(5), 20.

Earle, S.A. (2010). *The world is blue: How our fate and the ocean's are one.* Washington, DC: National Geographic.

Ebi, K.L., and Semenza, J.C. (2008). Community based adaptation to the health impacts of climate change. *American Journal of Preventive Medicine, 35*(5), 501–507.

Ebi, K.L., Kovats, R.S., and Menne, B. (2006). An approach of assessing human health vulnerability and public health interventions to adapt to climate change. *Environmental Health Perspective, 114*, 1930–1934.

Fisheries and Oceans Canada (2002). *Canada's Oceans Strategy: Our oceans, our future.* Ottawa, ON: Government of Canada. Available online at http://www.dfo-mpo.gc.ca/oceans/publications/cos-soc/pdf/cos-soc-eng.pdf

Fisheries and Oceans Canada (2005). *Canada's Oceans Action Plan: For present and future generations.* Ottawa, ON: Government of Canada. Available online at http://www.dfo-mpo.gc.ca/oceans/publications/cos-soc/pdf/cos-soc-eng.pdf

Fisheries and Oceans Canada (2010). *National Framework for Canada's Network of Marine Protected Areas.* Ottawa, ON: Government of Canada. Available online at http://www.dfo-mpo.gc.ca/oceans/publications/cos-soc/pdf/cos-soc-eng.pdf

Fleming, L.E., Broad, K., Clement, A., Dewailly, E., Elmir, S., Knap, A., Pomponi, S.A., Solo-Gabriele, H., and Walsh, P. (2006). Oceans and human health: Emerging public health risks in the marine environment. *Marine Pollution Bulletin, 53*(10–12), 545–560.

Glover, L.K., and Earle, S.A. (Eds). (2004). *Defying ocean's end: An agenda for action.* Washington, DC: Island Press.

Hoff, M., and McNutt, J. (Eds). (1994). *The global environmental crises: Implications for social welfare and social work.* Aldershot, UK: Ashgate.

Interagency Working Group on Climate Change and Health (2009). *A human health perspective on climate change: A report outlining the research needs on the human health effects of climate change.* Environmental Health Perspectives and the National Institute of Environmental Health Sciences. Research Circle, NC.

Interagency Working Group on Harmful Algal Blooms, Hypoxia, and Human Health (2008). *Interagency Oceans and Human Health Annual Report 2004–2006.* Washington, DC: Interagency Oceans and Human Health.

Interorganizational Committee on Principles and Guidelines for Social Impact Assessment (2003). US principles and guideline: Principles and guidelines for social impact assessment in the USA. *Impact Assessment Project Appraisal, 21*(3), 231–250.

Jarrett, M., Gale, S., and Kontgis, C. (2010). Spatial modeling in environmental and public health. *International Journal of Environmental Research on Public Health, 7,* 1302–1329.

Krieger, N. (2001). Theories of social epidemiology in the 21st century: An ecosocial perspective. *International Journal of Epidemiology, 30,* 668–677.

Laws, E.A., Fleming, L.E., and Stegeman, J.J. (2008). Centers for Oceans and Human Health: Contributions to an emerging discipline. *Environmental Health, 7*(Suppl2), S1. Available at http://ehjournal.net/content/7/S2/S1.

Loge, F.J., Arkoosh, M.R., Ginn, T.R., Johnson, L.L., and Collier, T.K. (2005). Impact of environmental stressors on the dynamics of disease transmission. *Environmental Science and Technology, 39,* 7329–7336.

Matthies, A.L., Närhi, K., and Ward, D. (Eds). (2001). *The eco-social approach in social work.* Jyvaskyla, Finland: SoPhi.

McKinnon, J. (2008). Exploring the nexus between social work and the environment. *Australian Social Work, 61*(3), 256–268.

Minister of Justice Canada (1996). Consolidation Oceans Act. Available at http://laws-lois.justice.gc.ca.

Moore, S.K., Trainer, V.L., Mantua, N.J., Parker, M.S., Laws, E.A, Backer, L.C., and Fleming, L.E. (2008). Impacts of climate variability and future climate change on harmful algal blooms and human health. *Environmental Health, 7*(Suppl.2). Retrieved February 10, 2012 from http://ehjournal.net/content/7/S2/S4.

National Oceanic and Atmospheric Administration (NOAA). (2003). *Social science research within NOAA: Review and recommendations.* Final Report of the Social Science Review Panel to the NOAA Science Advisory Board. Washington, DC: NOAA.

National Oceanic and Atmospheric Administration (NOAA). (2009). *Integrating social science into NOAA planning, evaluation and decisionmaking: A review of implementation to date and recommendations for improving effectiveness.* Report of the Social Science Review Panel to the NOAA Science Board. Washington, DC: NOAA.

National Research Council (1999). *From monsoons to microbes: Understanding the ocean's role in human health.* Committee on the Ocean's Role in Human Health. Washington, DC: National Academies Press,. Downloaded from http://nap.edu/catalog/6368.html.

O'Hara, T.M., and O'Shea, T.J. (2005). Assessing impacts of environmental contaminants. In J.E. Reynolds, Perrin, W.F., Reeves, R.R., Montgomery, S., and Ragen, T.J. (Eds). *Marine mammal research: Conservation beyond crisis.* Baltimore, MD: Johns Hopkins University Press. 63–85.

Ragen, T.J. (2005). Assessing and managing marine mammal habitat in the United States. In J.E. Reynolds, Perrin, W.F., Reeves, R.R., Montgomery, S., and Ragen, T.J. (Eds). *Marine mammal research: Conservation beyond crisis.* Baltimore, MD: Johns Hopkins University Press. 125–136.

Reynolds, J.E., Marsh, H., and Ragen, T.J. (2009). Marine mammal conservation. *Endangered Species Research, 7,* 23–28.

Reynolds, J.E., Perrin, W.F., Reeves, R.R., Montgomery, S., and Ragen, T.J. (Eds). (2005). *Marine mammal research: Conservation beyond crisis.* Baltimore, MD: Johns Hopkins University Press.

Reynolds, J.E., Perrin, W.F., Reeves, R.R., Montgomery, S., and Ragen, T.J. (Eds). (2012). *Marine mammal research: Conservation beyond crisis.* Baltimore, MD: Johns Hopkins University Press.

Sable, M.R., Schild, D.R., and Hipp, J.A. (2012). Public health and social work. In S. Gehlert and Browne, T. (Eds). *Handbook of health and social work* (2nd ed.). Hoboken, NJ: John Wiley and Sons. 64–99.

Sandifer, P., Sotka, C., Garrison, D., and Fay, V. (2007). *Interagency Oceans and Human Health Research Implementation Plan: A prescription for the future.* Washington, DC: Interagency Working Group on Harmful Algal Blooms, Hypoxia, and Human Health of the Subcommittee on Ocean Science and Technology.

Smalley, L. (1973). Proposal to establish the California Marine Mammal Center.

Stewart, J.R., Gast, R.J., Fujioka, R.S., Solo-Gabriele, H.M., Meshke, S., Amaral-Zettler, L.A., del Castillo, E., Polz, M.F., Collier, T.K., Strom, M.S., Sinigalliano, C.D., Moeller, P.D.R., and Holland, A.F. (2008). The coastal environment and human health: Microbial indicators, pathogens, sentinels, and reservoirs. *Environmental Health, 7*(Suppl2), S3. Available at http://ehjournal.net/content/7/S2/S3.

Van Dolah, F.M. (2005). Effects of harmful algal blooms. In J.E. Reynolds, Perrin, W.F., Reeves, R.R., Montgomery, S., and Ragen, T.J. (Eds). *Marine mammal research: Conservation beyond crisis.* Baltimore, MD: Johns Hopkins University Press. 85–100

VanLeeuwen, J.A., Waltner-Toews, D., Abernathy, T., and Smit, B. (1999). Evolving models of human health toward an ecosystem context. *Ecosystem Health, 5*(3), 204–219.

Wallace, R.L. (2003). Social influences on conservation: Lessons from U.S. Recovery programs for marine mammals. *Conservation Biology, 17*(1), 104–115.

Zinsstag, J., Schelling, E., Waltner-Toews, D., and Tanner, M. (2011). From 'one medicine' to 'one health' and systemic approaches to health and well being. *Preventive Veterinary Medicine, 101,* 148–156.

Acknowledgement

The author wishes to acknowledge and thank the Vet Crew – Joanne Handley, Lee Jackrel, Hanne Larsen, Jacquie Hilterman, Amy Miles, Joanne Lasnier, Tami Pearson, Bob Terrell, Ben Calvert, Chris Shields, Anne Bertaud-Pueto, Jean Criner, Siobhan Rickert, Jeff Robinson, Valerie Hershfield, Bill Van Bonn, Jeff Boehm, Frances Gulland, and Deb Wickham – and the Education Team – Ann Bauer, Adam Ratner, and Kathleen Hannah.

5 Climate change as a human rights issue

Frank Tester

Nobody ever told you that history was kind (Steve Earle, 2011).

Human rights not only protect individuals from discrimination and abuse but also, increasingly, ensure human survival, including access to food, water, shelter, and health. The right to health, as laid out in articles 12 and 25 of the Universal Declaration of Human Rights (UN, 1948), has received much attention, particularly in response to the global AIDS pandemic (Mann, Gruskin, Grodin, and Annas, 1999). Global climate change is increasingly recognized as another international crisis, with implications for positive human rights outlined in a long list of international covenants, declarations, treaties, and agreements. While this chapter focuses on the human rights dimension of climate change, understanding the chemistry and physics of climate change is important to appreciating the severity of the situation in which we – and that means all of us on the planet – find ourselves. A very readable introduction to all dimensions of the problem can be found in Danny Chivers' (2010) *No-Nonsense Guide to Climate Change.*

Human rights are also collective rights. For certain cultures finding 'ways of making sense' and surviving on the planet is considerably different from mainstream western-European traditions. Following the collapse of the Soviet Union in the early 1990s, these cultures with alternative relations to production and consumption have been under steady attack by Western capitalism working internationally, overseen by institutions created to manage the global economy: the World Bank, International Monetary Fund (IMF) and World Trade Organization (WTO) (Seabrook, 1993):

> Human rights are rights inherent to all human beings, whatever our nationality, place of residence, sex, national or ethnic origin, colour, religion, language, or any other status. We are all equally entitled to our human rights without discrimination. These rights are all interrelated, interdependent and indivisible.
>
> (Office of the United Nations High Commissioner
> for Human Rights, 2011)

The substance of these rights is found in texts and institutional mandates of the United Nations and other international organizations. Notable among them, with respect to environmental and human rights, are: The Universal Declaration of Human Rights (UN, 1948); International Covenant on Civil and Political Rights (Office of the High Commission for Human Rights, 1966); International Covenant on Economic, Social and Cultural Rights (UN, 1966); Convention on the Rights of the Child (UN, 1989); Declaration on the Rights of Indigenous Peoples (UN, 2008); American Convention on Human Rights (Inter-American Commission on Human Rights (IACHR), 1969); European Convention on Human Rights (Council of Europe, 1950); and the European Social Charter (Council of Europe, 1961). Also of importance are the American Declaration of the Rights and Duties of Man (IACHR, 1948) and the work of the Inter-American Commission on Human Rights (IACHR), the UN Economic and Social Council (ECOSOC), and the UN Human Rights Commission (UNHRC).

Article 3 of the Universal Declaration of Human Rights (UN, 1948) states: 'Everyone has the right to life, liberty and security of person'. Life, liberty, and security of person are recognized increasingly by environmentalists and social activists as inextricably tied to the quality of the environments in which people live. These are affected by the way in which production, consumption, and disposal are organized in capitalist economies. Climate change is a social and environmental cost of how society has organized the meeting – and creation – of human needs and wants. A report by the Special Rapporteur of the Commission for Human Rights Sub-Commission on Prevention of Discrimination and Protection of Minorities, submitted to the UN Economic and Social Council in July 1994, 'identified the right to a satisfactory environment as present in existing human rights covenants' (Johnston, 2011: 16). The report resulted from discussions preceding the 1992 United Nations Conference on Environment and Development (UNCED) held in Rio de Janeiro. Subsequently, a statement of Draft Principles on Human Rights and the Environment was presented to the Commission in 1995. It included the 'right to a secure, healthy and ecologically sound environment'. The Commission's members from the United States and European countries, lobbied heavily by corporate interests, rejected this articulation. This raises important questions about the fate of attempts to link human rights and environmental justice to economic development and growth in a globalized economy, given the power of international business elites (Corporate Europe Observer, 2001).

Climate change has serious implications for human health and access to food, water, and shelter (see Godrej, 2001). In some parts of the world, populations are vulnerable because of geographical location and a lack of the power and resources to address the conditions confronting them. While climate change poses the greatest threat to human rights and the meeting of basic human needs that modern civilization has ever faced, it is ignored in recently published social work texts dealing with human rights and social justice (Baines, 2007; Ife, 2002, 2008; Mapp, 2008). While alerting the profession to the relevance of environmental theory and practice to social work, in *Ecology and Social Work* Coates (2003) makes no mention of climate change as a human rights or environmental justice issue.

Social work has 'come late' to recognizing the importance of built and natural environments to the human condition. It remains focused largely on clinical practice, child welfare, hospital social work and, in Canada and Europe, community work often emphasizing empowerment and acting locally to build better communities and cooperative relations within global regimes of capital accumulation that are literally killing us (Harvey, 1996; Johnston, 2011; Seabrook, 1993).

Inuit Circumpolar Conference Petition

On December 7, 2005, the Inuit Circumpolar Conference (ICC), on behalf of all Inuit in Arctic regions of the United States and Canada, submitted a *Petition to the Inter-American Commission on Human Rights Seeking Relief from Violations Resulting from Global Warming caused by Acts and Omissions of the United States*. Unlike most bodies of the United Nations, under US law the Commission can receive petitions from individuals or nongovernment organizations. Its powers are investigative, generating reports recommending that governments take actions to remedy situations where the Commission's investigations have found in favour of a complainant. In extreme circumstances, where governments have repeatedly failed to respond to the Commission's recommendations, cases may be referred to the Inter-American Court of Human Rights, a body that, while limited in its jurisdiction, can award compensation to victims. The Inuit petition sought a determination that the United States had violated its obligations (those obligations potentially being many in relation to United Nations declarations, covenants, and treaties to which it is signatory) by failing to take action to limit greenhouse gas emissions.

Not unlike people in other parts of the world hard-hit by anthropogenic changes to the earth's upper atmosphere, Inuit find their cultural, physical, and social well-being subject to threats visited upon them by regimes, practices, and lifestyles located elsewhere and not of their making. The impact on Inuit – and other groups that the United Nations High Commission on Human Rights (UNHCHR) describe as living on the 'front line' of climate change – is considerable (Kasperson and Kasperson, 2001). These include people living on the low-lying islands of the Pacific and in sub-Saharan, and especially North Africa. But more than South countries are affected. While it is not certain that hurricane Katrina, devastating the city of New Orleans in August of 2005, can be attributed to climate change, erratic and extreme weather patterns in the past decade – in which the highest average earth surface temperatures in recorded history have been documented – have produced results visiting considerable misery on human populations in Northern as well as Southern countries. These include about 30,000 people who died in 2004 in a European heat wave (Giddens, 2008). Those who perished were not people privileged enough to have air conditioning. Nor were the most affected residents of New Orleans members of the US ruling or middle classes. They were, in fact, mostly poor and black. Climate change is a class – and racial – issue. It is the relation of these people, not only to their labour in environmentally challenging locations, but the nature of their relationship to power and resources, or the lack thereof – be it procuring furs or ivory for wealthy collectors while travelling on rotting sea ice, working in the sweatshop conditions of New Orleans hotels and bars behind levées in which those responsible refuse to invest adequate funds, or sweating it out in a Paris suburb with no means of relief from the sweltering heat – that defines their ties to places and circumstances that enhance their vulnerability.

The effect of climate change on Arctic environments and its human rights implications are well documented (Forbes and Stammier, 2009; Ford, 2009; Trainor, Chapin III, Huntington, Natcher, and Kofinas, 2007). A study in the community of Arctic Bay (Ikpiarjuk) on the northern tip of Baffin Island reveals a wide range of social, personal, and cultural impacts. Lives are more at risk. Traditional knowledge, used to assess weather conditions before venturing out on the land, is increasingly irrelevant in the face of changing conditions. Inuit are more at risk from poor ice conditions. Food security is affected. Access to hunting areas depends on the condition of sea ice and snow and the ability to use boats or snow machines. The use of snow machines has implications for how Inuit relate to their physical environment, posing particular risks in rapidly changing conditions with which operators are not familiar (Tester, 2011; Wenzel, 1991). Inland hunting of caribou is affected, as is access to seals, with implications for the rituals and meaning grounded in a hunting culture (Ford, Smit, and Wandel, 2006).

Articulating climate change as a human rights issue means documenting and articulating these complex relationships. Taken as a web of relationships originating with what is mandated – or not mandated – by government, and visited upon communities by the direct and systemic activities of global corporate interests, the generation of greenhouse gases by industrial activities – such as the production of oil from the Alberta tar sands – can be seen as examples of 'structural violence' (Farmer, 2004; Pellow, 2011). The implications for human health, well-being, and the capacity of people to adapt and protect themselves, are obvious. The concepts of social and environmental justice and human rights are intertwined.

Returning to the case the ICC put before the Inter-American Commission on Human Rights, the IACHR advised the ICC that it could not process its petition, noting that 'the information provided does not enable us to determine whether the alleged facts would tend to characterize a violation of [protected human] rights' (Letter from Ariel Dulitzky, Executive Secretary, IACHR to Paul Crowley, legal representative for Sheila Watt-Cloutier *et al.*, ICC, cited in Knox, 2009a, p. 482). The failure of the IACHR to hear the case points, on the one hand, to limits associated with the use of human rights *as law* in addressing what is arguably the most imponderable crisis human civilization has ever faced. On the other hand, the global attention focused on the petition has given impetus to human rights discourse in relation to climate change, *as a matter of international social concern* taken up by environmental and human rights activists around the globe. As Pellow (2011) illustrates in a case study of attempts by a Danish firm to incinerate pesticides at a cement plant in Mozambique, social organizing, social pressure, international communication, and a working knowledge of human rights and international agreements can be effective *as social power* in the delivery of environmental justice and respect for human rights (see Chapter 1).

Human rights, climate change, and the United Nations

The focus on the United Nations Commission on Human Rights (UNCHR) has served to further emphasize a human rights dimension to the global urgency of addressing climate change. The UNCHR was created by the United Nations Economic and Social Council (ECOSOC) in 1946 and was first chaired by Eleanor Roosevelt, wife of the former US President. Its mandate was to promote and protect human rights and fundamental freedoms. The initial context for its concerns was the holocaust and atrocities committed during the Second World War. In 1946 it created a Sub-Commission on the Promotion and Protection of Human Rights (replaced in 2006 by the Human Rights Council Advisory Committee) with a mandate to make recommendations addressing the prevention of discrimination of any kind relating to human rights and fundamental freedoms and the protection of racial, religious and linguistic minorities (United Nations Documentation, 2011). The Commission on Human Rights set about drafting what became the United Nations Declaration on Human Rights (UNDHR). The mandate of the Commission on Human Rights (UNCHR) has historically been broadly interpreted. In the past 20 years the Commission has increasingly paid attention to environmental issues in relation to Indigenous people, development issues and those related to science, technology, economic, social, and cultural rights. The Sub-Commission created a working group in 1982 that ultimately drafted the *United Nations Declaration on the Rights of Indigenous Peoples*, adopted by the General Assembly, 13 September 2007.

In 2006 the CHR was reconstituted as the Human Rights Council (HRC) with a somewhat different mandate: that of addressing human rights violations and making recommendations to address deficiencies. Of all the institutions, declarations and covenants found within the United

Nations, the HRC appears to have come closest to clearly defining climate change-related impacts as human rights issues. In 2009, in response to growing pressure from indigenous and other international organizations, the UNCHR published, after extensive public consultation, a *Report on the Relationship between Climate Change and Human Rights* (OHCHR, 2009). It concluded that people particularly vulnerable to climate change are those living on the 'front line [and that] vulnerability due to geography is often compounded by a low capacity to adapt, rendering many of the poorest countries and communities particularly vulnerable' (p. 30). The report went further to identify climate change in relation to considerations of gender, age, disability, and 'discrimination and unequal power relations' (p. 30). 'Unequal power relations' is a way of articulating social relations that can draw attention away from the structural and economic origins of these relations, suggesting that they can be addressed by tweaking democratic institutions or by administrative processes and procedures. The result is the de-politicization of social relations and what British playwright and author Jeremy Seabrook (2002) identifies as the impersonal formulation of class relations and differences 'with profound psychological implications for how social injustice is perceived' (p. 47). Social work has often done the same, attending to the measurement and documentation of inequalities with the lightest possible treatment of class and class differences. Reference to 'class' in the index of many social work texts amounts to little more than the word's appearance on a page. Class and class differences, in counter-distinction to discussions of inequality, suggest a population capable of being mobilized to address inequities because they have something in common; a deficit of social, political, and economic power.

The report of the OHCHR (2009) also noted that 'the physical impacts of global warming cannot easily be classified as human rights violations, not least because climate change-related harm often cannot clearly be attributed to acts or omissions of specific States' (p. 30). Proving that an act or omission by a national government is responsible for a climate change-related violation of human rights is a burden not likely to be met, even in the United States where a proclivity for litigation and the *Alien Tort Statute* allows non-Americans to bring claims to American courts against domestic and foreign corporations and government officials. Claims brought before American courts or courts mandated by the United States can be based on the violation of treaties or customary environmental law (Posner, 2007). But the difficulties likely to be encountered are many, as evidenced by the IACHR declining to hear the case brought forward by ICC. These problems have received considerable attention in recent works dealing with climate change as a human rights violation (Abate, 2007; Birnie, Boyle, and Redgwell, 2009; Churchill, 1996; Doelle, 2004; Halvorssen and Hovi, 2006; Knox, 2009a, 2009b; Picolotti and Taillant, 2003; Sinden, 2008; Zarsky, 2002). As noted, an overwhelming number of United Nations texts deal with human rights and the environment, but even in the case of treaties, their force in law is 'soft'. Their value to date has been as tools to be used internationally to bring pressure to bear on governments that claim one thing by signing international covenants and agreements, while practising another. Therefore UN documents have the power of embarrassment, persuasion, and reason.

Climate change and human rights: Challenges for social work

How might social workers and social work as a profession relate to the greatest threat to basic human rights to life, health, food, water, and shelter the world has ever seen? In Canada, the posture of the profession in supporting the kind of actions and commitments needed to address climate change and human rights has been modest in the extreme. As a profession, its interest in defining and protecting its status *within* the confines of state-mandated initiatives and services has often compromised its values and these commitments. This history has been well documented. Jennissen and Lundy (2011) present cases of faculty being dismissed for left-wing and Marxist views, and dissident front line workers losing their jobs over their political and social commitments. National and provincial associations are often guilty of offering them little or no support. The professionalization and codification of social work has given it a vested interest in state-mandated relations of power that recognize (and define) the norms that constitute professional behaviour. Requirements that agencies have on staff, someone with an MSW degree to supervise students who want to challenge the status quo, suggest that social work will remain a *status quo* profession, incapable of breaking into new terrain and working with activist organizations where skills of organizing, communicating, facilitating, and public engagement are required. Global realities require that accreditation standards for schools of social work be revised to reflect the need to address a rapidly changing world of environmental and social problems.

At the same time, since the 1970s some social work educators and scholars have contributed much to a better understanding of the dynamics of the culture, societies, and regimes that give rise to the problems absorbing much of the profession's attention (Corrigan and Leonard, 1978; Fook, 2002; Galper, 1975; Leonard, 1984; Lundy, 2004; London to Edinburgh Weekend Return Group, 1980). Nevertheless, in recent years much of the sharp analysis accompanying structural and social justice approaches to social work has been sidetracked by forms of anti-oppressive practice that subsume a long list of theoretical constructs – many of them contradictory and incompatible – under one roof, notable among them forms of cultural relativism that erect many hurdles for any workable concept of social and environmental justice (Harvey, 1996). Social work is often about 'job training', not to be confused with getting an education. Is social work a form of practice committed to a tradition of political, social, economic (and we must now add, radical environmental) change, or simply the palliative care of society's victims?

Climate change as an issue of human rights cannot be addressed without challenging the logic of the modern state and the corporate malfeasance that lies with it. This imperative emerges from any serious analysis of the root causes of climate change and the role of the state in creating the right conditions for capital accumulation, for which a rejuvenated Marxian analysis of the state and capital accumulation has much to offer. What concepts are useful and what, in this intellectual capital, needs to be reworked and rewritten? Historically, social work has been allied with the socialization of capitalism, but redistributive justice is far easier to achieve if the economic pie is growing. Unfortunately, climate change challenges the sustainability of current forms of economic growth. It invites considerable debate over whether or not there are forms of growth that are benevolent and that can be achieved without contributing further to greenhouse gas emissions. Evidence to date provides us with good reason to be sceptical (Kovel, 2009). Much hope has been pinned on the idea of sustainable development.

Sustainable development is a concept originating with the Brundtland report and popularized in 1987 by the publication of *Our Common Future*, the argument being that addressing environmental problems, including climate change, requires development to lift people out of poverty and provide resources necessary to fixing the problem. While the measurement of global poverty is fraught with logical and statistical problems, what has happened in the past two decades of development and economic growth is increasingly obvious (St Clair, 2006). Globally, the poor have become relatively poorer and the rich considerably richer. If growth (development), contrary to the logic of the Brundtland Commission, does not change poverty rates and if, as the Brundtland Commission argues, poverty is a contributing factor to environmental degradation, including climate change, the implications for the making of social policy are obvious and far-reaching (Fitzpatrick, 1998).

Taking climate change seriously means wading through the tenets, arguments, and 'logic' of what geographer David Harvey (1996) calls 'prevention and ecological modernism', against which Kovel (2009) mounts a sustained critique. Harvey (1996) describes prevention and ecological modernism as:

> a discourse [that] internalizes conflict. It has a radical populist edge, paying serious attention to environmental–ecological issues and most particularly to the accumulation of scientific evidence of environmental impacts on human populations, without challenging the capitalist economic system head on.
>
> (p. 382)

He cites Wolfgang Sachs (1993) who feared that as governments and big business made claims to ecological sensibility, environmentalism would change its face such that it would become 'sanitized of its radical content and reshaped as expert neutral knowledge, until it can be wedded to the dominant world view' (p. xv).

These concerns are not without substance. 'Greenwash' is a term describing the backlash to the success social and environmental movements have had in placing climate change, the concept of environmental justice and human rights, on the international stage. It includes the use of media in attempts to portray global polluters as good corporate citizens. In Canada, this is best illustrated by Alberta's tar sands, where the absence of appropriate environmental monitoring has emerged as an international scandal in the face of corporate media campaigns to portray tar sands operators as environmentally conscious (Nikiforuk, 2010).

Greenwash includes the creation of agencies that have all the appearance of being environmental organizations but that, in fact, are funded by corporations often with the expressed objective of lobbying for voluntary (meaning non-enforceable and non-monitored) compliance with industry-friendly standards and codes (Deal, 1993). It includes the branding and marketing of 'environmentally friendly products', including ethical mutual funds, intended to assuage the ethical consumer, but which make barely a dent – or less – in what corporate appetites are doing to the planet (Greer and Bruno, 1996). Challenging the lifestyle consequences and choices made not only by social workers but the communities with which they work is no easy matter. It requires a knowledge and awareness of issues that are not currently addressed within the curricula of most schools of social work.

Greenwash is one form of backlash to the relative success of environmental movements in making the environment, in countries like Canada, the number one concern of citizens in the late 1980s (Paehlke, 2000). The concept of sustainable development was part of a growing attempt to counter citizen concern. The Rio Conference on Environment and Development (1993) produced 27 principles, the majority of which, consistent with a backlash to the success of Indigenous people, scientists, the environmental and other social justice movements, focused on the *right to development*, tempering this with reference to 'sustainable' development. Few words have, in recent years, been more abused in the English language and what is often touted as 'sustainable' can, upon careful examination, be anything but (Luke, 2005). The neoliberal undertones of the Declaration are best captured by principle 16:

> National authorities should endeavour to promote the internalization of environmental costs and the use of economic instruments, taking into account the approach that the polluter should, in principle, bear

the cost of pollutions, with due regard to the public interest and without distorting international trade and investment.

(United Nations Educational, Scientific and
Cultural Organization, 1992: 4)

While heavy on a right to development, the Rio Summit did give impetus to creation of the United Nations Framework Convention on Climate Change (UNFCCC). The commitment in the convention to addressing climate change was strongly worded, calling for the stabilization of greenhouse-gas concentrations at a level that would prevent dangerous anthropogenic interference with the climate system. It called for this being done within a time framework that would allow ecosystems to adapt naturally (Parson, Haas, and Levy, 1992). The treaty led to the Kyoto Agreement of 1997. The United States, under the administration of George W. Bush, withdrew from the agreement in 2001. Levels of emissions set for participating countries under the Kyoto Agreement had been breached in all but a few cases. A subsequent 2009 attempt in Copenhagen to negotiate terms and conditions for a new climate protocol after Kyoto finishes in 2012 ended in failure. Faced with the reality that it was in serious breach of its commitments under Kyoto and major implications for future development of the Alberta Tar Sands, Canada withdrew from the Agreement in 2011 following the COP 17 (Convention of the Parties) on the United Nations Framework Convention on Climate Change meetings held in Durban, South Africa. These events suggest that an international class of business elites and lobbyists and institutions serving their interests – particularly those of the international oil and gas industry – currently dominate international discussions about how best to deal with global environmental problems, climate change paramount among them.

International human rights have been a focus of social work education and practice since the formation of the International Association of Schools of Social Work (IASSW) in 1928. The profession's commitment and interest in international human rights is centred on the work of the Association and the International Federation of Social Workers (IFSW). In 1994, the UNCHR produced, in cooperation with the IASSW and the IFSW, a manual for social workers addressing the role of human rights in social work practice. The manual made the following observation: 'Environment and development is a new field for social work which is being explored. Social workers active at the grass-roots level will have an important opportunity for awareness raising, advocacy and influence on lifestyles' (UNCHR, 1994: 34).

Social work is, therefore, a late-comer to the concept of environmental justice and human rights (see Chapter 1 in this volume). Until well into the 1980s, natural and physical environments were treated primarily as social environments within the confines of systems analysis (Tester, 1994). Commencing in the late 1960s and early 1970s, across Europe and North America, the relevance of natural, built and social environments to human well-being was articulated in newly founded programs of environmental science and environmental studies. Debates over concepts like Deep Ecology, ecofeminism, and humanism and environmental management were thick and heavy, generating an incredible volume of informative and controversial literature. Social work often appears to have discovered the importance of natural and built environments without fully appreciating the extent to which environmental philosophies have been debated in the fields of environmental studies and human geography. For example, some social workers look to Deep Ecology and an aesthetic redefinition of human–nature relations to address what humans are doing to natural environments (Besthorn and Canda, 2002; Coates, 2003, 2004). But without critical attention to aesthetic solutions in practice, social work runs the risk of contributing to the violation of human rights and the undermining of environmental justice. The pitfalls of Deep Ecology and considerations of nature as 'intrinsic value' – articulated by Norwegian eco-philosopher Arne Naess (Besthorn, 2011) – the non-instrumental appreciation of nature, cultural relativism, and the humanization of nature, have all been thoroughly worked over in the field of environmental studies (Hicks and Shannon, 2007; Tester, 1983). Deep Ecology, for example, has given rise to a Eurocentric misinterpretation of the relationship between Aboriginal people and nature that has visited on them considerable cruelty and hardship. For example, the European ban on the importation of seal pelts had a devastating impact on the economic as well as the cultural and spiritual well-being of Canadian Inuit (Pelly, 2001; Wenzel, 1991).

Conclusion

Why is climate change a class issue? Climate change has impacts that are greater on some populations because of their geographical location and poverty. Poverty inevitably results in populations depending heavily on local environments for subsistence, be it hunting – as in the case of Inuit – fishing, or agriculture. Poverty is increasingly globalized, with income disparities growing in North countries. As the case of New Orleans suggests, climate change may have impacts similar to those seen in South countries, on poor and disenfranchised populations in Europe and North America.

Climate change is the result of industrial processes that are controlled and owned internationally primarily by ruling elites. Having contributed most of the atmospheric carbon to planetary totals during their own decades of industrial development, the corporations of Europe and North America have now exported most of their dirty industrial activities to South countries. North Americans and Europeans continue to benefit from the imported products, carbon emissions now being blamed in large measure on the rapidly developing economies of countries like Indonesia, India, Brazil, South Korea and, of course, China. In many South countries, people and their governments have the least organizational and financial capacity to deal with the effects of climate change (Anguelovski and Roberts, 2011).

In Western countries, especially since the Second World War, class analysis has been complicated by the manner in which working people are implicated in the economic and social arrangements of a system from which they derive considerable benefit. The salaries, pensions, and other benefits of those employed in a modern capitalist economy are inextricably tied to the status quo. The rhetoric of prevention and ecological modernism has understandable appeal. We want to keep what we have, but do what we do 'smarter and better'. The refusal of the United States, the largest per capita emitter of greenhouse gases in the world and the country that is home to the vast majority of the world's global corporations, to participate actively in the Kyoto Agreement and to work to strengthen and expand its provisions, speaks loudly to what is at stake. In a globalized economy, class relations have been exported. They have not gone away. The world's poor are working in sweatshops and factories in the South, making what keeps the global economy functioning; more things for economies – notable among them that of the United States – centred on consumer spending and consumption. In North America and Europe, those who can afford to do so shop at organic food stores. Some have air conditioners and swimming pools. Others advocate for locally grown food. The poor shop at Wal-Mart, sourcing its goods from all over the world, anywhere labour is cheap, environmental standards are minimal, and costs as low as possible. That those who are poor in North countries, of necessity, contribute much to the environmental poverty of others is a tragic issue of social and economic justice, and human rights. Globalization has played a critical role in climate change as a human rights issue.

If climate change is a product of *how society organizes production, consumption, and disposal*, and not merely mistakes made *within* capitalist relations of production, then a serious re-think of the current social and economic systems governing our lives is in order. Economics is ideology masking as science. Its precepts and assumptions – and especially its goals and objectives – are ideological. There are ways of doing things that defy so-called economic logic. Such an exercise puts those who value family, community, social relations, creativity and quality of life – who take human rights seriously – against those whose interest is growth, development, and the terrible imperative of more, more, more. While Canadians, including social workers, want to believe in a culture and society where what people have in common is more important than their differences, climate change may seriously challenge this ideal, ultimately revealing just how different the interests of those currently directing our economic – and hence our social and political – affairs really are.

All over the world, class relations explain peasant movements, workers' struggles, and urban social movements fighting poverty, exclusion and environmental degradation. What they are fighting is the power of ownership and privilege. Harvey (1996) puts it this way:

> Issues like AIDS, global warming, local environmental degradation, the destructions of local cultural traditions, are inherently class issues and it needs to be shown how building a community in anti-capitalist class struggle can better alleviate the conditions of oppression across a broad spectrum of social action.

This, he notes, is not a 'plea for eclecticism and pluralism, but a plea to uncover the raw class content of a wide array of anti-capitalist concern' (pp. 431–432).

Social workers need to be educated with a new and invigorated set of analytical tools. Social workers need to organize around the environment and human rights in neighbourhood houses and community centres as well as in international forums. They need to present new realities and concerns in the classroom, on the street, in the theatre, in words, song and film, working *with* disaffected youth and adults at home and abroad. Climate change, as an issue of human rights, challenges theory, method, and practice unlike any issue social work has ever seen.

References

Abate, R.S. (2007). Climate change, the United States, and the impacts of Arctic melting: A case study in the need for enforceable international environmental human rights. *Stanford Environmental Law Journal, 26*, 4–76.

Anguelovski, I., and Roberts, D. (2011). Spatial justice and climate change: Multiscale impacts and local development in Durban, South Africa. In J. Carmin and Agyeman, J. (Eds). *Environmental inequalities beyond borders: Local perspectives on global injustices.* Cambridge, MA: MIT Press. 19–43.

Baines, D. (Ed.). (2007). *Doing anti-oppressive practice: Building transformative politicized social work.* Halifax,NS: Fernwood Publishing.

Besthorn, F. (2011). Deep Ecology's contributions to social work: A ten-year retrospective. *International Journal of Social Welfare,* Special Issue on Environmental Social Work. Article first published online: 9 DEC 2011. DOI: 10.1111/j.1468-2397.2011.00850.x.

Besthorn, F., and Canda, E. (2002). Revisioning environment: Deep ecology for education and teaching in social work. *Journal of Teaching in Social Work, 22*(1/2), 79–102.

Birnie, P., Boyle, A., and Redgwell, C. (2009). *International law and the environment* (3rd ed.). Oxford: Oxford University Press.

Brundtland, G.H. (1987). *Our Common Future: Report of the World Commission on Environment and Development.* New York: Oxford University Press.

Chivers, D. (2010). *The no-nonsense guide to climate change: The science, the solutions, the way forward.* Oxford: New Internationalist Publications.

Churchill, R. (1996). Environmental rights in existing human rights treaties. In M.R. Anderson and Boyle, A.E. (Eds). *Human rights approaches to environmental protection*. Oxford: Oxford University Press. 89–104.

Coates, J. (2003). *Ecology and social work: Toward a new paradigm*. Halifax, NS: Fernwood Publishing.

Coates, J. (2004). From ecology to spirituality and social justice. *Currents: New Scholarship in the Human Services*. Retrieved July 17, 2011 from http://wcmprod2. ucalgary.ca/currents/volumes#volume3_n2.

Corporate Europe Observer. (2001). *Rio+10 and the Corporate Greenwash of Globalisation*, Issue 9, June. Retrieved August 7, 2011 from http://archive. corporateeurope.org/observer9/greenwash.html.

Corrigan, P., and Leonard, P. (1978). *Social work practice under capitalism: A Marxist approach*. London: Macmillan.

Council of Europe. (1950). *European Convention on Human Rights*. Retrieved on January 9, 2012 from http://www.hri.org/docs/ECHR50.html#Convention.

Council of Europe. (1961). *European Social Charter*. Retrieved on January 9, 2012 from www.coe.int/socialcharter.

Deal, C. (1993). *The Greenpeace Guide to Anti-Environmental Organizations*. Berkeley, CA: Odonian Press.

Doelle, M. (2004). Climate change and human rights: The role of international human rights in motivating states to take climate change seriously. *Macquarie Journal of International & Comparative Environmental Law, 1*, 179–216.

Earle, S. (2011). *Little Emperor*. Detroit, MI: New West Records.

Farmer, P. (2004). An anthropology of structural violence. *Current Anthropology, 45*(3), 305–325.

Fitzpatrick, T. (1998). The implications of ecological thought for social welfare. *Critical Social Policy, 18*(1), 5–26.

Fook, J. (2002). *Social work: Critical theory and practice*. London: Sage.

Forbes, B., and Stammier, F. (2009). Arctic climate change discourse: The contrasting politics of research agendas in the West and Russia. *Polar Record, 28*, 28–42.

Ford, J. (2009). Dangerous climate change and the importance of adaptation for the Arctic's Inuit population. *Environmental Research Letters, 4*, 1–9.

Ford, J., Smit, B., and Wandel, J. (2006). Vulnerability to climate change in the Arctic: A case study from Arctic Bay, Canada. *Global Environmental Change, 16*, 145–160.

Galper, J. (1975). *The politics of social services*. Englewood Cliffs, NJ: Prentice-Hall.

Giddens, A. (2008). *The politics of climate change: National responses to the challenge of global warming*. A National Policy Network Paper. Retrieved August 4, 2011 from http://www.fcampalans.cat/images/noticias/The_politics_of_climate_change_ Anthony_Giddens%282%29.pdf.

Godrej, D. (2001). *The no-nonsense guide to climate change*. Toronto, ON: New Internationalist Publications and Between the Lines.

Greer, J., and Bruno, K., (1996). *Greenwash: The reality behind corporate environmentalism*. Penang, Malaysia: The Third World Network.

Halvorssen, A., and Hovi, J. (2006). The nature, origin and impact of legally binding consequences: The case of the climate regime. *International Environmental Agreements: Politics, Law and Economics, 6*(2), 157–171.

Harvey, D. (1996). *Justice, nature and the geography of difference*. Oxford: Blackwell.

Hicks, S., and Shannon, D. (2007). *The challenges of globalization: Rethinking nature, culture, freedom.* Oxford: Blackwell.

Ife, J. (2002). *Community development: Community-based alternatives in an age of globalization* (2nd ed.). Sydney: Pearson Education Australia.

Ife, J. (2008). *Human rights and social work: Towards rights-based practice* (2nd ed.). Cambridge: Cambridge University Press.

Inter-American Commission on Human Rights. (1948). *American Declaration of the Rights and Duties of Man.* Retrieved on January 9, 2012 from http://www.cidh.oas.org/Basicos/English/Basic2.American%20Declaration.htm.

Inter-American Commission on Human Rights. (1969). *American Convention on Human Rights.* Retrieved on January 9, 2012 from http://www.cidh.oas.org/basicos/english/Basic1.%20Intro.htm.

Jennissen, T., and Lundy, C. (2011). *One hundred years of social work: A history of the profession in English Canada.* Waterloo, Canada: Wilfred Laurier University Press.

Johnston, B.R. (Ed.). (2011). *Life and death matters: Human rights, environment, and social justice* (2nd ed.). Walnut Creek, CA: Left Coast Press.

Kasperson, R.E., and Kasperson, J. (2001). *Climate change, vulnerability and social justice.* Stockholm: Stockholm Environment Institute.

Knox, J.H. (2009a). Linking human rights and climate change at the United Nations. *Harvard Environmental Law Review, 33,* 477–498.

Knox, J.H. (2009b). Climate change and human rights law. *Virginia Journal of International Law, 50,* 164–218.

Kovel, J. (2009). The justifiers: A critique of Julian Simon, Stephan Schmidheiny, and Paul Hawken on capitalism and nature. *Capitalism Nature Socialism, 10*(3), 3–36.

Leonard, P. (1984). *Personality and ideology: Towards a materialist theory of the individual.* London: Macmillan.

London to Edinburgh Weekend Return Group. (1980). *In and against the state.* London: Pluto.

Luke, T. (2005). Neither sustainable nor development: Reconsidering sustainability in development. *Sustainable Development, 13*(4), 228–238.

Lundy, C. (2004). *Social work and social justice: A structural approach to practice.* Peterborough, Ontario: Broadview Press.

Mann, J.M., Gruskin, S., Grodin, M.A., and Annas, G.J. (1999). *Health and human rights.* London: Routledge.

Mapp, S. (2008). *Human rights and social justice in a global perspective: An introduction to international social work.* New York: Oxford University Press.

Nikiforuk, A. (2010). *Tar Sands: Dirty oil and the future of a continent.* Vancouver: Greystone Books.

Paehlke, R. (2000). Environmentalism in one country: Canadian environmental policy in an era of globalization. *Policy Studies Journal, 28*(1), 160–175.

Parson, E.A., Haas, P.M., and Levy, M.A. (1992). A summary of major documents signed at the earth summit and the global forum. *Environment, 34*(4), 12–15, 34–36.

Pellow, D.N. (2011). Politics by other Greens: The importance of transnational environmental justice movement networks. In J. Carmin and Agyeman, J. (Eds). *Environmental inequalities beyond borders.* Cambridge, MA: MIT Press. 247–265.

Pelly, D. (2001). *Sacred hunt: A portrait of the relationship between seals and Inuit.* Toronto, ON: Douglas and McIntyre.

Picolotti, R., and Taillant, J.D. (Eds). (2003). *Linking human rights and the environment.* Tucson, AZ: University of Arizona Press.

Posner, S.F. (2007). *Estate and gift tax handbook.* The Netherlands: Wolters Kluwer.

Sachs, W. (Ed.). (1993). *Global ecology: A new arena of political conflict.* London: Zed Books.

Seabrook, J. (1993). *Victims of development: Resistance and Alternatives.* London: Verso.

Seabrook, J. (2002). *Class, caste and hierarchies.* Oxford: New Internationalist Publications.

Sinden, A. (2008). Climate change and human rights. *Journal of Land Resources and Environmental Law, 27*(2), 255–271.

St Clair, A. (2006). Global poverty: The co-production of knowledge and politics. *Global Social Policy, 6*(1), 57–77.

Tester, F. (1983). *No weka, whale or kauri: Environmentalism, praxis and the human image.* Ocean Monograph No. 9, for the Waikato Workers Educational Association. Hamilton, New Zealand: Outrigger Publishers.

Tester, F. (1994). In an age of ecology: Limits to voluntarism and traditional theory in social work practice. In M. Hoff and McNutt, J. (Eds). *The global environmental crisis: Implications for social welfare and social work.* Aldershot, Hants: Avebury. 75–99.

Tester, F. (2011). Mad dogs and (mostly) Englishmen: Colonial relations, commodities, and the fate of Inuit sled dogs. *Études/Inuit Studies, 34*(2), 129–147.

Trainor, S.F., Chapin III, F.S., Huntington, H.P., Natcher, D.C., and Kofinas, G. (2007). Arctic climate impacts: Environmental injustice in Canada and the United States. *Local Environment, 12*(6), 627–643.

United Nations. (1948). *Universal Declaration of Human Rights.* Retrieved January, 2012 from http://www.un.org/en/documents/udhr/.

United Nations. (1966). *International Covenant on Economic, Social and Cultural Rights.* Retrieved on January 9, 2012 from http://www.un.org/millennium/law/iv-3.htm.

United Nations Centre for Human Rights. (1994). *Human rights and social work: A manual for schools of social work and the social work profession.* Professional Training Series No. 1. Geneva: UN.

United Nations Documentation: Research Guide. (2011). Dag Hammarskjöld Library. Retrieved October 6, 2011 from http://www.un.org/Depts/dhl/resguide/index.html.

United Nations Educational, Scientific and Cultural Organization (UNESCO). (1992). *Rio Declaration on Environment and Development.* Retrieved January 4, 2012 from http://www.unesco.org/education/information/nfsunesco/pdf/RIO_E.PDF.

United Nations General Assembly. (2008). *United Nations Declaration on the Rights of Indigenous Peoples.* New York: United Nations.

United Nations Human Rights Council. (2009). *Report of the Office of the United Nations High Commissioner for Human Rights on the relationship between climate change and human rights,* 15 January 2009, A/HRC/10/61. Retrieved on January 9, 2012 from http://www.unhcr.org/refworld/docid/498811532.html.

United Nations Office of the High Commissioner for Human Rights. (1966). *International Covenant on Civil and Political Rights.* Retrieved January 9, 2012 from http://www2.ohchr.org/english/law/ccpr.htm.

United Nations Office of the High Commissioner for Human Rights. (1989). *Convention on the Rights of the Child.* Retrieved on January 9, 2012 from http://www2.ohchr.org/english/law/crc.htm.

United Nations, Office of the High Commissioner for Human Rights. (2009). *OHCHR study on the relationship between climate change and human rights: Submissions and reference documents received.* Retrieved July 23, 2011 from http://www2.ohchr.org/english/issues/climatechange/submissions.htm.

United Nations, Office of the High Commissioner for Human Rights. (2011). *What are human rights?* Retrieved October 7, 2011 from http://www.ohchr.org/EN/Issues/Pages/WhatareHumanRights.aspx.

Wenzel, G. (1991). *Animal rights, human rights: Ecology, economy and ideology in the Canadian Arctic.* Toronto, ON: University of Toronto Press.

Zarsky, L. (Ed.). (2002). *Human rights and the environment.* London: Earthscan.

Part 2

Practice

Case studies of environmental social work practice

6 Community gardens, creative community organizing, and environmental activism

Benjamin Shepard

Community gardening is a way to fight the systemic injustice of poverty and other forms of structural oppression. Most gardens are in poor areas of the city, with much higher rates of asthma and lower rates of open space equity. Gardens offer a way for our community to heal itself and to recover a humanizing sense of itself in an otherwise very hard city.

(Friends of Brook Park, Gardener Ray Figueroa)

In recent years, a small core of social workers has highlighted the importance of attending to issues of social justice and sustainability in their work (Coates, 2003; Mary, 2008; Van Wormer and Besthorn, 2011). To do so, they have been forced to grapple with notions of social responsibility and environmental justice (Streeter and Gonsalvez, 1994); recognize the urban environment as a space for engagement and study (Park, Burgess, and McKenzie, 1925); and engage in practices to protect the environment through community organizing aimed at creating and preserving 'green space' (Carlsson, 2008; Dawson, Charley, and Harrison, 1997; Shepard, 2011). Community organizers recognize local neighbourhoods and their public spaces, including green spaces, as spaces for social engagement, community building, healing, personal growth, service learning, and social justice-based activism (Sherman *et al.*, 2005; Stocker and Barnett, 1998; Streeter and Gonsalvez, 1994). In New York City, much of this activism takes place within the context of community gardens (Carlsson, 2008; Shepard, 2011; Wilson and Weinberg, 1999).

This chapter considers the example of an innovative approach to creating and preserving green space by tracing the history of a successful campaign to save urban gardens in New York City. Through community gardening, citizens connect with community-supported agriculture, urban planning, and nutrition programs, and participate in the process of community regeneration by planning, planting, weeding, and harvesting in spaces once filled with garbage and rubble. Through a close engagement between the environment, social justice, and green space, gardeners tap into a space for difference, health, and creativity (Carlsson, 2008). In so doing, they build social capacity and bridge fields of micro, mezzo, and macro practice, while reimagining possibilities for creative community organizing.

Located mostly in low-income neighbourhoods, where high asthma levels and dense housing prevail, it is useful to consider the garden movement in relation to the politics of public space, uneven development, and neoliberalism (Carlsson, 2008; Schaper, 2007; Shepard, 2011). Community gardeners have brought safety, food, beauty, fresh air, and a 'sense of community' back to their streets and people. Given their orientation to civic – social – rather than commercial – economic – purposes, these public spaces have faced myriad threats from corporate globalizers, real estate agencies, and social pressures against unregulated open public space. Much of the garden struggle is a fight to preserve public space for those at the margins to find solace in post welfare neoliberal cities. Through creative community organizing, groups such as the Lower East Side Collective, More Gardens, and Times Up in New York, and more recently Harvest Gardens in Fredericton, Canada, have built a diverse coalition to defend community gardens. Their efforts represent a best practice in organizing against urban gentrification; it is an example of principles and techniques of community action. This qualitative case study builds on my voice as a reflective practitioner, observing participant and researcher to highlight the story of one campaign (Schön, 1987; Sherman and Reid, 1994).

In *Approaches to Community Intervention*, Rothman (1995) suggests that purposeful community change work can be divided into three distinct categories of practice: locality development, social planning, and social action. The term refers to direct action-based community practice. Social action has long been recognized as a vital, potentially transformative aspect of social work practice (Gray, Collett van Rooyen, Rennie, and Gaha, 2002; Mullaly, 1993). Much of this approach is witnessed in the case study of the community gardens in New York. Throughout the story of the gardens, activists, including this writer, rely upon any number of disciplines. Social action works well in combination with multiple methods of an organizing campaign, from ask, to research, mobilization, direct action, legal strategies, to media coordination and fun. Practising with an eclectic diversity of tactics, community action principles come to life and invigorate practice. This case study offers images of how neighbourhood residents can stake a claim, defend it, and create healthy communities. From this experience, the article seeks to garner a set of action principles for social workers to engage in environmental initiatives.

Urban space, sustainability, and social justice

New York City faces a range of challenges, including a lack of open green space, space for play, or opportunities for people to experience the natural environment. Conversely, asthma and obesity rates are increasing. In response, citizens created a network of community gardens, built out of the rubble of vacant lots, abandoned during New York's fiscal crisis of the 1970s (Lamborn Wilson and Weinberg, 1999). The benefits of community gardens are many:

> Community gardening is a way to fight the systemic injustice of poverty and other forms of structural oppression. Most gardens are in poor areas of the city, with much higher rates of asthma and lower rates of open space equity. Gardens offer a way for our community to heal itself and to recover a humanizing sense of itself in an otherwise very hard city.
>
> (Friends of Brook Park gardener Ray Figueroa,
> in Times Up!, 2010)

As well as providing much needed green space, community gardens function as park and play spaces: 'Successful parks are markers of healthy communities: children play; families spend time together; people of all ages exercise and relax; and the environment adds to the beauty, security, and economic value of the neighborhood' (Raya and Rubin, 2006: 1). Over the years, community gardens have come to serve as a practical solution to the challenge of open space inequity, including lack of access to parks and play spaces in low-income communities. In this way, they cultivate healthy communities.

In order to support these spaces, the New York City Department of Parks and Recreation has made use of community development block grants to fund 'Green Thumb', a municipal garden program that leases land to community groups to help them create gardens by providing workshops and supplies. However, with federal support for community block grants facing a range of challenges, the gardens are in precarious position (Kattalia, 2011). Many have come to see threats to gardens as a direct threat to spaces for healthy expression, such as play. Those who work with children and communities have long recognized that active play supports healthy communities (Shepard, 2011). Still, across the country, children have fewer opportunities for play, as recess time is challenged by calls for more time dedicated to study for standardized tests. Research on play highlights the implications of this turn, including increased obesity, with 69 per cent of parents in low-income communities suggesting there is no place to play in walking distance of their houses (Raya and Rubin, 2006). Free play supports childhood creativity, problem solving, executive function, resiliency, innovation, and space to exercise the body and mind (Shepard, 2011) and gardens are places where this expression thrives.

When the city of New York proposed easing protections on community gardens in 2010, community members spoke out: 'Don't destroy our gardens. Don't destroy our communities. Gardens help us connect with both the earth and our communities, in ways which parking lots, coffee shops, and other urban spaces fail to', declared long-time Lower East Side activist Paul Bartlett (in Times Up!, 2010). In making this point, Bartlett, a veteran of the Lower East Side Collective (LESC), harkened back to a history of community gardening and activism dating back to the 1990s in New York City when the Mayor announced plans to sell off over 400 community gardens. In response, community members cried foul, using every tool at their disposal to launch a multi-pronged sustained campaign to preserve the community gardens. Garden supporter Donna Schaper (2007) explained how growing gardens works in tandem with growing social change: '[G]ardening helps people with dynamite in their pants to change the world: it sustains us as we prod the world along' (p. xiv).

Change strategies

Service learning

Community gardens are ideal spaces to educate students about the environment, environmental research, planting, sustainable agriculture, and urban farming, as well as positive forms of community development and democratic renewal. They offer spaces for students to participate in organizing campaigns, service learning, education, and support for greener more sustainable urban spaces. Through participation in these spaces, social workers build on the lessons of service learning and the Settlement House Movement. The practice is rooted in the work of philosophers, John Dewey and William James, as well as Hull House founder Jane Addams: 'Hull House integrated service provision with community organizing. It became both a place for neighborhood political activity and a laboratory for applying social research to social problems', note Dolgon and Baker (2010: 10). Community gardens function in much the same way as Settlement Houses.

I bring a group of students to a garden every semester, and they love seeing these unique spaces. My kids love the gardens as a much needed space to play and explore outside of the asphalt of the concrete jungle of New York City. Community projects in gardens engage students through allowing them to connect with distinct communities, through planting and mapping. Through such projects, students connect campus with community, education with environment.

Social action

People came to New York from all over the world to become involved with the struggle. Through social action, those involved engaged in a range of tactics from civil disobedience to protest, to change institutions and alter the distributions of power in an effort to save these green spaces (Rothman, 1995). Much of the battle for public space alternated with the struggle over old-growth forests on the West Coast with Earth First. In a 2004 interview, activist L.A. Kauffman noted:

[Many] shuttled back and forth between the New York City community garden fight and old-growth forest blockades in remote Oregon ... The New York City community garden fight was one of the first times that Earth First!-style blockading techniques were used in an urban context ... And they worked really well here, putting the gardens issue onto the agenda.

(Kauffman, 2004: 377)

Gradually, a local issue connected with a global movement to reclaim public space for the people (Shepard, 2011). One of those activists drawn into the garden struggle was Tim Doody. Having dropped out of college, he was concerned about what was going on in his community outside of Pittsburgh, Pennsylvania: 'I started hearing people talking about the Allegany National Forest, which is in Northwestern Pennsylvania. And talking about it being clear cut'. As a result the entire composition of the forest was changing. Doody recognized the process threatened much of the biodiversity of the forest and was also aware the same process was taking shape throughout the ever-expanding urban sprawl of the United States, with corporate chains replacing mom and pop stores: 'We just get Walmart, Barnes and Noble, Starbucks – the thing that makes the most money. And everything else has to go.' Worried about what he was seeing, Doody started developing stills as an activist:

I went back and volunteered at Ruckus Camp (where activists are trained in direct action). Rainforest Relief was there ... 1999, I think. And some of the Ruckus climbers recommended this action. The benches there are made of rainforest wood from the Amazon as are most of the benches in Manhattan. We were going to repel down with a banner and crash Giuliani's opening of City Hall Park. And I thought, I'll do it, let's go.

Once in town, Doody heard the community gardens were under threat, in the same ways as the old-growth forests he had seen outside Pittsburgh. Yet, activists were fighting back and they were using many of the tools he had learned at Ruckus. Tools involved within the garden movement included a clear campaign, research, mobilization, direct action, fundraising, legal and sustainability strategies, and play to make the campaign fun and creative.

Groups involved included in community organizing, such as the Lower East Side Collective, Times Up, and the More Gardens Coalition noted: 'One of the most important steps toward defending your community garden is to have the support of your community ... After all, community gardens should be open to our communities!' (More Gardens! Coalition, 2002: 3). They gained the support of their communities through 'social' organizing: holding pleasurable events, such as parties, celebrations, and meetings, making them convivial public spaces. At their essence, gardens are social spaces. I first became involved with the movement as a member of the Lower East Side Collective. I was working in the South Bronx, where community members had looked to community gardening as a means for community revitalization in the years of Bronx burning in the 1970s. 'Improve don't move' was the slogan. Creating gardens was a vital part of the process of rebuilding the community. The same process took place in the Lower East Side. The organizing was very social. I recall running into members of the Lower East Side Collective after an early meeting in the streets of the Lower East Side and getting a hug from one of the organizers I had just met. That was when I knew LESC was a kind space for friendships as well as organizing. Many in the group appreciated the conviviality, the support system the group offered. It was all part of 'social' organizing. Through social organizing, LESC helped tap into the social capital of those in the Lower East Side: its people, their diverse experiences, and talents.

Throughout this period (from 1997 to 2000), key activists worked with members of LESC to develop strategies to preserve gardens as a dynamic component of public space and key community centres at a time when housing was being prioritized over environment and gardens. They effectively connected housing and gardens, arguing community gardens were both public spaces and smart alternatives to previous models of urban renewal. LESC and the other garden defenders, such as Ruckus, used a range of approaches, including street theatrics, media, and direct action, where people played an active role in advancing negotiations. Adrienne Maree Brown (2009) from Ruckus noted:

> At its best, direct action is where we advance the frontline of our movement work by visualising the change we seek. Direct action is how we first saw images of blacks and whites at lunch counters together in the south. Today, guerilla gardens are one example of a way to show that we know how to live more sustainably and we will push our leaders to catch up with us. It's about framing the issue in a way that inspires people to act, not just react. I think the key need of our movements today is visionary voices and actors who are living a viable future and making it accessible to our communities.

Direct action

As the garden movement escalated, garden activists made masterful use of direct action in their community organizing, including nonviolent civil disobedience involving actions such as lying down in or chaining oneself to spaces about to be bulldozed, refusing to disperse, or sitting in a tree in the space. They make a strong statement because they show that people are willing to use their bodies to stand up for what they believe in (More Gardens! 2002). These disruptive tactics are most useful when they include community outreach, media coverage, legal battles, and letter-writing campaigns. Direct action is a vital part of the practice of social action. Political participation and social action take multiple forms (Domanski, 1998). In this campaign, social action worked in coordination with multiple methods of practice, including a clear ask, research on the issue, mobilization, direct action, and legal and sustainability strategies. These strategies worked well in tandem and demonstrated the interplay of methods within a holistic organizing campaign.

One of the early examples of creative direct action in the movement to save the community gardens took place in July of 1998 when members of the Lower East Side Collective Public Space Group heard the city had plans to sell off a number of lots where gardens grew, as well as a community centre in the Lower East Side, Charas El Bohio. On July 20, 1998, twelve activists entered a public auction with envelopes full of crickets to disrupt proceedings in the hope they might prevent the sale of Charas and other community gardens (Shepard, 2011). Eventually Charas was sold, but LESC got their hands on one of the bidding forms and found out who had bought the property. The following day Charas supporters put up signs asking: 'Who sold Charas?' The newspapers were sympathetic to the case, supporting the neighbourhood argument that gardens support rather than hinder the neighbourhood (Shepard, 2011). Nevertheless, despite the protests, the city announced plans to sell off another hundred gardens the following spring.

After the announcement, plans were underway to delay and disrupt the scheduled auction of 119 garden sites. Interventions included demonstrations, protests, blocking streets with the consequent arrests of older women, grabbing media headlines, and using trusts and benefactors to purchase the land. Throughout this campaign, direct action and legal strategies worked effectively in tandem: 'I started calling the Attorney General's office', explained Howard. 'I had Foster Mayer from the Puerto Rican Legal Defense Fund, who had been on the CHARAS lawsuit.' It was the same case argument as had been used with Charas. This was public space: 'We sent in evidence, maps etc. They said they did not know. Yet, it was very compelling.' The plan was to get a temporary restraining order (TRO) on bulldozing gardens until legal arguments were resolved.

In the meantime, the city started moving in on a small garden on East Seventh Street called Esperanza, where members of More Gardens, LESC, and Times Up were holding a 24-hour vigil and bulldozer alert. This was in the winter of 2000. Throughout the campaign, direct action combined with a joyous approach played out through tactics including a 'sing out' to disrupt a public hearing, as well as an ecstatic theatrical model of organizing, which compelled many actors to participate in the story themselves. Thus groups made use of a range of crafty approaches that audiences found playful. This theatrical mode of civil disobedience lulled and disarmed audiences with stories that seduced rather than hammered, and shifted the terms of the debate.

The week after Howard's contact with the Attorney General's office, a phone tree from the garden put out the message that no parking signs were being put up all over East 7th Street: 'That means something in this long struggle', noted Howard, a veteran of the Lower East Side squatting and gardening scene. 'We assumed they were going for Esperanza. We started begging the cops not to participate, to back off. There is going to be a TRO from the Attorney General's office.' Police were surrounding the garden.

By this time, Tim Doody had made his way over to the garden, where he met those from LESC, More Gardens and anarchists from the neighborhood, including this writer, as police surrounded the space: 'The first street I've ever been to was the More Gardens! Blockade that we did together,' recalled Doody. 'All through that process, there was such a whimsical amazing element that combined the residents of the long time Puerto Rican homestead, who were caretakers of the Esperanza Community Garden.' Punk youth and grandmothers, kids and other neighbourhood characters got involved: 'People gravitated around the huge Coqui'. In a Puerto Rican legend, this tiny frog 'would let out a shrill cry rumored to scare the invaders away', noted Doody:

> In a very real sense, here was this huge massive frog, activists prepared to lock down, keeping up a vigil right there trying to scare away the developers. At the same time, it was a huge mystical thing looming over the gate, adding an element of play and spirituality into the struggle. It served as a galvanizing point, to get tons of media. And that had everything to do with creativity. If we just sat there, it wouldn't be the same. But instead there were picnics and parties and all night vigils.

The direct action strategy overlapped with media, policy, legal, and research strategies. The art of the campaign helped draw supporters and media. The research supported the claim that gardens should be preserved. Direct action helped draw media attention to the issue and legal action helped fortify short-term gains won from the media influence on public opinion, direct action, and mobilizing.

With Doody and company inside the garden holding the blockade, Howard leaped in a cab to go to the Attorney General's office. At the Attorney General's office Howard declared, 'There is a firestorm in the Lower East Side. They are going to bulldoze Esperanza Community Garden.' The receptionist was unable to help. Just then, the elevator opened and out came the lead attorney, Chris Amato. Howard tells him there are thirty people inside Esperanza holding off the police and bulldozers. He says 'follow me and tells some of the other lawyers what was going on'. The Attorney General's corporate counsel called the city and says: 'We hear you are going to bulldoze a community garden in the Lower East Side. Hold off until we hear from a judge.' A representative from the city retorted: 'we're going to go ahead unless we are delivered a stop work order'. By this time, the Attorney General's office was totally committed: 'They went out to find a judge to put on a TRO'.

While the Attorney General's office was out trying to find a judge, those inside the community garden on East 7th dug in. Activists locked themselves down in any way they could. It was the day after Valentine's, February 15, 2000. Garden defenders had been there all night: 'That's one of my favorite actions of all time', recalled Tim Doody: 'It was like a painting ... Everybody was in the garden playing drums, getting into their lock down positions and singing and chanting. And you just saw these hundreds of cops and like snipers on the roof tops.' Those inside the garden felt they were building the world they wanted to live in within the blockade, the garden and joy of resistance. The police said we were trespassing in an area that they had built a community around the day before. The city eventually did come in and bulldozed the garden, just as Richard Huttner of the State Supreme Court of Brooklyn was ruling. The Attorney General's office felt like the City had subverted the judicial process by going ahead with the bulldozing and did put on the TRO on bulldozing gardens. The whole city was furious with the Mayor. The city's actions and the community response eventually translated into a deal with the city to save the gardens for well into the next decade. 'Despite this ruling, the City continued seeking to destroy gardens, and in some cases, was successful', noted Howard.

In the summer of 2001, activists with More Gardens spent the summer collecting signatures to sponsor a ballot referendum to make the gardens permanent: 'The whole argument was to create a public campaign to have people support the gardens', explained Susan Howard, who took part in the signature collection process. Throughout the campaign, the activists brought a jigger of play: 'Bobby Lesko dressed as a rose bush. He danced around everyone for our tabling events.' The whole process generated support for the gardens. Years of organizing were followed by a September 17, 2002 deal by the Attorney General's office and the new mayor securing the gardens in New York City: 'The Stipulation of Agreement and Order was signed between the State of New York Attorney General Spitzer and the City of New York', noted Howard. 'The agreement covered only 546 gardens, with 100 of the gardens actually small open spaces. These gardens are supported by Green thumb.' Over the next eight years, the city budget would become more and more expensive. Many would be forced out as property values increased, placing more pressure on gardens as spaces for development.

With the 2002 garden agreement set to expire in September, 2010 the City Parks department published a draft of a new set of rules for the gardens, with few of the protections outlined in 2002. I had been going to New York City Community Garden Coalition meetings. A draft of the new rules was leaked to the *New York Times*. A subsequent article outlined many of these concerns (Moynihan, 2010a). Susan Howard gave me a call after the new garden rules were published in the *City Record*. Fearing the limitations of the rules, we called upon friends from More Gardens, Lower East Side Collective, and Times Up to attend a meeting at ABC No Rio. In mid-July, the group held a meeting to talk about strategies. Throughout the discussion, activists outlined a common goal: make the gardens permanent.

The meeting turned into a kind of focus group on the benefits of gardens, which are many. Keeping a space a garden provides the community with a significant return. A few of these benefits include: trees which reduce asthma and absorb carbon, increases in social cohesion and property value with a converse reduction in crime.

'The community gardens are up for review again and we need to come up with some strategies to save them,' wrote Bill from Times Up in an email blast after the meeting: 'One idea is to engage a full-fledged campaign using a community garden as a springboard, just like we did with Esperanza Community Garden years ago.' Those at the meeting looked to the strategies of the multifaceted organizing approach of a decade prior. Much of the struggle would take place through a battle over the story of the new rules. We wanted our version of the story to prevail, so we used a range of tactics, including creative direct action as well as media activism to push our version of the stories of the gardens and garden rules forward.

The working group from the meeting drafted a position statement in support of the gardens: 'Green Means Gardens: Preserve, Preserve, Preserve' read the first lines of the Times Up Statement on New Garden Rules:

> With the new parks and Housing Preservation and Development rules, the city has taken a huge step backward. Community gardens in New York have thrived since the 2002 Spitzer Agreement which preserved these precious green spaces. Yet, with the Preservation Agreement expiring on September 17, 2010, the city appeared to have abandoned its efforts to preserve green spaces. With the new rules, all the gardens may now be legally transferred for development, rather than preserved. In the end, those involved with Times Up and the garden movement urged the city to reject these rules and make a final commitment to a green city by making all the gardens permanent once and for all. The group plans to organize to defend these precious spaces using a wide range of means, from legal advocacy to direct action.

The final line was an invitation for the media. The Times Up Garden group sent these statements around the city, to lawyers, the Mayor's office, the Attorney General's office, and to the press. The following week the group held another meeting at ABC. There the group came up with a plan for three actions: a bike ride to the Mayor's house calling for him to make the gardens permanent, a trip to city hall for harvest day with crops from community gardens, and a tree climb in city hall park. By this point, the garden rules were becoming a large story. So the actions planned by

Times Up gave the press something to write about, connecting image with the story of policy changes.

The day of the Paul Revere Bike Ride to Save New York's Community Gardens, the press was already writing about the event (Weichselbaum, 2010). And much of the city knew what was in store. The rationale for the Paul Revere theme of the ride was simple. When Paul Revere rang his bell to warn that the British were coming during the American Revolution, all he had was his voice and his bell to sound the alarm: 'The Patriots are coming!' In the case of the July 29, 2010, Paul Revere bike ride, the group was aided by modern media – the internet, email, text messages, and newspaper reports. The point was to sound the alarm about the city of New York's new rules to eliminate protective status and endanger hundreds of community gardens.

The day of the action, members of Times Up planned to draw attention to the risk of the gardens by dressing up as Paul Revere and sounding the alarm, 'the developers are coming'. Cyclists planned to ride 'horse cycles' – bicycles with cardboard horse heads attached to the front – to several Lower East Side Gardens, before heading up to Mayor Bloomberg's house: 'We'll bring vegetables from gardens to Bloomberg's house to remind him that community gardens are precious resources for us all to treasure', I explained in a Times Up press release the day of the action.

Throughout the ride, garden supporters were forced to contend with a phalanx of police. Arriving at Bloomberg's townhouse on East 79th Street, a wall of the top brass of the police in white shirts walked toward the group of riders. It felt like a scene from the movie, *Shoot-out at O.K. Corral.* Rather than wait or be told to stop what we were doing, we rode past them. Walking straight up to the Mayor's door, a group of us delivered the flowers and a sign asking the Mayor and the city to please live up to his call to make this a green city: 'Bloomberg, please make the community gardens permanent for our children's children'. All that sound and fury about a simple bike ride (for a full overview, see Shepard, 2010). Media was there to photograph and tape the discussion and the story of activists pleading with the city to save the gardens went around the world.

The following Monday, word of the group's work had found its way back into the *New York Times* (Moynihan, 2010b). The group continued its push to highlight the plight of the gardens. At 10 a.m. on August 2, 2010 Jessica Sunflower climbed a tree in City Hall Park to call for the city to preserve the community gardens. Sunflower was surrounded by garden supporters with vegetables from the community gardens as well as signs declaring: 'Support the Gardens' and 'Make the Gardens Permanent'. Sunflower's gesture of direct action to affirm the need for community gardens harked back to decades of nonviolent civil disobedience, from Gandhi's Salt Sarataya to the Civil Rights era 'sit-ins' to ACT UP's campaigns against drug companies. The action garnered media attention city wide. The action helped demonstrate the point that garden activists were willing to use a range of creative tactics to make sure the city of New York preserves the community gardens.

Sunflower would spend the next 26 hours in jail. As we left the 'Tombs', the nickname for Central Booking at 100 Center Streets in downtown Manhattan, Jess Sunflower shared a statement about her 26-hour ordeal in custody and why she climbed the tree during the Time's Up Harvest Day Action for the Community Gardens: 'Heartening was being handed the NY Times editorial against the new rules when I walked out of the courthouse. The NY Times editorial seemed to echo our argument about the new parks rules, "The changes are troubling. The new rules talk mostly about transferring gardens – making them available for sale or development – and they remove the section of the 2002 agreement that creates a process for offering gardens to the city ... We urge the city to reconsider these rules and we urge the community gardeners to make their voices heard"' (quoted from 8/3/2010 NY Times Editorial). *The Times* editorial literally echoed the argument of activists. The city was starting to lose control of the story. 'I am very proud to take part in making our collective voice heard', Jess concluded (see Shepard, 2010).

The New York Garden Coalition held a press conference two days later. There activists from all over the city lambasted the new rules. By that time, the city was saying it might be interested in shifting its position. We hoped they would. It was clear that the city had lost the battle of the story. One by one, city politicians published comments critiquing the new rules, while calling for protections for the gardens. The Attorney General's chief of staff even helped Susan Howard and I meet with his legal staff, where we implored them to push the city to strengthen the rules. By early September the city published substantially improved rules for the gardens. In a later meeting, the Attorney General's office would concede that the city was angry that they had had to make so many changes. They made just as many as were necessary to avoid litigation. 'You got a lot', we were told. 'Go to court if they go after any of these gardens.'

Conclusion

The organizing used to build a coalition to defend the community gardens represents a best practice in the study of community organization. This case example highlights the use of a social action to propel a campaign. Here, a practical claim combined with a willingness to mobilize, use direct action and multiple media forms, including street theatre, social media, and play to support the campaign. Community gardens are places for neighbourhood members to meet, share a space, work on a common project, and to plant the seeds of community. These are spaces for people to be introduced, be creative, problem solve, and discuss issues of mutual interest. Yet, like many such spaces in the era of globalization, they are under attack – often because of this.

LESC, More Gardens, and Times Up each made use of sophisticated techniques to communicate a message and a policy solution. What started as small bits and pieces of organizing stories took on the dimensions as life-saving narratives. The gardens were created through direct action and sweat equity – creating a green space out of rubble. In the late 1990s, they were defended with direct action in combination with a well-organized campaign. In 2010, Times Up used direct action to sound the alarm about the limitations of the new rules and the city took notice. Today, gardens are ideal spaces for social work students interested in community practice to engage in service learning, community organizing, and sustainable development practices.

References

Brown, A.M. (2009). Interview with Adrienne Maree Brown: Voices of climate justice. *Race, Poverty and Environment: A Journal for Social and Environmental Justice, 16*(2). Retrieved July 13, 2011 from http://urbanhabitat.org/cj/brown.

Carlsson, C. (2008). *Nowtopia*. Oakland, CA: AK Press.

Coates, J. (2003). *Ecology and social work: Toward a new paradigm*. Halifax, NS: Fernwood Books.

Crane, D. (2006). Interview with the author.

Dawson, S.E., Charley, P.E., and Harrison, P. (1997). Advocacy and social action among Navajo uranium workers. In T.S. Kerson (Ed.). *Social work in health settings*. New York: Haworth Press. 391–407.

Dolgon, C., and Baker, C. (2010). *Social problems: A service learning approach*. Thousand Oaks, CA: Pine Forge Press.

Domanski, D.M. (1998). Prototypes of social work political participation: An empirical model. *Social Work, 43*(2), 156–167.

Doody, T. (2005). Interview with the author.

Figueroa, R. (n.d.). Friends of Brook Park. Retrieved February 27, 2012 from http://www.benjaminheimshepard.com/

Gray, M., Collett van Rooyen, C., Rennie, G., and Gaha, J. (2002). The political participation of social workers: A comparative study. *International Journal of Social Welfare, 11*, 99–110

Howard, S. (2006). Interview with the author.

Kattalia, K. (2011). A threat to local gardens. *New York Times, 27 April*. Retrieved April 27, 2011 from http://eastvillage.thelocal.nytimes.com/2011/04/27/a-threat-to-local-gardens/.

Kauffman, L.A. (2004). A short, personal history of the global justice movement. In E.Yuen, Burton-Rose, D., and Katsiaficas, G. (Eds). *Confronting capitalism: Dispatches from a global movement*. New York: Soft Skull Press. 375–388.

Lamborn Wilson, P., and Weinberg, B. (Eds). (1999). *Avant Gardening: Ecological struggle in the city and the world*. Brooklyn, NY: Autonomedia.

Mary, N.L. (2008). *Social work in a sustainable world*. Chicago, IL: Lyceum Books.

More Gardens! (2002). *How to save your community garden!* By the More Gardens Coalition. Zine.

Moynihan, C. (2010a). New rules worry community garden advocates. *New York Times, 6 July*. Retrieved July 15, 2011 from http://cityroom.blogs.nytimes.com/2010/07/06/impending-rules-worry-some-community-gardeners/?emc=eta1.

Moynihan, C. (2010b). 'The bulldozers are coming': Garden crusaders hop on their bikes. *New York Times*, 1 August. Retrieved July 15, 2011 from http://www.nytimes.com/2010/08/02/nyregion/02gardens.html?_r=1&ref=nyregion.

Mullaly, R. (1993). *Structural social work: Ideology, theory and practice.* Toronto, ON: McClelland and Stewart Inc.

NY Times Editorial. (2010). Keeping the gardens green. *New York Times*, 2 August. Retrieved July 15, 2011 from http://www.nytimes.com/2010/08/03/opinion/03tue4.html.

Park, R.E., Burgess, E., and McKenzie, R.D. (1925). *The city.* Chicago: University of Chicago Press.

Raya, R., and Rubin, V. (2006). 'Safety, growth, and equity: Parks and open space'. Policy Link. Retrieved July 14, 2011 from http://www.scribd.com/doc/34475582/Safety-Growth-And-Equity-Parks-and-Open-Space-Introduction

Rothman, J. (1995). Approaches to community intervention. In J. Rothman, Erlich, J.L., and Tropman, J.E. (Eds). *Strategies of community intervention* (5th ed.). Itasca, IL: F.E. Peacock.

Schaper, D. (2007). *Grassroots gardening.* New York: Nation Books.

Schön, D. (1987). *Educating the reflective practitioner.* San Francisco: Jossey-Bass.

Shepard, B. (2010). Paul Revere ride to save the community gardens. *Huffington Post.* Retrieved September 3, 2010 from http://www.huffingtonpost.com/benjaminshepard/paul-revere-ride-to-save_b_675671.html.

Shepard, B. (2011). *Play, creativity and social movements.* New York: Routledge.

Sherman, E., and Reid, W. (Eds). (1994). *Qualitative research in social work.* New York: Columbia University Press.

Sherman, S.A., Varni, J.W., Ulrich, R.S., and Malcarne, V.L. (2005). Post-occupancy evaluation of healing gardens in a pediatric cancer centre. *Landscape and Urban Planning, 73*(2/3), 168–183.

Stocker, L., and Barnett, K. (1998). The significance and praxis of community-based sustainability projects: Community gardens in Western Australia. *Local Environment, 3*(2), 179–189.

Streeter, C.L., and Gonsalvez, J. (1994). Social justice issues and the environmental movement in America: A new challenge for social workers. *Journal of Applied Social Sciences, 18*(2), 209–216.

Times Up! (2010). *Times Up Statement on the New Garden Rules.* Retrieved July 17, 2011 from http://www.times-up.org.

Van Wormer, K., and Besthorn, F.H. (2011). *Human behavior and the social environment: Groups, communities, and organizations* (2nd ed.). New York: Oxford University Press.

Weichselbaum, S. (2010). Cyclists' advocacy group Time's Up! plans to protest outside Mayor Bloomberg's townhouse: *New York Daily News.* Retrieved July 15, 2011 from http://www.nydailynews.com/ny_local/2010/07/29/2010-07 29_cyclists_advocacy_group_times_up_plans_to_protest_outside_mayor_bloombergs_townh.html.

Wilson, P.L., and Weinberg, B. (Eds). (1999). *Avant gardening: Ecological struggle in the city and the world.* New York: Autonomedia.

7 Social work practice with drought-affected families

An Australian case study

Daniela Stehlik

> [T]hose that are not directly involved in rural industry often do not understand the grief and loss suffered long term by farmers and rural communities. It is vital that services are available and easily accessed by rural people and that the people who are providing services have expert knowledge of the mental and physical effects of continual stress on people (DAFF, 2008a, Submission No.183. Drought Counsellor, Location withheld, Victoria)

Doing social work within an environmental context became a 'real-life' experience for many practitioners during the major Australian droughts of the past two decades. It is in the nature of such a crisis that social workers rarely, if ever, have an opportunity to reflect on the ways in which their practice deals with, or changes, during the crisis itself. A major Federal Government Review of the Drought Policy in 2008 gave practitioners and drought-affected families and communities a unique opportunity to consider how drought had impacted on their well-being, their businesses, their quality of life, and, for professional social workers, their practice, as the following statements from individuals who contributed to the Review summarize the issues raised in this chapter:

> Other natural disasters like fire and flood unite communities as we all draw together to help one another. Drought isolates us through a slow strangulation: leaving our moods bad, our self-esteem low and our decision-making difficult.
>
> (Farmer, Location withheld, Kenny *et al.*, 2008: 61)

> For me, the years of drought have been extremely sad, exhausting and frustrating. You may think we need *counselling*, but we don't want it. We will not use it. The most important issue for us is financial aid, especially for our children who do not choose this lifestyle.
>
> (DAFF, 2008a, Submission No. 246. Name and location withheld, New South Wales, emphasis in original)

[T]hose that are not directly involved in rural industry often do not understand the grief and loss suffered long term by farmers and rural communities. It is vital that services are available and easily accessed by rural people and that the people who are providing services have expert knowledge of the mental and physical effects of continual stress on people.

(DAFF, 2008a, Submission No.183. Drought Counsellor, Location withheld, Victoria)

This chapter draws on the contributions of the many people who, in 2008, made submissions to the Australian Federal Government Expert Social Panel chaired by the late Peter Kenny (Kenny *et al.*, 2008). It reflects on the need for an inclusive social work practice to deal with the inexorable nature of the drought crisis. It questions how the 'environment' might be considered from the point of view of 'practice' and how the external landscape and a crisis of nature, such as drought, directly impacts on the way in which social work practice is delivered. Two particular questions are explored: First, it asks how complex interrelationships between people and place influence practice and, second, how they affect agreed-upon norms of program delivery and practice. The chapter also includes the lived experience of a social worker (Sue, not her real name) interviewed as part of a larger project whose practice was challenged by the drought, and whose responses to it form part of this narrative (Stehlik, 2013).

The politics of the practice context

The Australian continent experiences severe droughts, floods, bushfires, and other 'natural' disasters, such as cyclones, on a regular basis. In early 2011, the nation experienced not only its worst floods in over 40 years but also severe bushfires in some states as well as the major continuing drought on the western side of the continent. It should be noted that many such disasters can be attributed as 'man made'; that the 'natural' aspect of the event is exacerbated by human decision making – for example, the recent floods in Queensland were far more extensive in their impact because of decisions made to locate houses on known flood plains (*The Guardian*, February 9, 2011). In this context, drought itself frequently becomes politicized as questions are raised about the need for governments to respond to ensure people can continue to manage their businesses despite the impact of the crisis. Such government responses are developed in the midst of the crisis, as it is very rare for policy to be developed in *anticipation* of a problem's occurrence (Graycar, 1979; Stehlik, 2012). In other words, policy on drought management is rarely developed when the country is not experiencing drought conditions, and it then follows that social work practice during drought is delivered within a politicized environment under highly pressurized conditions, often within policy frameworks that are stretched to 'catch up' with the reality on the ground.

The Australian political system includes a 'country-minded party', now named the National Party, whose 'natural' constituent group are those landowners who are most likely to be affected by drought. This party was in a Conservative coalition as the ruling party during both the 1990s drought and the drought of the early 2000s. The current ruling social democratic party – the Australian Labor Party – has tended historically to 'manage' the welfare side of drought impact and, in October 2007, it announced a total of $11 million (AUD) to extend and expand social and emotional counselling for drought-stricken farmers (Barnett, 2007). These funds were delivered partially through Centrelink (see below) and partially through existing NGOs. It was this government that established the Expert Social Panel (the Panel) as part of the 2008 Drought Review Taskforce. This chapter draws on that experience to reflect on the way in which social work practice is influenced during an environmental crisis.

Droughts expose underlying critical societal structural problems and they often occur at times when the nation is already under stress. They act to bring to the fore not only environmental impacts, but also political, institutional, or industrial weaknesses associated with responses to it. As a result, the long-term impacts of drought can also result in structural adjustment for farm industries and for many families and communities, as occurred, for example, with the Australian dairy industry in the 1990s (Harris, 2009). Consequently, the 1990s drought commenced at a time of national recession and unprecedented high interest rates, which added to the burden experienced by farm families and rural communities. The drought of the last decade extended over the period of the global financial crisis (2008–2009), again adding to already high levels of individual and family stress.

For Australian social work practitioners (and the related policy and program frameworks within which they are working), a major crisis – whether it be in a flood-ravaged community or the impact of a major bushfire – is usually dealt with according to agreed-upon systemic protocols between the three tiers of government – Federal, State or Territory, and Local – and between the nongovernment agencies responsible for service delivery. In some severe cases, such as the 2011 floods in Queensland and New South Wales, these government agencies worked together under such an agreed model, with the leader usually someone appointed by government, such as, for example, an ex-Army general. If any link were to be drawn between an environmental crisis and social work education, for example, it would likely be in the context of a locally responsive 'command-and-control' approach, which might then be related to similar approaches to international humanitarian or disaster relief work found within development studies. However, such an approach does not deal adequately with the issues associated with the drought crisis described later in this chapter.

The Federal Government's major agency responsible for the social aspects of such crises is Centrelink, which employs over 700 social workers.

Not only does this agency manage income-support payments but it also provides counselling. For example, it operates a national call centre and has a well-established reputation for the delivery of timely and professional services during such crises. One example of its innovative response is the 'drought bus' which was established during the height of the crisis to ensure that information reached even the most isolated communities (Centrelink, 2011).

However, what is unique and unusual about drought in Australia, and the social work response, is that it is *not* a named 'disaster' and is, therefore, *not* dealt with under emergency management framework, such as that described above. It is important to clarify the significance of this: The policies that enable responses to disasters, such as floods and bushfires, also determine the programmatic responses within which social work practice occurs. Federal and State government funding arrangements determine where, when, and how such responses are implemented. Individual social workers cannot prepare responses to such large-scale crises alone. Unlike the sudden, sharp shock of bushfires, drought has a creeping, long lead-time, so the mobilization of responses to clients is a matter of complex public policy decision making (see Stehlik, 2012). It can, therefore, often be months, sometimes even years, after the family and community has been affected, before a formal service response is instituted. A male local government member from western New South Wales who responded to the Drought Review put it this way:

> I was involved with the Thredbo landslide. A tragedy like that demonstrates the link between economic woes (no tourists) and social/mental issues, need for support, and need for interaction providing opportunities for mutual support. A *slower and more insidious* disaster like drought has the same effect, but lacks the immediate punch that gets media and political attention.
> (DAFF, 2008a, Submission No. 197. Nyngan, New South Wales)

This means that social work practice is also delivered differently in response to drought than in established emergency management frameworks. Thus social work practitioners, who became part of the Federal, State, and NGO responses to drought, 'entered into' the crisis *much later* than those who were experiencing it. It was not a crisis in which everyone participated simultaneously. Those who 'arrived late' were confronted with clients in serious need.

In 1989, drought was declared a farm management and planning issue – an issue of risk rather than a 'disaster'. This was over a decade before the now well-rehearsed media exposure about climate change, as governments, land managers, and environmentalists had already established that climate variability was a key factor in farming in Australia, and that such variability needed to be factored into on-farm management, as well as direct policy interventions. The concept which had historically framed the decision making of the newly arrived Europeans who settled this continent – that drought was an aberration to the 'natural' order of things – was overturned in 1989 when the Federal Government policy determined that drought would no longer be considered a disaster. Instead, 'drought [became] a normal part of the farmer's operating environment [and was to be] managed like any other business risk' and, at that time, then Prime Minister Paul Keating spoke of it as an Australian 'way of life' (Stehlik, 2003: 51).

The original purpose of the policy transition to 'managed risk' in the early 1990s supported the principle that the 'only welfare component … was aimed at encouraging non-viable farmers to leave the industry' (White, Botterill, and O'Meagher, 2003: 100). However, as the drought of the 1990s continued, pressure was brought to bear on governments, and 'significant welfare benefits' were introduced in 1994. With a change of government (see below) in 1996, 'the focus … was increasingly … on the human [especially the perceived welfare] impacts' (White *et al.*, 2003: 100).

This politicized transition to a 'welfare' response has had long-term consequences. As Stehlik (2003) noted, when reflecting on the impact of the major national drought of the 1990s (the so-called 100-year drought) and leading into the extended drought of the 2000s, this paradigm shift to personal risk management 'touched on issues of identity, community, [and] citizenship' (p. 66). It particularly impacted on those living in rural Australia and forced them to consider their 'place in society' more broadly.

As a result of this change in policy, responses to drought became a real challenge for social work practice. Within the 'managed risk' scenario, the call for support services for drought-affected individuals and families was expected to be 'managed' within existing resources and policies. In fact, the drought of the 1990s, and the extended drought of the subsequent decade, put critical pressure on the capacity of nongovernment and government agencies to respond, and this in turn placed additional pressure on individual social work practitioners to find and deliver solutions.

The Department of Agriculture, Fisheries and Forestry (DAFF) Drought Review (2008b) found that the responses provided were still predicated on a crisis model, primarily because of the process of drought declaration (see below). In other words, rather than adopting an early intervention approach, human services were mobilized *only when the situation was nearing a critical point*. The delivery of crisis programs within these policies remained fragmented and uncoordinated. In addition, when programs were finally funded, they needed start-up funding and establishment lead-in times, which only added to response delays. The report of the Expert Social Panel (Kenny *et al.*, 2008) strongly recommended that future social welfare services be developed within an early intervention and prevention policy framework.

Where the real 'tipping point' within previous drought policy was most visible was in its impacts on Federal service-delivery agencies, and consequently on their staff. The lead Federal agency responsible for matters associated with drought has always been (and remains) the DAFF. The service-delivery agencies, which include Health, Centrelink, Human Services, Transport, and Regional Development, among others, responded in their portfolio areas, but a national response to the crisis was *not* seen as the sole responsibility of any *one* particular agency. This meant that each agency 'did its own thing', funding crisis responses (and thereby specific social work practitioners) without much review or consideration as to what else was being funded and supported *in the same area*. In addition, as the Drought Review (Kenny *et al.*, 2008) found, coordination between agencies became even more challenging during the crisis. The involvement of state-based and funded agencies and the nongovernment sector then added further complexity. For example, the Expert Social Panel (ibid.) heard of many cases where individuals under extreme stress were being approached, in turn, by Federal, State, and local government services, nongovernment welfare agencies, church bodies, and sometimes even the media, in their uncoordinated desire to 'solve' the drought problem.

As the drought continued, years beyond any prior predictions, the attempts to resolve the crisis meant that some nongovernment services had not had any experience in working with farm families and rural communities, or, in specific crises, such as drought. One such agency was Relationships Australia, which received funding in early 2003 to provide 'free counselling [to people who had been] affected by the drought' (Johnson, 2003: 2). Johnson's (2003) evaluation report on this investment in counselling, and the time it takes to establish essential networks when an agency is unfamiliar with its targeted client group, makes salutary reading. The report makes two relevant points: first, there was a backlash against counselling as people wanted 'financial help'. They saw counselling as 'dealing with the cause rather than trying to manage the problem – there wouldn't be relationship breakdown if there weren't a drought, so help us with that' (ibid.: 12). Second, time was a critical barrier to counselling delivery, since funding was provided for a four-month period only in the hope that the drought would break in that time, and, in some cases, clients had been experiencing drought conditions for a considerable length of time with some still facing a further five to six years of drought:

> This [short-term funding] impacted upon the implementation of the counselling in a number of ways. Firstly, the difficulties in building relationships with the local community meant that much of the 4 months was *used just establishing the service*, rather than delivering actual counselling. Secondly, where many areas of need were identified, the short time frame meant that the counsellors were forced to choose between *competing possibilities of intervention*. Thirdly, a sense arose that the funding was ending but the drought certainly had not.
>
> (Johnson, 2003:10 emphasis added)

Place and the environmental complexities of practice

For international readers, it is important to contextualize not only the spatial but also the temporal nature of the two major droughts of the 1990s and early 2000s in Australia. At their height, these droughts extended over much of the country's arable areas, directly affecting production from most of the natural food bowl regions. For the first time, the drought of the early 2000s also entered into the nation's cities, as water became scarce, and, as a result, urban Australians began to take notice that drought was not just a 'farming issue'. Figures 7.1 and 7.2 map the extent of the drought in the 2000s, with Figure 7.1 focusing on the Australian 'food bowl', the Murray–Darling Basin.

The drought extended from the central and south of Queensland, across all of New South Wales, into Victoria and Tasmania and then west across to the once highly productive areas of the wheatbelt of Western Australia. Were this map to be overlaid with a population map of Australia, it would include nearly 80 per cent of the nation's population, as well as all of the nation's capital cities, except Darwin, and would, therefore, impact on all states and many local governments and NGOs, both large and small. Stafford-Smith (2003) has highlighted the 'cross-border solutions' that become an important component of the high transaction costs associated with managing a national drought. In the context of practice, it becomes yet another aspect of the complexity associated with on-the-ground service delivery.

Place is crucial to understanding the impact of drought on environmental issues more broadly and social work practice particularly (Stehlik, 2001, 2003). While the whole continent was experiencing a national drought, its *actual* impact was being experienced differently across different locations, depending on historical, cultural, and local factors, including localized funded supports. In some communities, this meant that decision making as to drought responses pitted neighbour against neighbour, as some land became drought declared. This resulted in support, including Federal and State government support, becoming available to that family, while other land, nearby, was not covered. The decision making as to who was, and who was not, in drought remains highly complex and, as White *et al.* (2003) point out, is highly subject to 'publicity and political point scoring':

> Farmers experiencing drought are required to make a case that the dry spell is more severe than could reasonably be encompassed within a risk management strategy. This case is then presented to the Commonwealth Government via the State Government. It is also reviewed by the [Federal] Government's advisory body ... which [then] recommends to the Minister [for Agriculture] whether exceptional circumstances exist.
>
> (p. 108)

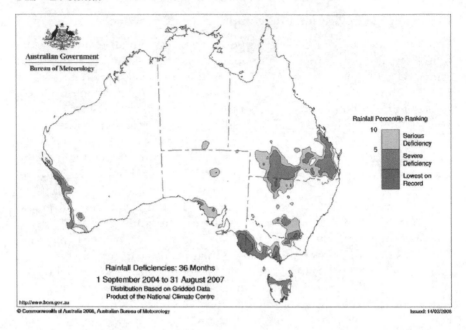

Figures 7.1 Australian Rainfall Deficiences (September 1, 2004 to August 31, 2007)

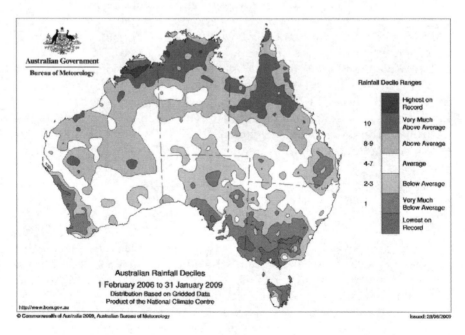

Figure 7.2 Australian Rainfall Deciles (February 1, 2006 to January 31, 2009)

The temporal aspect of these droughts extended over many years. Officially, the drought of the 1990s 'began' in 1991 and 'concluded' in 1995 (Stehlik, 2003) when, in some parts of the country, the drought had begun sooner and ended later. The drought of the 2000s officially 'began' in 2002 and, in many parts, concluded in 2009, remaining in Western Australia until May 2011 (Productivity Commission, 2009).

These 'official' declarations of drought (see White *et al.*, 2003), which trigger the formal mobilization of human service delivery, were significantly out of 'sync' with the lived experiences of those affected. Many families were already under a great deal of stress and had been making serious life decisions well before any formal support was offered to them. This meant that the demands on individual social work practitioners were greater when they finally connected with their clients. Again, the Relationships Australia experience, early in the 2000s drought, is revealing, as 'simply setting up an office, placing ads around town and waiting for clients to walk in the door did not always work' (Johnson, 2003: 13) even in areas where there had been drought for an extended period, but where the agency itself had not previously had a presence.

What does drought mean for the environment? Australia is understood to be a dry, ancient continent, with a highly variable climatic system. As Stafford-Smith (2003) points out, 'On top of the normal annual variability found in all semi-arid areas in subtropical to temperate zones ... Australia experiences additional multi-annual variability drivers such as El Niño' (p. 6). The nation is, therefore, very familiar with climate variability, and most farmers are well adjusted to managing such variability on their properties. Drought itself is complex and includes variables such as lack of rainfall and sub-soil moisture, and decision making based on past experience. The Australian Government Bureau of Meteorology (2008a) issued this complex definition:

> A drought is a prolonged, abnormally dry period when there is not enough water for users' normal needs. Drought is not simply low rainfall; if it was, much of inland Australia would be in almost perpetual drought. Because people use water in so many different ways, there is no universal definition of drought. Meteorologists monitor the extent and severity of drought in terms of rainfall deficiencies. Agriculturalists rate the impact on primary industries, hydrologists compare ground water levels, and sociologists define it on social expectations and perceptions (n.p.).

To this complexity could also be added that *policymakers determine it by an equally complex analysis of various localized data received from state and local governments.* Popularly, however, drought is still understood to mean a lack of rainfall. While Australia is becoming much more sophisticated in its ability to predict the El Niño or La Niña phenomena, it is still not possible to predict the temporal nature of such events, in other words of being able to say with any accuracy, when they begin, how long they are likely to last, and when they are likely to end.

This lack of predictability has had a direct impact on social work practice. As pointed out earlier, specific drought declarations are managed both locally (at local regional levels) and then at State and Federal levels. For any community, the responses managed by social workers are totally dependent on such declarations, as funding *is not made available* until they are confirmed. While individuals may be able to provide some localized responses early, this would largely be at the cost of some other form of grant, not identified specifically for drought-affected families. It is much more likely, therefore, that social work practitioners confronted with need are unable to respond.

Practice adaptation: The Expert Social Panel

Elected in 2007, at the height of the 2000s drought, the Federal Labor Government proposed a review of existing policy and program delivery. The Minister responsible for the review was then Minister for Agriculture, Hon. Tony Burke. It had become clear that responses developed (relatively *ad hoc*) during the drought of the previous decade were no longer meeting people's needs. Drought had come to cities, and people began demanding solutions.

The inexorable nature of drought makes it extremely difficult to predict how long it is likely to last, and this in turn means that responses which originally begin as 'short term', and crisis driven, quickly become systematized. This results in pressure to provide long-term funding. One characteristic of this pressure was that many programs were funded 'short term', sometimes for less than six months (such as, for example, the Relationships Australia program), and then had to be extended again and again. This meant that, by the time the new Federal Government began to understand the complex nature of the grant monies that were supporting many diverse and fragmented programs across the country, the drought had continued to impact on families and communities, and specifically, became critical as the Murray–Darling Basin area – the food bowl of Australia – dried up (see Figure 7.1).

The newly elected Federal Government's response was to establish a Review Taskforce with three distinct components: *meteorological* (to determine the latest predictive science), *economic* (to establish the most effective approach to using Treasury funds), and *social* (to determine the impact on families and communities and make recommendations for more effective human service responses). This three-strand approach was unique. Previously all national reviews, for example, the one in 2004, were primarily economic (Botterill, 2003a; Wood, 2004). This time, an opportunity to determine just how the proliferation of programs and policies was impacting at the community level, what was and was not working, would, it was argued, enable a policy formulation that was targeted to resolve these impacts, and which could then determine policy for the predicted drier future. A previous attempt had been made to summarize all the various responses in February 2008 (DAFF, 2008b).

The Taskforce was announced in April 2008, and the Australian Government Bureau of Meteorology Review Report (2008b) was issued in June that year. The Expert Social Panel and the Productivity Commission Review commenced in that same month, with both undertaking community consultations. The Expert Social Panel delivered its report to the Government in October 2008 (Kenny *et al.*, 2008) and the Productivity Commission in May 2009 (Productivity Commission, 2009). Throughout this period, Australia, along with the rest of the global community, was experiencing a severe financial crisis, while, at the same time, the impacts of drought remained extremely grave across the continent (see Figures 7.1 and 7.2). It was, therefore, an opportune time to review policy and evaluate, albeit across a number of jurisdictions, the drought responses to families and communities. Two questions guided the Expert Social Panel's community consultations:

1 How has drought impacted individuals' mental and physical health, family relationships and local communities?
2 What government and nongovernment support services are working well and how could their services be done better (i.e., what needs to be done that is not being done)?

Twenty-five fora were held across the six states and two territories attended by over 1,000 people. The Panel received 230 written submissions to its website, and meetings were also held with key industry and NGO stakeholders in most of the capital cities. These community fora were well advertised, held in easily accessible local venues, and attended by invited counsellors, usually social workers, drawn from local Centrelink offices. The Panel members also had an opportunity over morning or afternoon breaks to discuss issues informally with people from the community who perhaps were reluctant to speak in public. The community fora offered a 'snapshot' of the conditions facing rural or remote Australia, with drought as the major topic, and people shared their thoughts, fears, and anxieties about an uncertain future. At the beginning of each forum, the Chair asked those present to use one word to describe how they were feeling at that moment and share that with the rest of the audience (Stehlik, 2009, 2013).

Findings from the Social Panel Review included first, that for those affected, there was no respite from drought, as it permeated home and work, and its inexorable nature meant there could be no realistic future planning (the future remained uncertain) and so decision making became increasingly difficult. Second, these impacts rippled out beyond the individual families into their wider communities. Third, individual stress associated with drought increased with the time it was being experienced and children were found to be bearing much of that burden, despite their parents' best attempts to shield them from its consequences (for further details see DAFF, 2008a, Submission No 113, *beyondblue*, Victoria).

The Review also concluded that, despite heroic efforts in some cases, overall, human support services (in all levels of government) remained poorly coordinated and the 'crisis' response remained the framework through which much service delivery was undertaken, although not in a command-and-control approach. As a result, a submission from a female sheep grazier in Tasmania highlighted that the 'timeliness of rollout of services once declaration happened was poor and boundaries inflexible. A plan was lacking ... there is a disconnect ... [with] what is actually happening on the ground' (DAFF, 2008a, Submission No 124. Bothwell, Tasmania).

It was also a concern that many people, for various reasons, including a sense of stigma associated with 'welfare' (see below), were *not* accessing the supports made available to them. For Relationships Australia, this was an important lesson for their counsellors, as:

> Advertising free services in some cases led to the local community feeling they were being given charity, which was unwelcome. Even when clients did respond, some insisted on paying or at least making a contribution towards the cost. This usually translated into the clients being offered more sessions than the free counselling alone would have allowed.
>
> (Johnson, 2003: 11)

Learning for responsive practice

Personal 'stress' during times of crisis is now well documented, as is the relationship between ongoing stress and depression and emotional well-being (Beyondblue, 2008). In the case of drought, stress is extenuated as people experience a loss of control. It becomes increasingly difficult to anticipate any improvement in life circumstances. One submission to the Drought Review by a female sheep grazier from Tasmania put it this way:

> I had what was probably an old-fashioned nervous breakdown. I rang my neighbour in tears and asked her to take me to the doctor. I couldn't stop crying. I was completely physically and mentally exhausted. I spent two weeks in hospital whilst they stabilized my medication for depression, I slept most of the time and another two weeks at home mostly in bed. I gradually made the effort to get myself going again and now I am out there fighting for everyone like myself. I was amazed at the people who came up to me and said 'I know what you are going through'. I met [a human service worker] who was an inspiration and a great help. He gave us some groceries and vouchers to buy some clothes for our little boy.
>
> (DAFF, 2008a, Submission No 91. Baden, Tasmania)

A common theme throughout the Review, as well as evidence reported during prior research (Centre for Rural and Remote Mental Health (ACRRMH), 2008; Stehlik, 2003; Stehlik, Gray, and Lawrence, 1999), was that, while personal stress was acknowledged, seeking 'help' was not always the natural response, despite the many different ways in which it might be offered. In their submission to the Expert Panel, Beyondblue stated:

> We know that up to half of all residents living in non-metropolitan areas are significantly less likely to seek professional help for a mental health problem than their metropolitan counterparts and that if they do, they are less likely to have access due to a scarcity of rural services (DAFF, 2008a, Submission No 113).
>
> (*Beyondblue*, Victoria, p. 9)

In some cases, the stigma associated with calling on 'the welfare' was a more powerful driver for decision making than the need to accept help. This stigma has a long history. In a study conducted during the 1990s drought in Queensland, a female grazier responded as follows:

Q: Have you been emotionally stressed because of the drought?
I think people on the land are generally, in times of crises or droughts … usually stressed … answering all these questions about stress – stress counsellors are the last thing most of us need. It is just another bureaucracy brewing up.

Q: Has personal counselling been available to you and your family?
Yes, but we haven't used it.

Q: Do you want to comment on that?
Most people in the bush are resilient, independent and they want something tangible. There would be an odd case I suppose where counselling may help but they wouldn't have got to that stage if they had had some other assistance available before they got so emotional (Author's personal records).

The Panel heard that, in some cases, families limited their access to support and financial assistance and this created a challenge for social work practitioners keen to provide help. A female educational counsellor from Queensland put it this way: 'On many occasions I politely pointed out that funding was available, and was frequently told that "there were other people more deserving", that they did not really need it' (DAFF, 2008a, Submission No 243. Charleville, Queensland). Another common theme was that, while those who accessed support services found them useful, there was a sense that these agencies did not have enough resources to cope. In her submission to the Drought Review, a female sheep grazier made the following statement:

Personally, we have found rural financial counselling and Centrelink have been excellent with their support and the programs that they are associated with. They have responded in a helpful and timely fashion. Even they need more resources as their caseloads increase.

(DAFF, 2008a, Submission No 124. Bothwell, Tasmania)

In 2007, the Australian Institute of Family Studies conducted a national survey of 8,000 people living in rural and regional Australia in an ongoing study, 'Rural and Regional Families: The Impact of Drought and Economic and Social Change' (AIFS, 2007). The study found almost twice the rate of mental health problems in those areas where people reported being in drought when compared with those who had experienced drought in the previous three years (Kenny *et al.*, 2008, see also Edwards, Gray, and Hunter, 2009a, 2009b). Findings from an earlier historical analysis in New South Wales highlighted the correlation between an increase in suicide rates and a decrease in rainfall (see Nicholls, Butler, and Hanigan, 2006). It is now well understood that 'suicide is ... the tip of the stress iceberg' (Monk, 2000: 393).

As a component of the Social Impact Review (Kenny *et al.*, 2008, Appendices), two large-scale analyses were commissioned. First, an analysis of the social well-being of rural Australians was undertaken, drawing on existing datasets, such as the Household, Income and Labour Dynamics in Australia (HILDA) Survey – a longitudinal study (ibid., Appendix 10). This analysis found that rural people were less satisfied with their access to services than people in urban areas, and that their workplace stress was increasing. Second, in a survey conducted at the time of the Drought Review in June 2008 by the then Bureau of Rural Sciences, 3,300 primary producers were asked an array of questions about 'on-farm risks, self-efficacy, and social capital' (ibid., p. 114). The respondents (some 51 per cent) were then classified into one of two groups depending on whether or not they reported experiencing adverse weather conditions on their properties. One question was specifically aimed at the Review's terms of reference regarding access to government services and their usefulness. Findings from this survey revealed two primary sources of help: government relief payments through Centrelink and financial counselling through rural support services: 32 per cent of respondents who experienced adverse seasonal weather conditions and 13 per cent of those who did not accessed government relief payments while 13 per cent of those experiencing adverse conditions and 5 per cent of those who did not accessed rural financial counselling (ibid., Appendix 9).

The growth in rural financial counselling services in Australia can be charted across the two drought decades. Rural financial counsellors (often without any formal counselling training) were first employed during the 1990s drought, and rural financial counselling was then a primary frontline strategy during the drought of the subsequent decade. It was seen as the 'production' and structural readjustment side of the equation. In other words, rural financial counsellors were there largely to provide support and make difficult financial risk management decisions. They did '*not* provide family, emotional or social counselling, financial advice or succession planning services' (DAFF, 2011). In many cases, these 'counsellors' were not trained social workers, but accountants, ex-farmers, or people with agri-business experience.

The Expert Social Panel seriously considered the matter of mental health and lack of access to services. Subsequently, in Recommendation 31 of its Report, the Panel stated that there was an ongoing need to evaluate and enhance existing strategies aimed at overcoming farm families' reluctance to use health services in times of stress (Kenny *et al.*, 2008).

Critical issues in practice

Thus far this chapter has attempted to present the complexities of practice in times of drought. This next section considers two critical practice issues in this context: the first is the vital need for reflexivity in environmental crises and the second is the need to remain aware of the potential of practice to add to or minimize people's stress. Social workers might add to client stress through generalized judgements about people and their needs. Environmental crises, such as drought, are challenging and force social workers to confront issues for which they might be under- or even unprepared. Preconceived assumptions, too, might play a role if stereotypes such as the 'stoic farmer' or 'long-suffering wife' go unchallenged. Social workers caught up in the responses to the Australian droughts over the past two decades have shifted their practice response to people's needs. Just as individual farmers have learnt to adapt to climate variability, so too have individual practitioners learnt to adapt their practice reflexively to environmental crises, such as drought.

Reflective practice implies discernment and anticipation of appropriate responses from advocacy or 'speaking out' on behalf of clients to personal counselling, concrete advice, and appropriate referral. 'Appropriate responses' in times of crisis require sensitivity and diplomacy as people affected by drought have an acute sense that their identity and place is under threat, their known world has been turned upside down, and there are no certainties on which to rely. In this situation, people need to feel supported through the crisis.

The Expert Panel was left with no illusions about the complex interrelationships between 'the welfare' and people experiencing the stresses of prolonged drought. It was important to bear in mind that, if it were not for the environmental crisis, the majority of these 'clients' would *not* need or seek help. These were, therefore, not repeat users of what can be considered 'traditional' welfare assistance. In developing her new project, Sue was well aware of this: 'The project certainly was not generally working with [our] regular customers but rather new clients'. Nevertheless, the idea of 'welfare' raised issues of stigma and feelings of inadequacy for drought-affected people. For example, the Panel heard from people who had driven over an hour to join the Centrelink Drought Bus in another community, rather than have their neighbours see them entering the bus in their hometown; or who said they felt like 'second-class citizens' in Australian society; or who had been called 'environmental vandals' because media coverage had focused mainly on the deaths of their animals and the degradation of the landscape. Perhaps the most difficult aspect of environmental social work of this nature is that, unlike the familiar territory of problems with solutions, this is a predicament that cannot be 'solved' (see Chapter 10); social workers cannot make it rain.

Reflective practice, therefore, means understanding and appreciating that the drought might continue for some time, and that its end cannot be predicted. Our natural instinct to console and support others might be all that is possible at the individual level. Importantly though, our practice needs to consider that, while specific issues may be resolved, the underlying reason for stress and anxiety has not 'gone away'. However, the main problem reported to the Drought Review Panel was not a lack of help but an endless stream of people knocking on doors or calling to offer assistance. This uncoordinated response meant some people were overwhelmed by offers of 'help', while others had no support whatsoever. For Sue this manifested in her clients' failure to seek financial support even though they were 'under financial distress':

> When I was working with them it was clear to me that they were struggling but I utilized a problem solving framework working with them on the issues that they presented with and were comfortable talking about. [We found that the clients] didn't compare what was happening in [other places but] rather their experience was that they didn't want to deal with any more paperwork, and we endeavoured to look at strategies that were paperwork free, including handouts.
>
> (Author's personal records)

A fundamental characteristic of human services, reaching back historically to the early modern period, remains the moralistic distinction between the 'deserving and undeserving' because of government policy and the way resources are dispensed, hence deciding on 'deservingness' was a constant narrative in the aftermath of drought. As already mentioned, any official response only kicks into gear when the Federal Government officially 'declares the drought' and, by implication, all those affected are 'entitled' to – rather than deserving – of help. However, the Panel found that service distribution was neither planned nor equitable primarily because of the uneven population distribution and major concentration of services in urban areas. This, in turn, had direct implications for social workers caught up in implementing government decisions about the services dispensed. In this policy and practice context, several critical questions were raised relating to the complex interrelationships between people and places – with limited services to remote communities and an oversupply of services closer to large cities and regional centres.

Two examples highlight the centrality of 'place' or location during a crisis response. The second decade of drought, coming as it did hard on the heels of the drought of the 1990s, exposed an anecdotal fact now clearly identified as critical: Many farm families were able to reach regional centres, large rural towns, or even, in some cases, the fringes of larger cities, and it was their off-farm labour that kept their farms 'alive'. Alston and Kent (2004) found that, in the small NSW community of Condobolin (some 500 kilometres west of Sydney), nearly three quarters of those interviewed were working 'off-farm', often in casual, insecure positions and, in some cases, women had considered a move to regional centres, with their children, leading to 'involuntary family separation' (p. 97). This was confirmed over five years later, when the Drought Review was told by a female farmer that 'when you leave the farm to support it, you still have to work full time on the farm – full time, not part time as if it were a second job' (DAFF, 2008a, Submission No 201. Ardlethan, New South Wales).

Alston and Kent's (2004) research, undertaken very early in the drought of the 2000s, also highlighted that families living in remote communities, such as Bourke (800 kilometres north west of Sydney), were not able to procure alternative employment and this placed additional pressures on families faced with (in some cases) life-and-death decisions. This was again confirmed during the Drought Review, when the Panel heard from a rural financial counsellor in New South Wales that:

> Where properties are a considerable distance from town, off farm work can mean staying in town during the week and returning to the property at the weekend. I know of some cases where this has led to divorce. One client told me how she had obtained off-farm work but would never do it again or recommend it to anyone else, due to the effect on the family.
> (DAFF, 2008a, Submission No 170. Bourke, New South Wales)

This trend is unlikely to change in the near future given the 2006 Census reported that 3 per cent of farm families had negative or nil average weekly earnings compared with a national average of 1per cent and a median household income of $605 per week compared with a national median income of $649 per week (Kenny *et al.*, 2008). Botterill (2003b) has long pointed out the relationship between farming and poverty and warns that 'poverty on Australia's farms has not been studied in any detail since the mid-1970s' (p. 181).

The more remote the community, the more limited the available services to support families through drought. Resourcing remote Australian settlements has always been challenging to public policy and expenditure. A review of mental health services in Queensland found 'Services were unevenly distributed across drought-affected locations. In areas where there were multiple services, these ... were supplied by a combination of government, non-government or not-for-profit organisations' (Centre for Rural and Remote Mental Health, 2008: 15). However, where such services were available, the reality on the ground for families was that 'there was nearly a total lack of coordination' (p. 15). This leads to the second important question.

Norms associated with equitable service delivery are not only challenged by place in drought responses but also by the life-threatening nature of environmental catastrophes for which 'traditional' service delivery is ill equipped. Resource limitations in the face of a seemingly insurmountable problem are compounded by uncoordinated responses staffed by people on short-term employment contracts. In central west Queensland, the limitations of this short-term, crisis response were brought to the attention of the Expert Panel by a former school principal who asked:

> Can we have social counsellors on a long-term basis, adequately qualified, working in a preferred area that is a preferred career move, social counsellors who [work on a personal basis with families] and who can build a rapport?
>
> (DAFF, 2008a, Submission No 243. Charleville, Queensland)

The challenge of 'access' to services and the distances that needed to be covered to deliver them was highlighted in a report produced by the Centre for Rural and Remote Mental Health (ACRRMH, 2008), which found that states like Victoria (with shorter distances and larger populations) had more support workers available during the drought than did places like central western Queensland, where, for example, one community support worker had responsibility for an area of 700,000 square kilometres, nearly three times the size of Great Britain (ACRRMH, 2008: 15). For Sue, geography and distance became a real challenge:

> One of the outcomes required for [our] project was home visiting. We did not have the funding to visit homes in our Shires. One of our Shires is the size of Victoria, and with two staff and nine Shires and a short time frame we risk-managed project outcomes ... We utilized various strategies to reach into people's homes ... as we could not visit them ourselves.
>
> (Author's personal records)

Further, the situation would not return to normal when the rains came, yet programs would be quickly terminated and workers would be moved to other duties in other places at just the point where they were more urgently needed. As the Relationships Australia evaluation put it: 'For the most value for money, these networks need to be maintained. Otherwise, next time the process must start all over again' (Johnson, 2003: 11). Five years later, the ACRRMH Review Report (2008) also highlighted the extensive investment of resources that was subsequently abandoned, only to be raised again in the face of a drying future:

> Instead of losing these valuable resources and assets in the community, it is proposed that the [current human service professionals], who are clinically trained ... would be ideally placed to provide continuity and play a pivotal role in supporting the transitional strategies and recovering planning recommended by the [Federal Drought Review].
>
> (p. 16)

Conclusion

In conclusion, learning from this situation means first, national recognition that Australia faces a drying future. Despite the floods of summer 2010–2011, people are likely to be experiencing drought somewhere in the country that might again lead to a prolonged drought. Policies and programs need to recognize and prepare for this eventuality by mounting an early intervention and prevention strategy. Second, a collaborative, well-managed response is needed if resources are to be expended efficiently and effectively. Advocacy might ensure that NGOs push for resources to plan early intervention and prevention programs that do not operate on a stop-start model. Third, the logic of resource concentration, including social work services, in Australia's cities needs to be challenged given that most agricultural production occurs in rural and remote locations vulnerable to environmental and climate variations. While rural and/or environmental social work is yet to become a 'standard part' of the social work curriculum, social workers in Australia need to learn about the environment, Australia's drying future, and its implications for people providing food for the nation. In other words, they will need to be prepared for the next drought.

References

Alston, M., and Kent, J. (2004). *Social impacts of drought: A report to the NSW Department of Agriculture*. Charles Sturt University, Wagga Wagga: Centre for Rural Social Research.

Australasian Centre for Rural and Remote Mental Health (ACRRMH). (2008). *Mental Health and Drought in Rural and Remote Queensland*. Cairns: ACRRMH.

Australian Government, Bureau of Meteorology. (2008a). *Definition of drought.* Retrieved August 2, 2011 from http://www.bom.gov.au/climate/drought/livedrought.shtml.

Australian Government, Bureau of Meteorology. (2008b). *Drought: Exceptional Circumstances Report.* Retrieved February 2, 2012 from http://www.bom.gov.au/climate/droughtec/.

Australian Institute of Family Studies (AIFS). (2007). *Rural and regional families: The impact of drought and economic and social change.* Retrieved August 7, 2011 from http://www.aifs.gov.au/institute/research/projects/rrfidesc.html.

Barnett, D. (2007). Effective drought support. *The Drum Opinion.* Australian Broadcasting Commission. Retrieved December 14, 2011 from http://www.abc.net.au/unleashed/38842.html.

Beyondblue National Depression Initiative. (2008). *Research 2001–2007 Targeted research in depression, anxiety and related disorders,* February. Melbourne: Australia.

Botterill, L.C. (2003a). Late twentieth century approaches to living with uncertainty: The National Drought Policy. *From disaster response to risk management: Australia's National Drought Policy.* Dordrecht, the Netherlands: Springer. 51–64.

Botterill, L.C. (2003b). Lessons for Australia and beyond. In L.C. Botterill and Wilhite, D.A. (Eds). *From disaster response to risk management: Australia's National Drought Policy.* Dordrecht, the Netherlands: Springer. 177–183.

Centrelink. (2011). *Video about the Australian Government Mobile Offices.* Retrieved August 10, 2011 from http://www.centrelink.gov.au/internet/internet.nsf/individuals/drought_assist.htm.

Department of Agriculture, Fisheries and Forestry (DAFF). (2008a). *Online Submissions to the Expert Social Panel Drought Review.* Canberra: DAFF. Retrieved September 25, 2008 from http://www.daff.gov.au/agriculture-food/drought/national_review_of_drought_policy/social_assessment/submissions_received.

Department of Agriculture, Fisheries and Forestry (DAFF). (2008b). *Drought assistance: A summary of measures provided by the Australian State and Territory Governments.* Canberra: DAFF. Retrieved September 25, 2008 from http://www.farmpoint.tas.gov.au/farmpoint.nsf/downloads/E816C47E516A0081CA2574F20017E326/$file/Drought_assistance_summary.pdf.

Department of Agriculture, Fisheries and Forestry (DAFF). (2011). *Rural Financial Counselling Program.* Retrieved August 7, 2011 from http://www.daff.gov.au/agriculture-food/drought/rfcs/counsellors.

Edwards, B., Gray, G., and Hunter, B. (2009a). A sunburnt country: The economic and financial impact of drought on rural and regional families in Australia in an era of climate change. *Australian Journal of Labour Economics, 12*(1), 109–131. Retrieved February 2, 2012 from http://www.aifs.gov.au/institute/pubs/papers/2009/edwards4.pdf.

Edwards, B., Gray, M., and Hunter, B. (2009b). The impact of drought on mental health and alcohol use. Presentation at the Australian Social Policy Conference: 'An Inclusive Society? Practicalities and Possibilities', 10 July, Sydney. Retrieved February 2, 2012 from http://www.aifs.gov.au/institute/pubs/papers/2009/edwards2.pdf.

Graycar, A. (1979). *Welfare politics in Australia: A study in policy analysis.* South Melbourne: Macmillan.

Guardian (The). (2011). Editorial. Retrieved August 7, 2011 from http://www.guardian.co.uk/commentsfree/2011/feb/09/australia-disaster-zone-editorial.

Harris, D. (2009). *Agricultural industry support and structural adjustment.* RIRDC Publication No 09/010. RIRDC Project No DAH-6A. Canberra: Rural Industries Research and Development Corporation.

Johnson, I. (2003). *Drought counselling funding evaluation: Implementing services in rural and regional areas.* A Report to Australia: Relationships (National) November.

Kenny, P., Knight, S., Peters, M., Stehlik, D., Wakelin, B., West, S., and Young, L. (2008). *It's about people: Changing perspectives on dryness.* Retrieved February 2, 2012 from http://www.daff.gov.au/__data/assets/pdf_file/0008/889946/dryness_report.pdf.

Monk, A. (2000). The influence of isolation of stress and suicide in remote areas. *Rural Society, 10*(3), 393–403.

Nicholls, N., Butler, C.D., and Hanigan, B.I. (2006). Inter-annual rainfall variations and suicide in New South Wales, Australia. 1964–2001. *International Journal of Biometeorology, 50*(3), 139–143.

Productivity Commission. (2009). *Government Drought Support.* Inquiry Report No. 46. 27th February. Retrieved December 7, 2011 from http://www.pc.gov.au/projects/inquiry/drought.

Stafford-Smith, M. (2003). Living in the Australian environment. In L.C. Botterill and Wilhite, D.A. (Eds). *From disaster response to risk management: Australia's National Drought Policy.* Dordrecht, the Netherlands: Springer. 5–13.

Stehlik, D. (2001). 'Out there': Spaces, places and border crossings. In S. Lockie and Bourke, L. (Eds). *Rurality bites: The social and environmental transformation of rural Australia.* Annandale, NSW: Pluto Press. 30–42.

Stehlik, D. (2003). Managing risk? Social policy responses in time of drought. In L.C. Botterill and Wilhite, D.A. (Eds). *From disaster response to risk management: Australia's National Drought Policy.* Dordrecht, the Netherlands: Springer. 65–83.

Stehlik, D. (2009). Australian women: Still flourishing in a changing environment. In Australian Technology Network (ATN). (Ed.). *The promise and the price. Ten years of the Clare Burton Memorial Lectures.* Sydney: University of Technology. 236–249.

Stehlik, D. (2012). Social science as evidence in drought policy. In L.C. Botterill and Cockfield, G. (Eds). *Drought, risk management and policy: Decision-making under uncertainty.* London: Taylor and Francis.

Stehlik, D. (2013 forthcoming). *Drought, climate variability and change: An Australian case study.* London: Taylor and Francis, Drought and Water Crises Book Series.

Stehlik, D., Gray, I., and Lawrence, G. (1999). *Drought in the 1990s: Australian farm families' experiences.* Canberra: Rural Industries Research and Development Corporation.

White, D., Botterill, L.C., and O'Meagher, B. (2003). At the intersection of science and politics: Defining exceptional drought. In L.C. Botterill and Wilhite, D.A. (Eds). *From disaster response to risk management: Australia's National Drought Policy.* Dordrecht, the Netherlands: Springer. 99–111.

Wood, E (2004). (Chair). *Consultations on national drought policy: Preparing for the future.* Australian Department of Agriculture, Fisheries and Forestry: Canberra. (Can be found as e-version on http://catalogue.nla.gov.au/Record/3097527 – Retrieved 23rd April, 2012.)

8 Social work, animals, and the natural world

Thomas Ryan

At first glance one could easily be led to believe that moral consideration of the non-human world has nothing whatsoever to do with social work, that the discipline's rationale and function is unreservedly and properly human centred. This view would, however, be in stark contrast to the reawakened concern and respect for the non-human world in Western societies during the twentieth and twenty-first centuries, which has been the seminal catalyst in the generation of contemporary environmental and social movements, placing considerations for the natural world onto the political agenda (Hay, 2002). From fringe beginnings, these concerns have gradually come to be embraced by the mainstream, to the extent that it is now increasingly rare to find individuals who do not consider themselves to be solicitous about the natural world. Human understanding and appreciation of the natural environment and non-human animals has been significantly enhanced and elevated by the disciplines of ecology and ethology respectively.

The moral community

At heart these concerns involve a reassessment of moral rights and status, as well as the criteria for membership of the moral community, the conceptualization of which is of great consequence since it circumscribes the boundaries of moral considerability. Regan (1982) states that a 'basic moral right is itself the ground of a moral obligation' (p. 117) and Warren (1997) argues that moral status 'is a means of specifying those entities towards which we believe ourselves to have moral obligations, as well as something of what we take those obligations to be' (p. 9). Pluhar (1995) claims that to be 'morally considerable, is to be the sort of being to whom others can have duties' (p. 166) and 'maximum moral respect is due any being, human or nonhuman, who is capable of caring about what befalls him or her' (p. xiii). In short, all concepts refer to those individuals to whom *direct* duties are owed. By way of contrast, Passmore (1974) contends that membership of the moral community and moral obligations are dependent upon shared interests and mutuality and, accordingly, it makes no sense to apply such concepts beyond the human community.

Analysis of the root cause of indifference toward the non-human world in Western thought tends to attribute culpability predominantly to the Christian tradition (Passmore, 1974; White, 1967). Others argue that notions of stewardship of nature have evolutionary plausibility (Midgley, 1983a), and beliefs in a covenant between God, and *all* creation, and a common origin points to an inclusive moral community (Attfield, 1991; Linzey and Cohn-Sherbok, 1997). Furthermore, the basis for the contemporary notion of balance in nature was theological well before it was scientific (Thomas, 1983). However, it can be argued that it is an *exclusive* humanism, one that conceives humankind to be the measure of all things, which is the more likely cause of a pervasive anthropocentrism:

> that has expanded the notion of 'humanism' from a modest, honorable respect for what is good in humanity into a disreputable quasi-religion, exalting us into substitute gods ... degrading all other creatures into mere material for our free activity.
>
> (Midgley, 1992b: 10, 8).

Closely allied to it is the restrictive contractual notion that rights and duties are essentially correlative. Not only does this make it well-nigh impossible to conceive that humans have duties to the non-human world (Midgley, 1983b), but it also belies the reality that in everyday life vulnerability and weakness impose *greater* duties. The anthropocentric beliefs that the natural world has only utilitarian value and exists merely to serve human needs and designs, that only humans possess moral standing, represent a philosophical worldview that Callicott (1980) terms *ethical humanism*. It is seen as axiomatic that human interests are constitutive of ethics and morality. As Schweitzer (1955) observes:

> European thinkers watch carefully that no animals run about in the fields of their ethics ... Either they leave out altogether all sympathy for animals, or they take care that it shrinks to a mere afterthought, which means nothing. If they admit anything more than that, they think themselves obliged to produce elaborate justifications, or even excuses, for so doing.
>
> (pp. 228–229)

In contrast, the concept of community takes on a radically expanded and inclusive character in deep ecology, comprising not only human beings, but all species, plants, and ecosystems (Johnson, 1993; Leopold, 1949), entailing that humans are 'enfolded, involved, and engaged within the living terrestrial environment' (Callicott, 1989:. 51). Such an understanding owes much to Darwin's worldview which has profoundly shaped the way humans view their place within the natural world, and other creatures. Human biological continuity entails that differences among humans and other animals are a matter of degree rather than kind, for 'We are not just rather like animals, we *are* animals' (Midgley, 1996: xxxiv). Darwin (1936) envisaged a progressive evolution of human moral and ethical sensibilities, prophesying 'a disinterested love for all living creatures' (p. 494), whereby all sentient beings would eventually come to be included in the moral community. That said, the moral implications of this continuity, grounded in the 'discovery of the law of evolution, which revealed that all organic creatures are of one family, shifted the centre of altruism to the whole conscious world collectively' (Hardy, 1930: 138), are only beginning to be grasped (Rachels, 1999).

All this is a salutary reminder that the natural world does not exist merely to environ the human animal, and an acknowledgement that respect is not something that is owed only to creatures of the human kind. And more to the point, the health and well-being of ecosystems is inseparable from the flourishing of *all* their members. It ought to matter to social workers, for instance, that the communities within which they practise have access to clean water and good air quality, that their waterways, neighbourhoods, and environs are free from pollution and toxic chemicals, that as much as humanly possible people have access to organic and nutritious food. Invariably, consequences flowing from the absence of any of the aforementioned disproportionately impact upon the poorest and most disadvantaged in society, this being often more pronounced in many non-Western nations. Therefore, it is obvious that such concerns are not only legitimate but also essential components of a holistic understanding of the nature of social justice. In addition, it is a salient example where evident self-interest is not contrary to the interests of the non-human world. Moreover, animals, domesticated or otherwise, have similar vested interests. An abiding concern for habitats and ecosystems self-evidently includes the interests of non-domestic animals, and it ought to be seen as a legitimate role of social workers to add their voices to campaigns to ensure that wilderness areas are protected, as this is indispensable to the flourishing of those animals. All creatures, if moral rights mean anything, are entitled to their natural spaces and places in the sun (Clark, 1985).

Transforming social work's moral scope

There is a growing social work literature addressing broader concerns for the natural world, and the ways in which they have direct relevance to the well-being of human beings (Coates, 2003; McKinnon, 2008; Zapf, 2009). The increasing recognition that the human species is deeply embedded within the natural world is a most gratifying development, serving to redress the anthropocentrism that has characterized social work's worldview. The discipline's best traditions consider individuals within the context of their wider environment – families, relationships, and communities – the key concepts being *person-in-situation* and *person-in-environment*. A widening of social work's moral scope, so as to extend consideration from the social environment to individuals in the context of their natural environment, appears to be a rather obvious and sensible augmentation. As humans inhabit three worlds – the natural, the social, and the world of self – reality is better understood as the whole of creation (Wilkes, 1981). Conceptual bridges to such a widened view can be seen to be provided by the life model, and systems and transpersonal theories (Turner, 1996).

Nonetheless, the moral claims of the non-human animals, with whom humans share the world, remain largely unacknowledged. While there are exceptions (Hanrahan, 2011; Loar, 1999; Wolf, 2000), this is conspicuously the case with domesticated animals even in the social work literature that does take the natural world into account, apart from one notable exception (Gray and Coates, 2011), and in this regard it remains steadfastly anthropocentric. Such pervasive disregard and indifference stems in large part from the conviction that *any* consideration extended to them would invariably divert attention and resources away from far more deserving subjects – in a word, humans. Both practitioners and senior academics have expressed exactly those sentiments to the author, who has argued elsewhere that animals have legitimate moral and ethical claims against humans in general, but more specifically against social workers (Ryan, 1993, 2011). There is also the suspicion that animal companions are merely a compensation for the companionless or the socially inept. Midgley (1983a) remarks that the accusation that human affection for animals represents a 'gratuitous perversion' (p. 116) makes as little sense as suggesting the same about our interests in machines and music, for '[e]xperience of animals is not essentially a substitute for experience of people, but a supplement to it – something more which is needed for a full human life' (p. 119). There are signs that this orthodoxy is beginning to be challenged, with a growing empirical and qualitative literature making explicit the interrelationship and linkage between the abuse of animals and humans (Ascione and Arkow, 1999; Linzey, 2009), and a burgeoning human–animal bond literature (Anderson, 2008; Beck and Katcher, 1996; Podberscek, Paul, and Serpell, 2000; Risley-Curtiss, 2010). In addition, the health benefits of animal companionship and their use in therapeutic settings is increasingly acknowledged (Fine, 2010; Sable, 1995; Tedeschi, Fitchett, and Molidor, 2005). Whilst not for a moment diminishing these valuable contributions, animals need to be considered as ends in themselves, not merely as serving human needs and well-being.

Reconceptualization of social work's moral and ethical framework

The difficulty in getting social workers to conceive and acknowledge the moral claims and standing of animals, notwithstanding their relationships with their own animals, is at once metaphysical and philosophical. In large part, it is the consequence of the key principles underpinning and informing the discipline's moral and ethical imagination (see below). It will be instructive to reflect further upon the conceptualization of human relationships with the natural world, in addition to the ways in which environmental philosophies understand the nature of moral community and value. Both are essential in the articulation of a social work respect for the natural world *and* the non-human creatures dwelling within it, and the nature of humans' moral obligations and duties to both. As Midgley (2003) observes, 'The way in which we imagine the world determines what we think important in it' (p. 2). Particular attention will be accorded to the writings of the environmental philosopher J. Baird Callicott, for their illuminative contributions to the question as to whether environmental and animal ethics can be moral bedfellows. As such they provide a pertinent blueprint for social work's engagement with, and moral consideration of, the non-human world.

The aforementioned diametrically opposed understandings of the relationship between humans and the natural world, Fox (1991) argues, reflect a *discrete entity ontology* and a *continuity ontology* respectively. In the former, the world is pictured as being constituted by discrete entities, with emphasis accorded to differences, whereas while the latter acknowledges a degree of independent existence, it nevertheless conceives beings as fundamentally characterized by interrelationship and connectedness. For Leopold (1949) 'the individual is a member of interdependent parts' (p. 203), while for Clark (1983) all individuals 'exist as patterns of relationship ... as elements within modes of a continuing community' (p. 195).

A further distinction is made between a shallow environmentalism and a deep ecology (Naess, 1973), between what might, for convenience sake, be characterized as conservationism (in large part for reasons of human self-interest), and a respect for the intrinsic and independent moral value of the natural world respectively. The message of the latter is 'there is a world out there, embodying more beauties than our own imaginations can create' (Clark, 1995a: 6). In essence, we are not the world and the world is not made for us. Contrary to anti-realists, the world is not what humans say it is, for 'words are not the world ... changing the way we speak of things does not change the way things *are*' (Clark, 1986: 53) for the very good reason that the 'universe is wider than our views of it' (Thoreau, 1968: 282). It would be more truthful to say that we are truly made *for* the world.

Given the foregoing, Nash (1990) argues that the 'emergence of this idea that the human–nature relationship should be treated as a moral issue conditioned or restrained by ethics is one of the most extraordinary developments in recent intellectual history' (p. 4). Nevertheless, such concerns are not revolutionary in the sense that they represent an unparalleled phenomenon or a unique feature of the modern world (Preece, 2005; Thomas, 1983).

Environmental versus animal ethics?

The aforementioned divergence between shallow environmentalism and Deep Ecology is paralleled by what some see as a fundamental incompatibility between environmental and animal ethics. Leopold's (1949) assertion that a 'thing is right when it tends to preserve the integrity, stability, and beauty of the biotic community. It is wrong when it tends otherwise' (p. 203) informed Callicott's (1980) initial conviction as to their irreconcilability given that the demands of the biotic community represent 'the ultimate measure of moral value' (p. 320). However, this ignores the reality that holism represents but a part, not the whole, of morality (Sapontzis, 1984).

The incompatibility is derived from what Callicott (1980) saw as the clash between Leopold's (1949) holistic ethic, and the individualistic and atomistic orientations of deontological and utilitarian perspectives. The former, termed *ethical holists*, contend that the good of biotic community takes moral precedence, whereas the latter, termed *humane moralists*, locate moral value in individuals according to metaphysical attributes that determine moral inclusion or exclusion. Callicott (1980) castigated the latter for what he depicted as their 'world-denying or rather a life-loathing philosophy... [and] anti-natural prophylactic ethos' (pp. 333–334). From the former perspective, rare and endangered species have moral priority, and misanthropy was seen as *the* yardstick of environmentalism's biocentrism.

In contrast, the welfare and well-being of domesticated animals was considered of minimal moral significance, especially given that pain and pleasure are deemed irrelevant from the perspective of an ecological biology. As well as obscuring the moral issue of human-caused pain and suffering in animals, his condemnation of factory farming and vivisection as 'immoral' had less to do with either the suffering or killing of animals than outrage at 'the transmogrification of organic to mechanical processes' (Callicott, 1980: 336). In response to claims that factory-farmed animals have frustrated natural behaviours, Callicott (1980) retorted that it 'would make almost as much sense as to speak of the natural behavior of tables and chairs' and domesticated animals are best conceptualized as 'living artifacts ... bred to docility, tractability, stupidity, and dependency' (p. 330).

This failure to recognize suffering as imposing more urgent moral duties, and as an intrinsic evil always requiring justification, invariably blurs understanding of the reasons why it is immoral to subject human beings to certain forms of treatment (Warren, 1983). And as with humans, the only moral justification for the infliction of suffering on animals is if it is in *their* best interests. As Bentham (in Singer, 1976) famously insisted, the question is not can they *reason* or can they *talk* but *can they suffer?* (p. 8). Given that consciousness is the 'fundamental mode or form of moral being' (Murdoch, 1993: 171), a creature's subjectivity and sentience, rather than human sympathy toward it, ought to determine its moral considerability (Darwin, 1936).

Kheel (1996) argued that environmental ethics perpetuates dualism, with the bulk of the literature insisting the establishment of hierarchies of value was essential in enabling humans to make moral choices concerning their interactions with the natural world. The Platonic consequences of this dualism are:

> The whole is greater than the sum of the parts ... As for the actual role-players, as long as they are self-renewing, as long as they keep coming forward, we need pay them no heed ... Our eye is on the creature itself, but our mind is on the system of interactions of which it is the earthly, material embodiment. The irony is a terrible one. An ecological philosophy that tells us to live side by side with other creatures justifies itself by appealing to an idea, an idea of a higher order than any living creature.
>
> (Coetzee, 1999: 53–54)

This drowning of animals in a sea of indiscriminate cosmic identification results in a failure to respect their otherness and individuality (Plumwood, 1992): 'What is loved and admired is not the individual organism as something that can be harmed or hurt, but the pattern, the form of life' (Clark, 1994: 236). It is the philosophy that deems it morally permissible to always override the interests of the individual, for the good of the whole, that Regan (1983) labels 'environmental fascism' (p. 362). It has implications for both animals *and* human beings: 'If the biotic community would benefit, abortion, infanticide, and the killing of certain adults would all be justified. Measures routinely taken with non-human animals would be extended justifiably to humans' (Pluhar, 1983: 120). In contrast ethology has been instrumental in correcting misconceptions of the lives of animals, and in confirming their individuality:

> Learning to recognize individual animals under natural conditions... has led to the discovery of previously unsuspected patterns of behavior that could not be appreciated when the animals were treated as interchangeable units. One discovery has been that not only the ethologist but the animals themselves often recognize their companions as individuals and treat them accordingly.
>
> (Griffin, 1984: 165)

Callicott (1988, 1998) later came not only to acknowledge but also to make the case for the compatibility of concerns for the biosphere and domesticated animals, even arguing for the moral necessity of vegetarianism for environmentalists. While this chapter does not explore the latter in any detail, human consumption of animal products has profound environmental impacts (Singer and Mason, 2006). Callicott's critique of the evils of factory farming and research laboratories extends beyond his earlier outrage at their mechanization, to a moral revulsion at their depersonalization, and the denial or ignorance of their subjectivity. The basis for this compatibility derives from a shared concept of community – Leopold's (1949) *biotic community* and Midgley's (1983a) *mixed community*. Midgley's (1983a) claim that 'hardly any of us, at heart, sees the social world as an exclusively human one' (p. 118) is underpinned by Hume's (1998[1777]) conviction that morality is founded on personal attachment, altruistic sentiment, and a diffuse sympathy rather than rationality and self-interest. Leopold's (1949) land ethic ought to be seen as a component of what Callicott (1988, 1998) terms a *biosocial theory* of morality, whereby social and biological relationships determine the nature of moral obligations. This Humean understanding is allied with Darwin's conviction that social instincts are what made human morality possible in the first place. As social animals, human beings inherit tendencies to assist and protect their fellows, and in common with other animals, are impelled by mutual love and sympathy. It is these co-evolved tendencies 'that attend upon and enable sociability ... [and] intersubjective interaction between species' (Callicott, 1988: 165). As Midgley (1984) observed, the Darwinian understanding of social instincts:

> is not just one more set of impulses among others, but a whole way of regarding those around us, based on sympathy, which involves imagining them as subjects like oneself, experiencing life in the same way, and not essentially different in status.
>
> (p. 90)

In their natural state, animals are members of the biotic community, not the mixed community. Callicott (1988, 1998) argues that human obligations to them are markedly different from those owed to domesticated animals. Whereas humans and domesticated animals belong simultaneously to biological and social communities, animals in the wild 'should not lie on the same graded moral standing as family members, neighbors, fellow citizens, fellow human beings, pets, and other domestic animals' (Callicott, 1988: 168). Callicott (1985) concedes rights to the latter, given that 'many domestic animals often actually seem to understand not only their rights as honorary participants in a human civil order, but their obligations as well' (p. 372). This concurs with Hearne's (1987) belief that our relationships with animals are constituted by a complex, albeit fallible, moral understanding.

Rowlands' (2002) distinction on the one hand between the natural and negative duties of humans toward animals in their natural environments, and the positive and acquired duties owed to domesticated animals, can be seen to shed light upon social workers' specific duties. In their natural state, what humans principally owe animals is the right to be left alone so as to live their lives with nil, or at worst minimal, human interference. We do best when we do no, or at worst least, harm. By contrast, human obligations towards domesticated animals are more complex and compelling. That said, human duties to animals outside their immediate households are not as restrictive as Callicott's (1988) delineation of the mixed community. As such, it is expressly contrary to Midgley's (1983a) expansive conceptualization. She argues that compassion 'is not a rare fluid to be economized, but a capacity which grows by use' (p. 119). Human compassion and sympathies – linked as they are to the presence of consciousness – for all humans and animals are extensive because the same moral psychology is in play (Fisher, 1982), and moral considerability holds regardless of our relationships to others (Pluhar, 1995). Were it conditional upon our capacity for emotional connection, we would have no moral obligation to care for those to whom we are indifferent. That one is unfailingly solicitous about the animals in one's mixed household should give pause for reflection as to why one might consider the moral status of distant animals an arbitrary or discretionary matter.

Animals and human beings share a social *and* ecological inter-dependency (Benton, 1993), and are, to varying degrees, constitutive of all human societies (see also Serpell, 1986). Sharpe (2005) observes:

> throughout the world, animals are not restricted to the outer fastnesses beyond the rim of the circle but are at its hub as part of the family, forming the nucleus from which our 'benevolent affection' must develop before it can expand to cope with concern at an impersonal level.
>
> (p. 62)

Benton (1993) insists that any adequate portrayal of societies and social relationships must, of necessity, take account of animals as embodying social *and* moral relationships. While admitting that species bonds are genuine and strong, and that an emotional preference for our own kind might be to a degree natural, Midgley (1983a) asserts they are not invariably exclusive, possessing neither the force nor authority to accord justification for the absolute dismissal of other species, as there is 'no reason to think it an impenetrable social barrier, cutting us off from other creatures in a way that makes them none of our proper concern' (p. 124).

The purported incompatibility of concerns for the natural world and animals is thus not borne out, for the 'whole environment cannot be served except through its parts' (Midgley, 1992a: 63) and 'it is not necessary to choose between regarding biological communities as unified systems, analogous to organisms, and regarding them as containing many individual sentient creatures' (Warren, 1983: 131). Both philosophies share in common an opposition to anthropocentrism and can surely concur with Callicott's (1979) observation that a distinctly environmental ethic needs to be founded 'upon love and respect, upon an expanded moral sentiment' (p. 79). Such a conceptual model is congruent with social work's respect for individuals and their subjectivity, as well as the communities within which they are embedded, and facilitates an extension of moral concern to the natural environment and *all* animals. As such, it represents a genuinely holistic and non-anthropocentric worldview.

Relationship between animal companions and social work

The fact that domesticated animals are part and parcel of the social environment – the world within which social workers practise – should, of necessity, serve to widen the scope of social work's moral compass. Indeed, animals are routinely regarded as family members by many of those people with whom social workers work, and by social workers themselves in their private lives. As noted by Sorabji (1993), the animals who share our lives 'are literally *oikeioi* – members of the household' (p. 215). For these reasons, the remainder of this chapter concerns itself with the relationship between animal companions and social work. To facilitate reflection upon the nature of social work's direct duties to animals and the moral impediments that invariably frustrate such considerations, a practice scenario is provided.

> Pat, an elderly single male, with no close relatives, has to find new accommodation for himself and his beloved 13-year-old dog Tess. The house he has been renting for many years was recently sold, and he needs to vacate within the month. His income means that he can now only afford a unit, and he has been referred to a community social worker after having no success in obtaining a new rental property. All owners have stipulated that no animals are permitted. It has been suggested that he needs to find a new home for the dog, or failing that, given her age and frailty, that the kindest thing may be to have Tess euthanized.

Animals are conspicuously absent from social work ethical literature and codes of ethics, with Banks (1995) effectively speaking for the discipline when she unequivocally and emphatically states: 'Moral judgements are about *human welfare*' (p. 10). Where fleeting mention of animals is made in the literature, it is invariably cursory and unsympathetic, sending the unmistakable message that they are of no meaningful moral consequence (Clark, 2000; Clark and Asquith, 1985; Beckett and Maynard, 2010).

The chief culprit for this moral indifference is the principle of *respect for persons*, seen by many as the cardinal social work principle, from which all others are derived. Emanating from Kant's categorical imperative that *persons* must always be treated as ends in themselves, it makes a crucial moral distinction between *subjects* – to whom direct duties are owed – and *things* – to which indirect duties are owed. Rationality, not consciousness, is held to determine unconditional and absolute value, and tellingly Kant (1989[1775]) declares: 'Our duties towards animals are merely indirect duties towards humanity' (p. 23). Given the discipline's philosophical indebtedness to Kant, it is unsurprising that moral value is conceived as a human-only affair.

That said, *respect for persons* is seen by not a few as highly problematic for many human beings given the pre-eminence accorded to rationality – for example, babies and young children, and adults with profound cognitive impairment – and one more and more viewed as fundamentally incongruent with social work's moral imagination. Increasingly, the principle of *respect for human beings* is embraced as a way around these substantial objections, with respect linked to taking decisive account of the interests of each human being, and a far wider range of capacities (Watson, 1978).

While acknowledging that the expanded characteristics of value are not exclusive to humans, Watson (1978) puzzlingly pays it no moral heed, in spite of the fact that there is no capacity that is possessed by *all* humans, and by *no* animals. In rescuing all humans, it simultaneously sidelines all animals from moral consideration. While our common humanity has its foundation in a natural sympathy, it does not follow that the latter is peculiar to the human species (Clark, 1995b; Midgley, 1983a).

Both principles, informed as they are by an exclusive humanism, are patently inadequate to ground and guide notions of duty and obligation beyond the human sphere. Neither provides any reasons to consider the interests of Tess in the practice scenario. At best, any duties to her would be construed by any social worker using either principle as *indirect* duties to Pat. For instance, consider Clark and Asquith's (1985) observation:

> it is possible that personhood is extended to domestic pets. When people say their dog is one of the family they may be speaking more literally than metaphorically. The pet may well receive every possible care and comfort, denied to arguably more deserving persons away from the family orbit.
>
> (p. 18)

This tells us a number of important things. First, the admission of the possibility of personhood is patently inconsistent with either principle. Second, Pat – as most people with animals are – *is* literal when he says that Tess is family, for mixed communities are not merely metaphorical. His initial incredulity at the supposedly helpful suggestions that he either find a new home or seriously consider euthanizing Tess quickly gives way to his incredulity that anyone would have the audacity to propose such a thing, pointedly asking how *they* would feel if it were suggested in respect of one of their human loved ones.

Third, the final sentence captures the systemic anthropocentrism of social work, the prejudice that the love, care, and attention given to individual family members, while understandable at one level, is at another to be condemned as it comes at the expense of more deserving humans outside the family. Pat's solicitude for Tess is ultimately a counterfeit of the genuine article. Not only is such an interpretation deeply insulting to him, but it also completely ignores the interests of his dog. The social worker's duties to Tess will be framed indirectly, whereas Pat gives greater priority to Tess's interests, as most would routinely do when it comes to our loved ones. He is moved by her particularity and preciousness, and contrary to the social worker, unabashedly conceives that he has compelling direct duties to her. To Pat, Tess *is* an end in herself.

Apart from the obvious fact that most social workers would be deeply offended if their relationships with *their* animals were similarly trivialized, it fundamentally misrepresents the very nature of mixed communities. Humans routinely enter into deep and abiding relationships with other animals, relationships nurtured and sustained by emotional fellowship:

> What makes creatures our fellow beings, entitled to basic consideration, is surely not intellectual capacity but emotional fellowship. And if we ask what powers can justify a higher claim ... those that seem to be most relevant are sensibility, social and emotional complexity of the kind which is expressed by the formation of deep, subtle lasting relationships.
>
> (Midgley, 1985: 60)

Furthermore, Pat would most likely heartily concur with Clark's (1997) observation:

> The first charge upon our moral account is to care for those who are in our care, to be loyal to those with whom we have bonds of affection and familiarity. Only a doctrinaire humanism can ignore the obvious fact that among those domestic ties are ties of friendship and family loyalty to animals not of our species ... treating them [human strangers] 'like animals' is not always a bad idea.
>
> (p. 106)

One of the more heartening, and morally serious, social work contributions considers that duties to animals can have a moral priority over the claims of humans. Just as the rights of the weak and vulnerable take priority in human communities, Ife (2001) maintains there will be occasions where the weakness and vulnerability of animals will give moral precedence to their interests over those of humans.

Although written specifically about our moral duties to fellow humans, Gaita's (1991) reflections on their preciousness and irreplaceability have relevance to human relationships with animals: 'They must be treated on every occasion in ways which reflect that their individuality conditions the way they limit our will' (p. 154). Apart from having obvious implications for the animals that literally share our lives and homes, it should apply to domesticated animals at large. Their individuality ought to limit the many ways in which humans currently see fit to use them as mere means to human ends, be that in factory farming, research laboratories, or the live-export trade. That very same individuality should also serve to limit our will so that vegetarianism, as Callicott (1988) argues, becomes morally obligatory. Humans need to reflect upon:

> what justifies the totally disproportionate cost of our presence? Ask it for once without presupposing the answer of the egotism of our species, as God might ask it about his creatures: Why should a dog or a guinea pig die an agonizing death in a laboratory experiment so that some human need not suffer just such a fate? ... Why, in the perspective of eternity, should the life of a human be more precious than that of a dog? Why should the dog's suffering weigh any less in the moral balance of the cosmos?
>
> (Kohak, 1987: 92)

A principle of *respect for individuals* would allow for respect to be extended not exclusively to *persons*, nor more inclusively to all human beings, but to *all* subjective and sentient creatures (Ryan, 2011). A social work concern for the non-human world, and a desire to be holistic, cannot but include animals within its moral circle, given that the essence of morality is 'attention to individuals, human individuals or individual realities of *other* kinds' (Murdoch, 1996: 38 emphasis added).

References

Anderson, P.E. (2008). *The powerful bond between people and pets: Our boundless connections to companion animals.* Westport, CT: Praeger.

Ascione, F., and Arkow, P. (Eds). (1999). *Child abuse, domestic violence, and animal abuse: Linking the circles of compassion for prevention and intervention.* West Lafayette, IN: Purdue University Press.

Attfield, R. (1991). *The ethics of environmental concern.* Athens, GA: University of Georgia Press.

Banks, S. (1995). *Ethics and values in social work.* London: Macmillan.

Beck, A., and Katcher, A. (1996). *Between pets and people: The importance of animal companionship.* West Lafayette, IN: Purdue University Press.

Beckett, C., and Maynard, A. (2010). *Values and ethics in social work: An introduction.* London: Sage.

Benton, T. (1993). *Natural relations: Ecology, animal rights and social justice.* London: Verso.

Callicott, J.B. (1979). Elements of an environmental ethic: moral considerability and the biotic community. *Environmental Ethics, 1,* 71–81.

Callicott, J.B. (1980). Animal liberation: A triangular affair. *Environmental Ethics, 2,* 311–338.

Callicott, J.B. (1985). Review of 'The case for animal rights'. *Environmental Ethics, 7,* 365–372.

Callicott, J.B. (1988). Animal liberation and environmental ethics: Back together again. *Between the Species, 4,* 163–169.

Callicott, J.B. (1989). The metaphysical implications of ecology. In J.B. Callicott (Ed.). *Nature in Asian traditions of thought: Essays in environmental philosophy*. New York: State University of New York Press. 51–64.

Callicott, J.B. (1998). 'Back together again' again. *Environmental Values, 7*, 461–475.

Clark, C. (2000). *Social work ethics: Politics, principles and practice*. Basingstoke: Palgrave Macmillan.

Clark, C., and Asquith, S. (1985). *Social work and social philosophy: A guide for practice*. London: Routledge & Kegan Paul.

Clark, S.R.L. (1983). Gaia and the forms of life. In R. Elliot and Gare, A. (Eds). *Environmental philosophy: A collection of readings*. St. Lucia: University of Queensland Press. 182–197.

Clark, S.R.L. (1985). Rights of the wild and tame. *Chronicles of Culture, 9*(8), 20–22.

Clark, S.R.L. (1986). *The mysteries of religion*. Oxford: Basil Blackwell.

Clark, S.R.L. (1994). New issues: Genetic and other engineering. *Journal of Applied Philosophy, 11*(2), 233–237.

Clark, S.R.L. (1995a). Objective values, final causes: Stoics, Epicureans, and Platonists. *Electronic Journal of Analytical Philosophy, 3*, 1–7.

Clark, S.R.L. (1995b). Enlarging the community: Companion animals. In B. Almond (Ed.). *Introducing applied ethics*. Oxford: Basil Blackwell. 318–330.

Clark, S.R.L. (1997). *Animals and their moral standing*. London: Routledge.

Coates, J. (2003). *Ecology and social work: A new paradigm*. Halifax, NS: Fernwood.

Coetzee, J.M. (1999). *The lives of animals*. Princeton, NJ: Princeton University Press.

Darwin, C. (1936). *The origin of species and the descent of man*. New York: Modern Library.

Fine, A. (Ed.). (2010). *Handbook on animal-assisted therapy: Theoretical foundations and guidelines for practice*. London: Academic Press.

Fisher, J. (1982). Taking sympathy seriously: A defence of our moral psychology toward animals. In E. Hargrove (Ed.). *The animal rights/environmental ethics debate: The environmental perspective*. Albany, NY: State University of New York Press. 227–248.

Fox, W. (1991). Self and world: A transpersonal, ecological approach. *Revision: Journal of Consciousness and Change, 13*(3), 116–121.

Gaita, R. (1991). *Good and evil: An absolute conception*. Basingstoke: Macmillan.

Gray, M., and Coates, J. (2011). The environment and social work: An overview and introduction. *International Journal of Social Welfare, 21*, 1–9. Article first published online: 13 DEC 2011 | DOI: 10.1111/j.1468-2397.2011.00851.x.

Griffin, D. (1984). *Animal thinking*. Cambridge, MA: Harvard University Press.

Hanrahan, C. (2011). Challenging anthropocentrism in social work through ethics and spirituality: Lessons from studies in human–animal bonds. *Journal of Religion and Spirituality in Social Work: Social Thought, 30*(3), 272–293.

Hardy, T. (1930). *The later years of Thomas Hardy: 1892–1928*. New York: Macmillan.

Hay, P. (2002). *Main currents in western environmental thought*. Sydney: University of New South Wales Press.

Hearne, V. (1987) *Adam's task: Calling animals by name*. New York: Knopf.

Hume, D. (1998[1777]). *An enquiry concerning the principles of morals*. Oxford: Oxford University Press.

Ife, J. (2001). *Human rights and social work: Towards right-based practice*. Cambridge: Cambridge University Press.

Johnson, L. (1993). *A morally deep world: An essay on moral significance and environmental ethics.* Cambridge: Cambridge University Press.

Kant, I. (1989[1775]). Duties in regards to animals. In T. Regan and Singer, P. (Eds). *Animal rights and human obligations.* Englewood Cliffs: Prentice-Hall. 23–24.

Kheel, M. (1996). A liberation of nature: a circular affair. In J. Donovan and Adams, C. (Eds). *Beyond animal rights: A feminist caring ethic for the treatment of animals.* New York: Continuum. 17–33.

Kohak, E. (1987). *The embers and the stars.* Chicago: University of Chicago Press.

Leopold, A. (1949). *A sand country almanac.* New York: Oxford University Press.

Linzey, A. (Ed.). (2009). *The link between animal abuse and human violence.* Brighton: Sussex Academic Press.

Linzey, A., and Cohn-Sherbok, D. (1997). *After Noah: Animals and the liberation of theology.* London: SPCK.

Loar, Lynn (1999). 'I'll only help you if you have two legs': Or why human service professionals should pay attention to cases involving cruelty to animals. In F. Ascione and Arkow, P. (Eds). *Child abuse, domestic violence, and animal abuse: Linking the circles of compassion for prevention and intervention.* West Lafayette, IN: Purdue University Press. 120–136.

McKinnon, J. (2008). Exploring the nexus between social work and the environment. *Australian Social Work, 61*(3), 256–268.

Midgley, M. (1983a). *Animals and why they matter.* Athens, GA: University of Georgia Press.

Midgley, M. (1983b). Duties concerning islands. In R. Elliot and Gare, A. (Eds). *Environmental philosophy: A collection of readings.* St. Lucia: University of Queensland Press. 166–180.

Midgley, M. (1984). On being terrestrial. *Royal Institute of Philosophy Lecture Series, 17,* 79–91.

Midgley, M. (1985). Persons and non-persons. In P. Singer (Ed.). *In defence of animals.* Oxford: Basil Blackwell. 52–62.

Midgley, M. (1992a). A problem of concern. In R. Ryder (Ed.). *Animal welfare and the environment.* London: Duckworth/RSPCA. 62–67.

Midgley, M. (1992b). Is the biosphere a luxury? *Hastings Center Report, 22*(3), 7–12.

Midgley, M. (1996). *Beast and man: The roots of human nature.* London: Routledge.

Midgley, M. (2003). *The myths we live by.* London: Routledge.

Murdoch, I. (1993). *Metaphysics as a guide to morals.* London: Penguin.

Murdoch, I. (1996). *The sovereignty of good.* London: Routledge.

Naess, A. (1973). The shallow and the deep, long-range ecology movement: A summary. *Inquiry, 16,* 95–100.

Nash, R. (1990). *The rights of nature: A history of environmental ethics.* Leichhardt: Primavera Press.

Passmore, J. (1974). *Man's responsibility for nature: Ecological problems and western traditions.* London: Duckworth.

Pluhar, E. (1983). Two conceptions of an environmental ethic and their implications. *Ethics and Animals, 4*(4), 110–127.

Pluhar, E. (1995). *Beyond prejudice: The moral significance of human and nonhuman animals.* Durham, NC: Duke University Press.

Plumwood, V. (1992). Sealskin. *Meanjin, 1,* 45–57.

Podberscek, A., Paul, E., and Serpell, J. (Eds). (2000). *Companion animals and us: Exploring the relationships between people and pets.* Cambridge: Cambridge University Press.

Preece, R. (2005). *Brute souls, happy beasts and evolution: The historical status of animals.* Vancouver: University of British Columbia Press.

Rachels, J. (1999). *Created from animals: The moral implications of Darwinism.* Oxford: Oxford University Press.

Regan, T. (1982). *All that dwell therein: Essays on animal rights and environmental ethics.* Berkeley, CA: University of California Press.

Regan, T. (1983). *The case for animal rights.* London: Routledge & Kegan Paul.

Risley-Curtiss, C. (2010). Social work practitioners and the human–animal bond: A national study. *Social Work, 55*(1), 38–46.

Rowlands, M. (2002). *Animals like us.* London: Verso.

Ryan, T. (1993). *The widening circle: Should social work concern itself with nonhuman animal rights?* Unpublished Honours Thesis, James Cook University, Townsville, North Queensland.

Ryan, T. (2011). *Animals and social work: A moral introduction.* Basingstoke: Palgrave Macmillan.

Sable, P. (1995). Pets, attachment, and well-being across the life cycle. *Social Work, 40*(3), 334–341.

Sapontzis, S. (1984). J. Baird Callicott, animal liberation: A triangular affair. *Ethics and Animals, 5,* 113–121.

Schweitzer, A. (1955). *Civilization and ethics.* London: Adam & Charles Black.

Serpell, J. (1986). *In the company of animals: A study of human–animal relationships.* Oxford: Basil Blackwell.

Sharpe, L. (2005). *Creatures like us? A relational approach to the moral status of animals.* Exeter: Imprint Academic.

Singer, P. (1976). *Animal liberation: A new code of ethics for our treatment of animals.* London: Jonathan Cape.

Singer, P., and Mason, J. (2006). *The way we eat: Why our food choices matter.* Emmaus, PA: Rodale.

Sorabji, R. (1993). *Animal minds and human morals: The origins of the western debate.* London: Duckworth.

Tedeschi, P., Fitchett, J., and Molidor, C. (2005). The incorporation of animal-assisted interventions in social work education. *Journal of Family Social Work, 9*(4), 59–77.

Thomas, K. (1983). *Man and the natural world: Changing attitudes in England 1500–1800.* London: Allen Lane.

Thoreau, H.D. (1968). *Walden.* London: Dutton.

Turner, F.J. (1996). *Social work treatment: Interlocking theoretical approaches.* New York: Free Press.

Warren, M.A. (1983). The rights of the nonhuman world. In R. Elliot and Gare, A. (Eds). *Environmental philosophy: A collection of readings.* 109–134.

Warren, M.A. (1997). *Moral status: Obligations to persons and other living things.* Oxford: Oxford University Press.

Watson, D. (1978). Social services in a nutshell. In N. Timms and Watson, D. (Eds). *Philosophy in social work.* London: Routledge & Kegan Paul. 26–49.

White, L. (1967). The historical roots of our ecologic crisis. *Science, 155,* 1203–1207.

Wilkes, R. (1981). *Social work with undervalued groups.* London: Tavistock.

Wolf, D. B. (2000) Social work and speciesism. *Social Work, 45*(1), 88–93.

Zapf, M. (2009). *Social work and the environment: Understanding people and place.* Toronto, ON: Canadian Scholars Press.

9 Restoration not incarceration

An environmentally based pilot initiative for working with young offenders

Christine Lynn Norton, Barbara Holguin, and Jarid Manos

> Those who dwell among the beauties and mysteries of the earth are never alone or weary of life (Rachel Carson, 1965 as cited in Lewis, 2012)

In many Western industrial societies, human and environmental concerns have been considered separate problems. This modern dualistic view, based on the idea that humans are separate from nature, may actually worsen social and environmental problems (Roszak, 2001). Nowhere has this view been more pronounced than in the United States criminal justice system. Here humans are literally separated from nature, imprisoned in built structures, sometimes in solitary confinement, and often under inhumane conditions (Ross, 2011). In fact, the US has the largest prison population in the world with 650,000 people being released from State and Federal prisons each year (Harrison and Beck, 2005), 100,000 of whom are juveniles discharged from locked facilities (Snyder and Sickmund, 2006). This large prison population is due to a variety of complex issues, including violent crime related to gun accessibility, harsher sentencing laws, especially regarding drug use and possession, as well as American values and moral judgements focusing on accountability of the individual (Whitman, 2003).

On reentering society, these former inmates often drift from one place to the next, experiencing homelessness, substance abuse, and physical and mental health problems as well as significant challenges in housing, education, employment, and family and community reintegration (Gibbons and Katzenbach, 2006; Solomon, Palmer, Atkinson, Davidson, and Harvey, 2006). According to the Commission on Safety and Abuse in America's Prisons (in Gibbons and Katzenbach, 2006), 67 per cent of former prisoners were rearrested and 52 per cent were reincarcerated within three years of their release. While there is no national recidivism data for juveniles, Snyder and Sickmund (2006) reported an average recidivism rate of 55 per cent. These statistics demonstrate how ill-equipped society is to deal with the reintegration and rehabilitation of offenders.

Though many different approaches to offender reentry and recidivism reduction have been attempted (Blechman, Maurice, Buecker, and

Helberg, 2000; Warren, 2007), only a few have considered the role of the natural environment in the rehabilitation process (Ulrich and Nadkarni, 2008; Thigpen, Beauclair, and Carroll, 2011). If integrated and effective solutions to these problems are to be reached, it is important to move towards prisoner reentry and recidivism reduction programs built on reciprocal models of human and ecological restoration (Geist and Galatowitsch, 1999).

This chapter describes an environmentally based pilot initiative that sought to address the complex problems surrounding offender reintegration by using this type of reciprocal model. Called *Restoration Not Incarceration (RNI)*, it was developed by the Great Plains Restoration Council (GPRC) in the USA. This initiative engages formerly incarcerated young men and women in ecological restoration of Houston's (Texas) prairies, bayous, wetlands, and Gulf Coast shore in partnership with the Harris County Corrections System and Bread of Life shelter. RNI proactively promotes prosocial values and productive work in nature – restoration – as an avenue for young adults to reintegrate into society and improve their life outcomes – rehabilitation.

The purpose of this chapter is to provide an example of grassroots program development using an environmental social work approach. It is our hope that social work students, practitioners, and community providers who read this chapter will gain insight into the connection between theory and practice in environmental social work with former offenders, as well as the concrete steps needed to implement an initiative like RNI. In the end, we would like the reader to be able to grasp the benefits and challenges to developing and implementing this type of initiative, and we would like this chapter to spur meaningful dialogue about the viability of initiatives like this, as well as the implications for social work practice and research.

Incarceration and recidivism

Given the high costs of incarceration, as well as overcrowding in US prisons, there has been a strong push to implement evidence-based programs that will reduce recidivism and promote the reintegration of former offenders into society (Janetta, 2011). According to Warren (2007), recidivism reduction programs that are implemented and designed properly are more cost effective than incarceration in reducing crime. In particular, cognitive behavioural interventions (Harper and Chitty, 2004) and life-skills training (Blechman *et al.*, 2000) have been shown to be most effective in reducing recidivism.

Janetta (2011) reviewed 26 different recidivism reduction programs and found similar evidence of what constitutes best practices: 'the principles of effective intervention are program design elements that have a demonstrated relationship to program success in reducing recidivism' (p. 6). These program elements include:

- use of risk and needs assessment information
- clarity of the program's theoretical model
- existence of a program manual or curricular material
- use of cognitive-behavioural or social learning methods
- responsiveness to important differences among offenders such as in learning styles
- use of positive reinforcement
- use of motivational enhancement techniques
- establishment of continuities with other programs and prosocial support networks
- staff attributes
- collection and use of program data (Janetta, 2011).

These critical components of properly designed and implemented recidivism reduction programs are often supported through group work. While little research has been done on its impact on formerly incarcerated young adults, the Substance Abuse and Mental Health Services Administration in the United States (SAMHSA, 2011) recommends the use of psychoeducational and support groups to assist former offenders who were arrested specifically because of substance abuse issues. Psychoeducational and support groups offer members the opportunity to learn new skills, build mutual aid, share resources, develop leadership ability, and create a sense solidarity (Shulman, 2009). SAMHSA believes that targeted programs for ex-offenders, in particular those with substance abuse problems, should offer respect, hope, positive incentives, clear and accessible information, consistency, compassion, information about the career ladder, and assistance with skills transfer. In keeping with the last two SAMHSA guidelines, many recidivism reduction programs focus on employment. According to Visher, Winterfield, and Coggeshall (2005):

> Stable, satisfying employment is a critical predictor of post-release success for individuals released from prison. However, former prisoners typically have poor work histories and a limited range of skills. These deficits, coupled with a recent felony conviction and period of incarceration, often lead to difficulty finding and keeping a job that will allow these individuals to provide financial support for themselves, and for many of them, their families.
>
> (p. 17)

For this reason, employment interventions are often implemented with former offenders and 'can include a range of services such as job-readiness classes, vocational education, GED certification, job training, job placement, and job monitoring by a case manager for some time period' (Visher *et al.*, 2005: 17). Despite the need for these programs, however, the community employment programs for ex-offenders surveyed in Visher *et al.*'s (2005) study did *not* reduce recidivism. While it is clear that employment interventions are needed, they are not sufficient in and of themselves in reducing recidivism. Rather, Harper and Chitty (2004) believe that successful community reintegration may be the most important factor for reducing recidivism. However, this is often hardest to achieve due to what SAMHSA (2011) refers to as offender alienation, which can occur from substantial time spent in prison away from societal norms and prosocial relationships. This alienation, and the subsequent culture shock that can sometimes occur when a person is released from prison, requires holistic, community-based responses, such as environmentally-based initiatives (SAMHSA, 2011).

Environmentally based initiatives

More relevant to this chapter are the emerging US initiatives using life-skills training in the context of environmental sustainability and conservation (Ulrich and Nadkarni, 2008; Thigpen *et al.*, 2011). For example, the 'green prison reform' initiative has been enacted in the state of Washington through the Sustainable Prisons Project, a partnership between the Washington State Department of Corrections, the Evergreen State College, and the Nature Conservancy. Through the creation of partnerships between ecologists and prisoners, its goal is to reduce the environmental, economic, and human costs of imprisonment by training prison staff and offenders to understand and appreciate the science of sustainability and develop skills for the emerging green economy (Ulrich and Nadkarni, 2008). Beginning as an initiative to create a more sustainable prison system, the program has expanded to include organic gardens producing healthy food grown by and for inmates, while at the same time promoting prairie restoration and related biological research. Though the 'greening of corrections' has become a national movement in the US (Thigpen *et al.*, 2011), the main focus has been on sustainability, green workforce development, and life-skills training for those who are currently incarcerated, rather than for inmates who are released.

The importance of these initiatives notwithstanding, recidivism reduction programs that incorporate the natural world are also needed for inmates who are released from prison to address mental and physical health issues and help former offenders reintegrate with their community in meaningful ways. Given the proven benefits of human contact with nature, environmentally based recidivism reduction programs may be even more effective than traditional programs (Berman, Jonides, and Kaplan, 2008; Groenewegen, van den Berg, De Vries, and Verheij, 2006; Mitchell and Popham, 2008). Based on the reciprocal ecosystem restoration model (Geist and Galatowitsch, 1999), *Restoration Not Incarceration* uses environmental restoration work in nature as a therapeutic modality for promoting mental and physical health, guided by principles of ecology and social work. The program also works to promote successful community reintegration by working collaboratively with other agencies and engaging participants to give back to the community through land restoration work.

Reciprocal ecosystem restoration model

The reciprocal ecosystem restoration model arose from the ecological and social needs present in human communities. Spurred by the loss of biodiversity and the devastation of fragile ecosystems, the need for ecological restoration of the land has emerged as an important strategy in conservation biology (Geist and Galatowitsch, 1999). However, the role of humans in contributing to this loss and devastation, as well as being able to reverse it, has long been neglected. This disconnection between human and environmental issues limits prior ideas about restoration, which must be redefined and expanded 'to include humans in a reciprocal relationship with the natural environment' (Geist and Galatowitsch, 1999: 971). According to Geist and Galatowitsch (1999), the reciprocal ecosystem restoration model 'integrates the essential elements of both ecological and human restoration' and aims to increase 'human commitment to restoration by restoring relationships with the environment' (p. 971). In other words, the model considers what humans might contribute to meet ecological restoration needs, while examining what nature provides for human needs based on research on the human benefits of having a relationship with nature (Berman *et al.*, 2008; Groenewegen *et al.*, 2006; Mitchell and Popham, 2008). According to Wilson's (1993) biophilia hypothesis, human beings have an innate connection to nature, and this relationship has affective qualities. Kaplan and Kaplan's (1989) work reaffirms this hypothesis by documenting some of the restorative benefits to humans that come from being in nature, including, but not limited to, improved focus and attention, elevation of mood, and a sense of belonging. It is important to note that exposure to nature has physiological, psychological, and spiritual benefits, and some environmental psychologists have gone so far as to label these 'Vitamin G', referring to green spaces that can lead to improved health (Groenewegen *et al.*, 2006).

While this research certainly supports the use of the reciprocal restoration model as a means of promoting positive mental and physical health, why should it be applied to recidivism reduction programs for former offenders? We believe the answer can be found in the fact that nature is a therapeutic setting (Berger and McLeod, 2006) and a 'connection between humans and the natural environment is integral to developing a sense of place' (Geist and Galatowitsch, 1999: 973) to ensure successful community reintegration, which Harper and Chitty (2004) found to be a key factor in preventing recidivism. If former offenders feel a deeper connection to their communities by helping to restore the land, a case can be made that they will experience personal restoration as well. The motto of *Restoration Not*

Incarceration, 'Heal the earth and self', draws upon the reciprocal ecosystem restoration model, as does the program itself.

Applying the model: Restoration Not Incarceration

The Great Plains Restoration Council (GPRC, 2011) was founded on the belief that protecting wild nature is a public health matter because of its potential to restore human lives. *Restoration Not Incarceration* (RNI) is one of GPRC's pilot initiatives developed to help previously incarcerated youth to reintegrate into society through participating in an ecological restoration project in Houston's shattered prairies. This section describes the program's development, collaboration, participants, staffing, framework, curriculum, and goals.

Program development

Program development in social work is informed by a range of considerations, including research, resource availability, organizational support, and practice experience. In community contexts, it is also driven by community concerns and needs and successful community programs often succeed through the passion and drive of those involved. *Restoration Not Incarceration* is no different. RNI was started by GPRC Founder and CEO Jarid Manos, who had previously applied the ideas of reciprocal restoration with youth in the Dallas Fort Worth area in a program called Plains Youth InterACTION, which:

> engages children in discovering the values of leadership and personal responsibility for their own health, their life's direction and their environment … the active process of hands-on ecological restoration and protection is threaded into self restoration and protection so both are healed at the same time, and deeper, richer, healthier lives are engendered.
>
> (GPRC, 2011: 4)

Manos believed this approach would also work well with other populations. Based on his practice and life experience, Manos decided to adapt the reciprocal restoration model for young offenders. He discovered that Harris County Corrections in Houston, Texas had previously piloted a Corrections Conservation Corps in which inmates performed community service projects in local parks and recreational areas (GPRC, 2011). However, the Sheriff's office had not yet gotten behind a restart of similar and enhanced efforts, despite the strong support of the Harris County Attorney's Office. Manos realized that a pilot initiative like RNI would probably not be equipped to work with incarcerated inmates and considerable staffing and security measures would have to be in place for that to happen.

Instead, Manos reached out to formerly incarcerated young offenders who had been released from prison and were participating in the Bread of Life After Dark Program providing the Downtown-Midtown Houston homeless community with low-impact shelter, consistent service linkage, and case management support. While RNI was not affiliated directly with the criminal justice system, Harris County Corrections helped Manos identify participants who had recently been released into the community. Even though the initiative was not an official diversion program affiliated with the criminal justice system, Manos chose the name *Restoration Not Incarceration* to highlight the two very different paths or life choices available to participants. He also garnered support for the initiative from the criminal justice system and other agencies. Harris County Corrections and Bread of Life were glad to have RNI's assistance in helping these formerly incarcerated young people 'walk through the process of re-entry' (Fairman, 2010: 7) and provide them with additional support. In this way, RNI responded to the overwhelming need of the criminal justice system in Houston, faced with overcrowded jails and prisons and high numbers of incarcerated individuals, who often face daunting challenges, such as homelessness, upon reentry into the community.

RNI also responded to the ecological needs of the Houston community. The native Gulf Coastal Prairie is among the most severely damaged and least protected of any major ecosystem. Less than 1 per cent of native Gulf Coastal Prairie remains, mostly in Texas. Many native prairie wildlife and plant species are threatened with extinction due to human encroachment on wild habitats necessary for their survival. The coastal prairie region is home to 700 species of birds, animals, and reptiles at risk of losing their habitat. Protecting and restoring native prairies conserves the habitat of other prairie wildlife like prairie dogs and grassland nesting birds. RNI offered one means of restoring native coastal prairie in the Houston area, while providing special rehabilitative work opportunities and psychosocial support to formerly incarcerated young people.

Collaborative approach

As with any grassroots social work program, a collaborative approach is the best way to ensure meaningful community engagement in a new project. In order to pilot the *Restoration Not Incarceration* initiative, key stakeholders were identified to recruit participants and staff, and to pool resources to develop an ecological restoration project *and* meet the psychosocial needs of the participants. Key stakeholders in the project included Harris County Corrections, the Bread of Life shelter, and St John's Downtown United Methodist Church. As previously mentioned, Harris County Corrections helped identify potential formerly incarcerated participants who were living at Bread of Life shelter. By partnering with Bread of Life, RNI ensured that participants had access to hot meals, laundry services, showers, case management, anger and stress management, medical services and referrals, and substance abuse counselling, services which were not provided by RNI, but were essential to the reintegration process. Bread of Life also collaborated with other local agencies to provide RNI participants with mental health counselling and legal aid when needed. St John's donated the land for the project and RNI consulted with a local ecologist from the Bayou Preservation Association in planning the land restoration project. The ecologist helped RNI develop strategies for the removal of non-native species and minimized recovery time, two important components of successful land restoration (Geist and Galatowitsch, 1999). Likewise, funders for the project were needed to cover work stipends, meals, staff salaries, promotional materials, and so on. Funders for the project included several prominent local foundations.

Participants

Participants were identified by Harris County Corrections and recruited at the Bread of Life shelter. Residents were introduced to the program as an opportunity to develop job and life skills, while contributing to the environment. RNI staff conducted screening interviews to determine the appropriateness of the program for participants and vice versa. During these interviews, the Coordinator explained that the program was strictly voluntary and participants would receive incentives for their work, such as nutritious meals, a small stipend, and individual and psychosocial group work support at no cost. Participants were informed that, even if they signed up for the program, they were allowed to leave at any time if they wished.

The Criminal Justice Coordinator, a Master's level sociologist trained in criminal justice, conducted screening interviews using the Level Service Inventory Review (LSI-R), which is utilized by professionals in the social service field to assess client need and risk. According to Andrews and Bonta (2011):

> The LSI-R™ assessment is a quantitative survey of offender attributes and offender situations relevant for making decisions about levels of supervision and treatment. The instrument's applications include assisting in the allocation of resources, helping to make probation and placement decisions, making appropriate security level classifications, and assessing treatment progress ... LSI-R scores are proven to help predict parole outcome, success in correctional halfway houses, institutional misconduct, and recidivism.
>
> (pp. 1–2)

By using this tool, the Criminal Justice Coordinator was able to assess the program's appropriateness for the participants. The pilot group of RNI participants thus recruited comprised three men and a woman. All were formerly incarcerated African-American young adults, aged between 19 and 25 years, who were living at the shelter. The information gained during the pre-screening interviews also yielded important information about the participants' prior offences, as well as their substance abuse and mental health histories. Their prior offences included the unauthorized use of a motor vehicle, misdemeanour assault charges, Federal interstate drug trafficking, possession of marijuana, a terroristic threat, illegal possession of a firearm, and theft. Three participants reported problems with substance abuse and two with a prior history of serious mental health issues. The Criminal Justice Coordinator determined that all participants could take part in the program, especially given their willingness to be involved and the fact that they would be receiving multiple levels of support from RNI and Bread of Life.

Staff

According to Janetta (2011), staff attributes are a key aspect of successful recidivism reduction programs. Participants are more likely to relate to staff with a similar life history and racial and ethnic identity. This was certainly true for RNI. Visionary founder and CEO, Jarid Manos, provided participants with an African-American role model of someone who had once lived on the streets, been incarcerated, and struggled in many of the same ways that they had, yet had risen above those challenges to make something of himself and give back to the community. This made him very accessible to participants, especially since he worked alongside them every day of the challenging land restoration project.

In addition to GPRC administrative staff, Manos hired a Criminal Justice Coordinator who provided psychosocial group work and case management services in conjunction with Bread of Life staff, and monitored participants' weekly progress through self-reporting and assessments. Not only was the Criminal Justice Coordinator professionally qualified for this role, she was also a tangible role model for program participants. As a young Hispanic woman, who came from a 'tough upbringing and poor background', she was kicked out of her house, left to fend for herself, and had put herself through school. In several instances, she chose to share elements of her life story with participants not only to build trust, but also to create a sense of hope that they, too, could rise above the challenges they were facing. The Criminal Justice Coordinator made herself accessible to participants, who could contact her at any time, which they found helpful. Many times during the program a participant called to express concern for another's well-being. Sometimes calls came from a participant unable to connect with family or access needed resources. In this way, the Coordinator provided case management and crisis support.

Along with the RNI staff, members of the business community volunteered their time as mentors to work with participants on an individual basis. The goal was to give participants a chance to think about their aspirations and how to reach them, and how they might create a network in the community to help them in this endeavour. While a weekly 'mentoring hour' was available to those who chose to attend, only one participant took advantage of this opportunity. This was not surprising given that initially participants were very closed and distrusting of others, especially if they were from different backgrounds.

Program framework

Restoration Not Incarceration is an ecological health initiative targeting the restoration of Greater Houston's prairies, bayous, wetlands, and Gulf Coast shore while assisting young adults and juveniles in the Harris County Corrections System in their reintegration into society (GPRC, 2011). It offers a brief, intensive intervention comprising a structured ecological health curriculum, bi-weekly psychoeducational group work, and land restoration work. Facilitated over a 12-week period, participants were together for four days a week, when they met on-site, restoring the land while reflecting on their lives in nature. Twice a week, the group would meet at the RNI office or another forum, to allow for a more comfortable learning environment (the public library was often used) for a two-hour psychoeducational group to build life skills while reflecting on the concepts and values taught in the ecological health curriculum. The program's dual focus aimed to restore nature while equipping participants with valuable life skills.

Ecological health curriculum

Janetta (2011) highlighted the importance of a clear theoretical model and structured curriculum to work effectively with former offenders. For this reason, the RNI program focuses on the concept of ecological health and the development of related life skills. Ecological health is defined as the interdependent health of humans, animals, and ecosystems and aims to improve the health of all three interlocking social 'ecosystems':

1   *Self:* physical, mental, emotional, and spiritual
2   *Community:* relationships with others
3   *Native prairie ecosystems:* the living, breathing, and damaged natural world (GPRC, 2011).

This integrated ecosystems model is not new to social work but has been broadened to an eco-social approach, which redefines the central person-in-environment concept to include the natural world and seeks a deeper connection between humans and nature (Coates, 2003; Norton, 2011). The ecological health model has much in common with the eco-social. The core

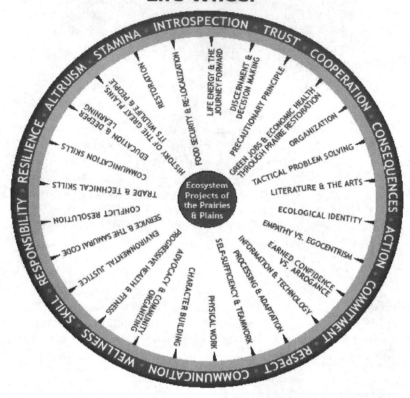

Figure 9.1 Life Wheel

concepts of the ecological health curriculum are taught via the Life Wheel, a trademarked tool developed by Manos (GPRC, 2011) to promote prosocial behaviours (see Figure 9.1). The Life Wheel was modelled on the Indigenous medicine wheel (Dapice, 2006) used for healing and teaching purposes. The framework of the Life Wheel served as a guide for the psychoeducational group sessions and land restoration fieldwork. Each spoke of the Life Wheel was accompanied by a set of exercises to promote discussion on prosocial values, thoughts, and behaviours.

Psychoeducational group work

Through exposure to prosocial values, relationships, and life skills in psychoeducational groups, participants were helped to understand and cope with mental health and substance-abuse issues, as well as other challenges in their lives. The group provided opportunities for participants to practise their newfound communication and problem-solving skills. At the beginning of the group sessions, participants created group rules and norms with the help of the Criminal Justice Coordinator, who facilitated the groups. Each week, the group reviewed these norms and discussed progress in the 'on-site' fieldwork component of the curriculum. The group engaged in hands-on activities in the classroom and field that promoted the development of communication, relationships, decision making, problem solving, conflict resolution, time management, and basic employment skills, such as how to complete an application form, appropriate dress, and follow up following a job interview. Participants were able to explore difficult emotions, deal with conflict, and assertive rather than aggressive communication. Participants engaged in ongoing reflection on group process and dynamics and the ecological health curriculum content.

Ecological land restoration

Given the voluntary nature of the program, by agreeing to participate, the participants gave their commitment to give back to the community, especially since the shelter was closed during the day until four in the afternoon. Through education and deeper learning in the areas of ecology, sustainability, and personal growth, participants learnt about the history of the Great Plains and developed awareness of their environment, its wildlife and people. By understanding the 'big picture' it was hoped that participants would get a sense of their own unique place in history and develop a deeper commitment to playing a positive role in this story. However, a true commitment to restoration relies on the development 'of significant human relationships' (Geist and Galatowitsch, 1999: 972). As relationships developed between staff and participants in the program, the motivation to maintain consistent attendance and punctuality increased. As the work project began to take shape, participants could see the impact of their labour and noticed the ways in which the natural world responded. In the first year of being opened, native coastal prairie plants like rattlesnake master, Maximillian sunflower, slender gayfeather, and little bluestem grass emerged from remnant seeds in the ancestral soil, all because of the hard work of the program participants in removing non-native species.

The land restoration work involved cutting down more than a thousand invasive and non-native trees, bushes, and vines, without the aid of heavy machinery, to transform the donated tract of land, an unkempt unnatural forest, into an inhabitable site for coastal prairie wildlife and humans alike. This work took place in the gruelling Texas heat, and was difficult physical labour. There were many times when participants wanted to throw in the towel but they were encouraged by Manos, who continued to work alongside them. The tough work environment led to group conflict and feelings of frustration and despair. At these times, Manos looked for opportunities to point to the lessons of the Life Wheel. Manos encouraged introspection, an important aspect of the ecological health model. Self-reflection was critically important as participants processed their group experiences and reentry into society following incarceration. Participants gradually developed the physical, mental, and emotional stamina and perseverance to complete the land restoration work, in the process developing into a tight knit, trusting, and supportive group, and finding time for quiet contemplation in nature (Norton, 2010). In connecting with nature, participants were encouraged to ponder: What do I know about the place where I live? How do I connect to the earth? What is my purpose as a human being? These questions are central to the development of an *ecological identity*: 'a profound sense of oneself in relationship to natural and social ecosystems' in which the individual uses 'the direct experience of nature as a framework for personal decisions, professional choices, political action, and spiritual inquiry' (Thomashow, 1996: xiii).

Individual, group, and program goals

The goal of the program is to reduce recidivism by educating formerly incarcerated young offenders on how to take ownership of their personal development, while engaged in environmental restoration. The ecological health curriculum, group involvement, and hands-on fieldwork experience provided opportunities for participants to use these life skills to improve their social relationships and connection to the community. Participants' personal goals included the following:

- *Participant A*: learn how to do nails, go to school, and get a job.
- *Participant B*: become a business owner, go to school, and support my family.
- *Participant C*: complete GED, go to cosmetology school, and get a job.
- *Participant D*: go to school, become a zoologist, and work with animals.

In order to achieve these larger personal goals, it was critical for participants to work through the ecological health curriculum and land restoration project from start to finish as a first step. All four participants completed the program.

Evaluating the impact of the program: Participant feedback[1]

At the end of the three-month program, all of the participants had completed the restoration project, which culminated in an open house for the community. Community members came to tour the rehabilitated land, now known as Esteban Park in honour of Esteban the Moor, known to be the first African-born person to have come to what is now the United States (Arrington, 1986). During this open house, participants had a chance to speak to the public about what they had learned through their participation in the program. The participants gave tours of the new park and had a sense of pride and ownership for the work they had done.

Along with the completion of the land restoration project, we assessed the program's impact on the participants' lives in terms of the program and personal goals outlined above at the end of the pilot phase through follow-up interviews. Participants were asked what they had gained from the program; what had made the biggest impact on them during the program; whether there was a moment they remembered most; and whether their life was different now and, if so, how. These open-ended questions yielded rich narratives from participants about the positive impact of the program on them. Participants requested that their answers were not recorded or videotaped due to privacy concerns. However, they were written down as accurately as possible. Interestingly, participants talked most about their group experiences during the restoration work, and less about the other aspects of the program. Very few spoke about the ecological health curriculum directly though they appreciated the support of the Criminal Justice Coordinator who had facilitated the psychoeducational group. They also reported having a very positive relationship with GPRC Founder, Jarid Manos, who worked alongside them in the park, and served as a role model to the young participants. As they talked about the impact of the program, however, participants did share some of the prosocial values and ideas that were a part of the ecological health curriculum, especially as they related to the restoration work. For example, participants reported positive feelings of being associated with the Esteban Park project related to a sense of pride in giving back to the community.

> When we're out here working, people stop by and ask us what we're doing, and it feels good to talk with people in the community and tell them what we're doing. It feels important (Participant B).

> No one thought we'd do this. It's about letting people know that just because we were in jail doesn't mean we don't care about our community. We worked hard to make this a place people could come and get away from the craziness of the city (Participant D).

---

1   Parts of this section have been reprinted with the permission of the journal *Ecopsychology* (see Norton and Holguin, 2011).

The ecological restoration work made the most impact with participants reflecting on how hard, yet meaningful, the work was, and how it brought them together as a group:

> It was so hot and there were days I didn't want to be there, but I kept coming because I didn't just want to wander around the streets. The shelter closes during the day, and a lot of folks don't have a place to go, but we had a place to go and work to do. We fought with each other, but we became like a family (Participant A).

> We all live in the shelter, we all work at the park, and we all meet in the group. We together all the time, so we know what's up with our lives and we all going through the same thing (Participant D).

> Sometimes we had fun. We'd laugh and throw mud at each other. We worked hard though too to help out this forgotten piece of land (Participant C).

Reaffirming Geist and Galatowitsch's (1999) finding, the ecological restoration work also provided participants with direct healing experiences in nature. As they worked to eradicate non-native species and restore the land to its original state, they watched how quickly the land was able to heal itself. This became a metaphor for renewal and transformation in their lives:

> I can't believe what we did. You should've seen this place. It was a dump. But then we started cutting and digging, and we even filled up that pond with water. You know what happened, all of a sudden a crawfish came out of the ground ... like it had been just waiting for that water, and dragonflies started flying around. It was like creating life, and I knew if that land could get better, then so could I (Participant B).

> Fixing the land made me feel like I was giving life, instead of taking it (Participant A).

> It's amazing how when you fix up the land, life just suddenly appears (Participant D).

The work in nature as a group also promoted a deeper sense of connection to the land and to one another:

> For the first time, I feel connected to a place. I've moved around so much, but this is a place I can bring my kids to, and my kids' kids (Participant C).

Being out here, it made me have respect for all life. It's just a beautiful thing (Participant D).

I've become more open. I can't explain it, but I'll talk to people now. Before this program, I wouldn't have even talked to you (Participant C).

Most importantly, when asked about whether or not their lives were different since completing the program, participants reported a deeper awareness of their personal strength and resilience:

My life is not that different – but I'm different (Participant B).

I used to be a very violent person, but the work helped me release my anger into nature (Participant C).

I lost my son, and my whole life, I've wanted revenge. I let that go. I mean, my life is still hard, but I'm stronger (Participant D).

Overall, participants conveyed a deeper respect for life, development of empathy, pride in giving back, increased connection to community, openness to others, spiritual growth and renewal, a sense of purpose and future, enhanced motivation, and clearer goals. It became evident that even though the challenges and hardships in participants' lives had not disappeared, the program had helped participants to face these challenges with a greater sense of internal strength and clarity.

These insights reflect attitudinal rather than behavioural change. At the follow-up interviews, participants reported an increase in prosocial decision making, and none had reoffended or were incarcerated again. Participants reported taking steps towards employment and continuing education, and increased self-esteem and confidence. The group felt deeply connected to one another, to the RNI staff and to the larger community, reflective of aspects of successful community reintegration.

Critical analysis of the RNI initiative

While the program was a profound life experience for the participants, they still struggled with poverty, homelessness, mental health issues, and deficiencies in education, and remained unemployed. In particular, the stipend provided by RNI was not enough to live on, and while it did not allow them to 'break out of life on the streets', it did give them motivation but not the means to do so. Living wage green jobs and intensive case management services are needed in the future should this program continue to work with formerly incarcerated individuals. Until these opportunities are in place, it will be hard for participants to sustain the shifts in attitude that were achieved through this positive experience.

One of the primary limitations for RNI was the staffing challenges and limited budget, with case management functions outsourced to social workers at Bread of Life shelter. While in some ways, this collaborative approach worked, it also limited the accountability of program staff to the participants despite the close relationships forged. Increased program resources and a more formal contract with Bread of Life may be needed for the program to continue. Another limitation was the challenge of developing 'indigenous' leadership to sustain the program. As the program progressed and the group became more cohesive, it became evident that it would be important to keep some of the program 'graduates' involved as peer leaders to work with a new group of participants in the future. However, 'graduates' continued to face their own life challenges and required ongoing support and mentoring. RNI was unable to follow up with participants after the program though follow-up services were provided by Bread of Life. Nevertheless, RNI has remained in contact with those who completed the pilot restoration project. They have on-site reunions where the participants can return to the land and reconnect, perform maintenance on the trails, or just talk with staff. The program is hoping to reengage 'graduates' of the pilot phase of the program to come back and teach and mentor new participants.

Finally, there is a need to develop more systematic, longitudinal methods for evaluating program efficacy. If the program is going to increase and expand to work directly with Harris County Corrections, quantitative as well as qualitative data on recidivism, employment, education, and life skills acquisition would need to be collected. As Janetta (2011) discovered, data of this nature is essential to effective intervention with prison reentry populations.

Implications for social work practice and research

The reciprocal ecosystem restoration model and ecological health framework reflect a shift away from the conventional social work approach, which focuses solely on helping people cope with and adapt to the stressors of modern life, instead of promoting a new, interconnected paradigm of existence or structural change. This is especially true for traditional recidivism reduction programs, which address behaviour change and skills training, but do not attempt to foster a sense of global consciousness through connection to the natural world. RNI's framework reflects a holistic social work approach that involves the body, the soul, and the spirit, as shown in Figure 9.2.

BODY
Physical work (in nature)
Native prairie grass and land restoration

SOUL
Group work (in nature and in an agency setting)
Psychosocial and life skills

SPIRIT
Spiritual work (in nature)
Reflection, contemplation, ecological identity

Figure 9.2 Ecological Health Framework

This importance of physical work in nature to the development of an ecological identity reflects a new paradigm of social work practice built upon a global consciousness in which the connectedness of all things is understood and valued. Social work can and should:

> nurture the development of a personal and collective global consciousness by supporting people in their transformation and by providing opportunities for people to critique and understand their personal stories and relationships in light of their understanding of wholeness and creativity.
>
> (Coates, 2003: 101)

RNI does this in the hope that helping participants to develop a deeper ecological identity in which they feel more connected to one another, their community, and the natural world, might decrease their risk of committing future offences (Harper and Chitty, 2004). The preliminary evaluation revealed that the program had had a positive impact on participants but in order to better understand how environmentally based initiatives, such as the RNI program, work to reduce recidivism, it is important to begin to measure *specific outcomes* and their long-term sustainability. According to Masters (1994), empathy is a key factor in reducing recidivism along with improved life skills, increased prosocial attitudes and behaviour, and access to resources (Solomon *et al.*, 2006). While programs like RNI might enhance personal growth and change, social workers need to work at multiple levels to promote social change through, *inter alia,* advocacy, community organizing, and workforce development. By engaging in ecosystem restoration projects (the centrepiece of the Life Wheel), participants contributed to making their community a better place, while learning about environmental justice (see Chapter 1) and the disproportionate consequences of environmental injustice and racism on black and minority communities (Shrader-Frechette, 2002). Participants began to understand the reality of environmental oppression and the power of environmental activism.

Conclusion

Restoration Not Incarceration provides one model of an environmentally based initiative to address social and ecological needs in the Houston community, to reduce recidivism and ecological degradation respectively, and promote the healing of people and restoration of the land. Through a multidimensional approach, the program integrated prosocial values and productive work in nature as an avenue for reintegration into society and the improvement of life outcomes. Though small in scale, the pilot initiative showed promising methods for helping formerly incarcerated youth find a way to reenter society that can be replicated in social work practice.

References

Andrews, D., and Bonta, J. (2011). *Notes: LSI-R Level of Service Inventory-Revised.* Retrieved June 22, 2011 from http://www.assessments.com/catalog/LSI_R.htm.

Arrington, C. (1986). *Black explorer in Spanish Texas: Estevanico.* Austin, TX: Eakin Press.

Berger, R., and McLeod, J. (2006). Incorporating nature into therapy: A framework for practice. *Journal of Systemic Therapies, 25*(2), 80–94.

Berman, M., Jonides, J., and Kaplan, S. (2008). The psychological benefits of interacting with nature. *Psychological Science, 19*(12), 1207–1212.

Blechman, E.A., Maurice, A., Buecker, B., and Helberg, C. (2000). Can mentoring or skills training reduce recidivism? Observational study with propensity analysis. *Prevention Science, 1,* 139–155.

Coates, J. (2003). *Ecology and social work: Toward a new paradigm.* Halifax, NS: Fernwood Press.

Dapice, A. (2006). The medicine wheel. *Journal of Transcultural Nursing, 17*(3), 251–260.

Fairman, D. (2010). *Reintegrating ex-offenders into communities.* Cambridge, MA: Consensus Building Institute. Retrieved January 10, 2012 from http://cbuilding. org/publication/case/reintegrating-exoffenders-communities

Geist, C., and Galatowitsch, S.M. (1999). Reciprocal model for meeting ecological and human needs in restoration projects. *Conservation Biology, 13*(5), 970–979.

Gibbons, J.J., and Katzenbach, N. de B. (Co-Chairs). (2006). Confronting Confinement: A Report of the Commission on Safety and Abuse in America's Prisons. New York: Vera Institute of Justice. Republished in *Federal Sentencing Reporter, 24*(1), 36–41 by University of California Press on behalf of the Vera Institute of Justice. DOI: 0.1525/fsr.2011.24.1.36. Retrieved January 20, 2012 from http://www.jstor.org/stable/10.1525/fsr.2011.24.1.36.

Great Plains Restoration Council (GPRC). (2011). *Helping youth rebuild their lives.* Retrieved June 20, 2011 from http://www.gprc.org.

Groenewegen, P.P., van den Berg, A.E., De Vries, S., and Verheij, R.A. (2006). Study protocol Vitamin G: Effects of green space on health, well-being, and social safety. *BMC Public Health, 6*(149), 6–149.

Harper, G., and Chitty, C. (2004). *Impact of Corrections on Reoffending: A Review of 'What Works'*. London: Home Office. Retrieved January 10, 2012 from http://www.ncjrs.gov/App/publications/abstract.aspx?ID=208430.

Harrison, P.M., and Beck, A.J. (2005). *Prisoners in 2004*. Bureau of Justice Statistics Bulletin, NCJ 210677. Washington, DC: U.S. Department of Justice.

Janetta, J. (2011). *CPAP assessment of CDCR recidivism-reduction programs*. Irvine, CA: University of California, Center for Evidence-Based Corrections. Retrieved January 10, 2012 from http://ucicorrections.seweb.uci.edu/files/CPAP%20 Assessment%20of%20CDCR.pdf.

Kaplan, R., and Kaplan, S. (1989). *The experience of nature: A psychological perspective*. New York: Cambridge University Press.

Lewis, J.J. (2012). 'Rachel Carson quotes'. About Women's History. URL: http://womenshistory.about.com/od/quotes/a/rachel_carson.htm. Date accessed: (2/20/12).

Masters, R. (1994). *Counseling criminal justice offenders*. Thousand Oaks, CA: Sage.

Mitchell, R., and Popham, F. (2008). Effect of exposure to natural environment on health inequalities: An observational population study. *Lancet, 372*(9650), 1655–1660.

Norton, C.L. (2010). Exploring the process of wilderness therapy: Key therapeutic components in the treatment of adolescent depression and psychosocial development. *Journal of Therapeutic School and Programs, 4*(1), 24–46.

Norton, C.L. (2011). Social work and the environment: An ecosocial approach. *International Social Welfare Journal*. Article first published online: 9 DEC 2011. DOI: 10.1111/j.1468-2397.2011.00853.

Norton, C.L., and Holguin, B. (2011). Restoration not incarceration: Preliminary evaluation of an eco-social work intervention for formerly incarcerated young adults. *Ecopsychology, 3*(3), 205–212.

Ross, J.I. (2011). Moving beyond Soering: U.S. prison conditions as an argument against extradition to the United States. *International Criminal Justice Review, 21*(2), 156–168.

Roszak, T. (2001). *The voice of the Earth: An exploration of ecopsychology*. Grand Rapids, MI: Phanes Press.

Shrader-Frechette, K.S. (2002). *Environmental justice creating equality, reclaiming democracy*. New York: Oxford University Press.

Shulman, L. (2009). *The skills of helping individuals, families, groups and communities* (6th ed.). Belmont, CA: Brooks/Cole.

Snyder, H.N., and Sickmund, M. (2006). *Juvenile Offenders and Victims National Report (JOVNR)*. Washington, DC: National Center for Juvenile Justice. Retrieved June 20, 2011 from http://www.ojjdp.gov/ojstatbb/nr2006/downloads/NR2006.pdf.

Solomon, A., Palmer, T., Atkinson, A., Davidson, J., and Harvey, L. (2006). *Prisoner reentry: Addressing the challenges in weed and seed communities*. Urban Institute Justice Policy Center: Winston Salem State University Center for Community Safety.

Substance Abuse and Mental Health Services Administration (SAMHSA). (2011). *SAMHSA/CSAT Treatment Improvement Protocols*. Rockville, MD: Center for Substance Abuse Treatment. Retrieved 1/10/12 from http://www.ncbi.nlm.nih.gov/books/NBK14119/.

Thigpen, M., Beauclair, T., and Carroll, S. (2011). *The greening of corrections: Creating a sustainable system.* Washington, DC: U.S. Dept. of Justice National Institute of Corrections.

Thomashow, M. (1996). *Ecological identity: Becoming a reflective environmentalist.* Cambridge, MA: The MIT Press.

Ulrich, C., and Nadkarni, N.M. (2008). Sustainability research and practices in enforced residential institutions: Collaborations of ecologists and prisoners. *Environment, Development and Sustainability.* DOI 10.1007/s10668-0089145-4. Retrieved January 18, 2012 from http://blogs.evergreen.edu/sustainableprisons/files/2009/09/Springer-Ulrich-and-Nadkarni_Sustainability-Research-and-Practices-in-Enforced-Residential-Institutions_3-08.pdf.

Visher, C.A., Winterfield, L., and Coggeshall, M.B. (2005). Ex-offender employment programs and recidivism: A meta-analysis. *Journal of Experimental Criminology, 1,* 295–315.

Warren, R.K. (2007). *Evidence-based practice to reduce recidivism: Implications for state judiciaries.* Washington, DC: National Institute of Corrections.

Whitman, J.Q. (2003). *Harsh justice: Criminal punishment and the widening divide between America and Europe.* Oxford: Oxford University Press.

Wilson, E.O. (1993). Biophilia and the conservation ethic. In S.R.Kellert and Wilson, E.O. (Eds). *The biophilia hypothesis.* Washington, DC: Shearwater Books/Island Press. 31–41.

Author Disclosure Statement

Christine Lynn Norton is on the Advisory Council for RNI and has been asked to serve in that role to consult on program development and evaluation. In that sense, her research has stemmed directly from this role. Barbara Holguin served as the Criminal Justice Coordinator during this project. Jarid Manos is the Founder and CEO of Great Plains Restoration Council.

10 Social work and the struggle for corporate social responsibility

Dyann Ross

> Power and ethics are inseparable and socio-environmental justice efforts need to embrace this complexity in: relationships in context, within specific historical situations, over time, with the people involved, and differently situated in the controversy (Dyann Ross).

As a profession, social work stands for human rights and social justice for individuals, communities, and societies. This chapter examines how social workers might engage in the struggle between multinational corporate mining companies and neighbouring communities directly affected by mining activities. This examination is based on the belief that social work's invaluable knowledge and skills can inform debates and practice in the area of corporate social responsibility toward adjacent communities. Drawing on research about the tensions between social, health, and environmental concerns associated with alumina mining in a rural community in Australia, the chapter explores the quest for social justice for local people and sustainability for the local environment. It argues that profit unhinged from the parallel considerations of 'people and place' threatens environmental sustainability as well as social justice. A key insight is the importance of engaging the powerful parties – the mining company and senior government officials and politicians – in any attempt to assist surrounding communities to have their concerns addressed in fair and substantial ways. To further social justice and environmental sustainability, power dynamics must be grasped and relationship tensions held. This needs to occur within a strongly supported logic of limits being set on corporate profits through, for example, compensation paid for adverse community, social, and environmental impacts arising from mining operations. This is unlikely without the mining company holding to a very robust sense of its corporate social responsibility.

How then might social workers engage in the struggle between competing interests of multinational corporate mining companies and neighbouring communities? First, social work needs to position itself as a key player in socioenvironmental conflicts by extending its practice beyond its ameliorative and reactive focus on caring and support for vulnerable populations. In this instance, social workers need to engage with powerful mining interests and their profit-driven agendas that prevail over their social responsibilities towards community and environmental well-being. Further, they need to do this in the absence of satisfactory international legal strategies and federal and state government regulations (Higgins, 2010) to ensure the fair treatment of communities, landscapes, and ecosystems directly affected by mining operations. Here there is potential for social work to participate actively in building ethical norms in civil society and effective strategies for just and sustainable mining practices.

In building this argument, the chapter presents a case study positioning social work in the struggle for corporate social responsibility through an Australian research study involving the multinational mining corporation Alcoa World Alumina (Wagerup) and the Yarloop community in Western Australia. Importantly, Alcoa (2002) claims to use its values to build financial success, environmental excellence, and social responsibility in partnership with all stakeholders, while social work claims to promote social and environmental justice. The chapter describes learning from the experience which sought to align these two value systems and advance knowledge of how social workers might engage with corporate social responsibility in the interests of promoting social and environmental justice (see Chapter 1).

Repositioning social work

In Australia and globally, social work has committed itself as a profession to working with socially, economically, and culturally disadvantaged, marginalized, and oppressed people (Australian Association of Social Workers (AASW), 2010; International Federation of Social Workers (IFSW), 2011, with the International Association of Schools of Social Work (IASSW)). Despite its clear normative statements about human rights and social justice, this is an ethical minefield given powerful *social* interests in maintaining the status quo. This is especially so where the *natural* environment is being degraded and local citizens are being negatively affected (Besthorn, 2002; Coates, 2003). The relationship between social and environmental injustice has not been part of mainstream social work education or practice in Australia (Ife, 2008; Hawkins, 2010). Additionally, and perhaps because of the absence of the natural environment as a matter of social work concern, it remains less obvious that socioeconomic injustices are directly related to environmental degradation and unsustainable mining practices, as demonstrated in this chapter.

Long associated with anti-oppressive social work practice is Marxist originator of critical pedagogy Paulo Freire's (1970) argument that change is best leveraged through bringing the oppressed into a – resistant – relationship with their oppressor. Through this political process the oppressed are conscientized as to their rights and interests and how they were being compromised or exploited (Leonard, 1997; Mullaly, 1997;

Young, 1990). This overly reductive binary of 'oppressor and oppressed' belies the complex power relations between corporate mining conglomerates and local mining communities. Nonetheless, it is a useful starting point for critical engagement with powerful financial mining interests that are beyond the control of national boundaries and their local effects. This is a new area for social work given the dearth of concrete evidence as to its effectiveness not only in relation to corporate social responsibility but also issues of socioenvironmental justice. There is little prior guidance, therefore, in how social work might influence corporations whose operations threaten local economies and ecosystems (Ross, 2002a, 2009).

Social work at the edge of corporate social responsibility

Corporate social responsibility (CSR) refers to the desire of corporations to pursue their business interests giving due regard to social, economic, legal, ethical, and philanthropic expectations at a given point in time (Carroll and Buchholtz, in Crane and Matten, 2010). However, corporations 'self-define' the nature and extent of their social responsibility. For the most part, corporate social responsibility employs a philanthropic or charity model (Porter and Kramer, 2006), 'voluntarily committing to social actions and programs ... [to] forestall legislation and ensure greater corporate independence from government' (Moon and Vogel, in Crane and Matten, 2010: 51). A report in *The Economist* found that more than 50 per cent of global business leaders engaged in CSR primarily as a marketing exercise to establish better 'brand reputation':

> For companies with a strong global brand, consumer pressure can be a key driver towards more responsible practices ... and employees might be attracted to work for and even be more committed to a corporation perceived as being socially responsible.
> (Green and Truen, in Crane and Matten, 2010: 51)

With the growth of the environment movement, environmental sustainability has become an increasing aspect of corporate social responsibility so in successive annual reports of major mining corporations it is not uncommon to find claims that mining is sustainable (Holliday, Schmidheiny, and Watts, 2002). For example, extensive rehabilitation of mine sites or investment in initiatives like land care in Australia are cited as evidence of mining's environmental sustainability (Alcoa, 2008). This weak definition of sustainability, while the same company clear cuts unique jarrah forests to extract bauxite, belies the deeply contradictory use of language by many multinational mining companies to obscure social upheaval and environmental degradation. According to MacDonald (2011), Alcoa's claims of being socially responsible are more rhetoric than reality. From an anti-oppressive social work perspective, CSR reinforces 'relations of domination and subservience' under the guise of 'doing good' for the community and ecosystems and there is little evidence of social justice for communities adjacent to mining operations or of sustainability for local ecosystems under the pervasive influence of corporate skies (Brueckner and Ross, 2010). Internationally, there is a deeply troubling pattern of exploitation and degradation of sovereign homelands, usually legally sanctioned by the peoples' own governments (Higgins, 2010). It is simply not sufficient for social work as a collective of people who understand the importance of social justice to patch up those displaced and exploited by mining corporations (Global Social Agenda, 2011).

Hence an invitation from a multinational mining company to assist in resolving an issue that was affecting their good standing in the local area arose in 2002 when Alcoa Wagerup commissioned Edith Cowan University to undertake research to discover how to respond to an aggrieved community's pollution concerns. Alcoa's Wagerup mine site and alumina refinery is situated south-east of Perth in Western Australia in close physical proximity to several small towns, in particular, the town of Yarloop. Over a two-year period, this study provided an opportunity to bring the corporation and community into a relationship to resolve an environmental concern. The research became a crucial space for re-framing the problem as a socioenvironmental issue for a local community concerned about the sustainability of the local environment. Given the complex power dynamics alluded to above, Alcoa had the advantage but, in light of its commitment to financial success, environmental excellence, and social responsibility, the corporation wanted to pursue its profit-driven interests in a socially and environmentally responsive manner. At the same time, practising social work at the edge of corporate social responsibility presented a professional challenge. This was unfamiliar territory and the limited mandate for holding Alcoa accountable through the research was clear from the outset: What might a social work researcher committed to socioenvironmental justice achieve in these circumstances?

The Wagerup controversy: A struggle between people, place, and profit

Before answering this question, a brief account of the controversy is provided. The case study centres on a particularly intractable conflict in the mining industry in Western Australia. The conflict involves Alcoa World Alumina, one of the largest producers of aluminium in the world, and residents of the adjacent rural community of Yarloop. Many of Yarloop's 600 residents believe that the polluting effects of Alcoa's operations have adversely affected their health and socioeconomic well-being (Community Alliance for Positive Solutions, 2011). Additionally, overlaying these concerns was the social upheaval arising from the intrusive and divisive effects of Alcoa's purchase of private properties to protect its commercial interests (Ross, 2002a, 2002b). The extent and persistence of the controversy has been highlighted by a Parliamentary Inquiry (2004), ongoing media attention (Flint, 2005), including the Australian Broadcasting Corporation's (ABC) 'Four Corners' television program (McDermott, 2005), and Brueckner and Ross's (2010) book documenting the issues. At the heart of the controversy are claims of harm and disadvantage resulting from Alcoa Wagerup's failure to contain emissions and noise within its footprint and to provide a legal 'buffer' area between the refinery and the nearby town without buying up private properties and displacing local people:

> My skin, I get burnt. It's like a radiation thing ... You also have bladder problems and it affects your bowel, it affects your moods, it affects your skin, see my skin is horrible ... I went to a naturopath and he told me I had chemical liver poisoning, that my liver was not coping with all the toxins in my blood.
>
> (Brueckner and Ross, 2010: 67)

While Alcoa consulted local people, they proceeded to create a buffer without formal government planning approval and refused to admit the property buy-ups would cause problems in the community (Alcoa, 2001/2002). Rising alarm about the health risks from the refinery emissions led many people to sell their properties and move out of the community. This created a domino effect as residents lost friends and family and, in turn, sold to Alcoa and left Yarloop as a ghost town where the quality of life disintegrated:

> Well it's almost no town now. I feel it's a dying town (resident)
>
> It's a beautiful place ... But I wish to God I had never moved here (former resident)
>
> (Brueckner and Ross, 2010: 65)

Alcoa is on the public record as saying it is very sorry for the disruption it has caused to people in the Yarloop area (Sharp, 2004). Nevertheless, it denies any responsibility for the collapse of the town or the individual health issues. After denying their extension plans for some time (Alcoa, 2003), Alcoa pushed ahead with gaining government approval for a substantial expansion of its Wagerup refinery. It did so despite calls from the Wagerup Medical Practitioner's Forum (2005) and an unprecedented number of public submissions to the government concerning the increased risk of further adverse impacts from the refinery operations and Alcoa's adversarial public relations behaviour. In 2012, the situation remains unchanged, though the expansion has not proceeded yet due to the global financial crisis. A number of local residents are pursuing a class action against Alcoa for knowingly causing a range of health, social, and environmental problems. Higgins (2010) would describe Alcoa's dogged pursuit of its development agenda in the face of continued human and ecological distress as 'ecocide', which she defines as the 'extensive destruction, damage to or loss of ecosystem(s) of a given territory, whether by human agency or by other causes, to such an extent that peaceful enjoyment by the inhabitants of that territory has been severely diminished' (p. 63). Since the parties involved in the conflict do not agree on the issues, and who should be responsible for fixing them, a major power struggle around irreconcilable interests continues:

1   The Western Australian state government has a pro-development agenda to support job creation and economic prosperity.
2   Alcoa has profit-driven corporate and legal imperatives to satisfy its shareholders.
3   The Yarloop people are differently positioned but collectively constitute a range of claims for guarantees of a safe environment, fair treatment in property sales, compensation for losses, and non-intrusion in their lives and town.
4   The public at large consume Alcoa's aluminium products.
5   Australian society overall wants the jobs Alcoa provides and less obviously and more cynically is content with a social contract that ensures the negative trade-offs of corporate profit making do not affect the silent majority.

At the same time, to some extent these irreconcilable interests can be addressed through negotiated trade-offs (Brueckner and Ross, 2010) and this points to the interconnected nature of each party's interests and the reasons why the conflict has been so protracted and not finally winnable for any particular party. Through the work of the research team, each of the three main parties – the government, company and community – has gained respect for and awareness of the interests and rights of the others involved (see Brager and Holloway, 1978). This would constitute an important juncture in any socioenvironmental change effort.

Despite the impasse reached, Alcoa has continued to position itself as a leader in corporate social responsibility and to claim that its operations are socially just and environmentally sustainable (Alcoa, 2008; Donoghue and Cullen, 2007). Yet the social and environmental consequences at Wagerup and the long-running conflict suggest otherwise. CSR theory suggests the best outcomes ensue when corporate agendas align with government and community interests (Brueckner and Ross, 2010).

Social work in relation to corporate moral pressure and legislative influence

Earlier it was claimed that building ethical norms in civil society was necessary for just and sustainable mining practices. Many corporations place value on local community endorsement of their activities giving them a 'licence to operate' (McKibben and Waters, 2010). This approval is often tacit and follows transparent processes surrounding local development. However, for many residents, Alcoa lost its 'operating licence' when it went ahead with private land purchases while denying pollution concerns without government approval or sufficient local community endorsement and support. Alcoa's values of building financial success, environmental excellence, and social responsibility were jeopardized (Alcoa, 2002). Clearly, Alcoa's ethical stance as to the nature of a 'good' company meant 'good for profits and appeasing shareholders', thus privileging financial success. Financial success could not be compromised by social responsibility and environmental sustainability.

Environmental advocates like Mackenzie (2004) argue that society needs to exert greater moral pressure on corporations to make them accountable for the negative impacts of their profit-making activities on neighbouring communities and environments. This is in line with calls for corporations to be held accountable for the externalized costs of production – costs such as polluted air and water, poisoning of plants and animals, and exposure of people to toxins (see Coates, 2003). Mackenzie (2004) asks how pressure groups and other elements of civil society might effectively regulate corporate behaviour 'without access to legal or market means' (p. 50), especially when corporations deny responsibility and injury to both the environment and to victims in neighbouring communities' (Anand, Ashforth, and Joshi, in Crane and Matten, 2010: 167). Brueckner and Ross (2010) reported residents were caught in a double bind and made to appear 'bad and wrong' for raising their health concerns while Alcoa reacted as if it were being unfairly accused and attacked. This insidious abuse of power by Alcoa has the ripple effect of hiding the human rights abuses perpetrated on people in local communities through pollution, water contamination, and other environmentally unsustainable and health-degenerating industrial practices (Cosier in Flannery, 2009: 120).

No amount of appeals to good ethical behaviour by corporations such as Alcoa can be relied upon to address significant power inequalities between the corporation and the impacted community and the interrelated environmental degradation. The limits of voluntary self-regulation by corporations are well documented (Walker and Howard, 2002): corporations will not typically act to support legislation that curbs their current operations or profits. Social workers need to know, therefore, how to address the power dynamics that are intricately interconnected with the ethical and legal dynamics in conflicted situations. For example, the opportunity to influence government behaviour on the Alcoa issue was afforded by invitations to the research team, supported by Alcoa, to address the state government's Ministers' Council, which also comprised senior government officials. Recommendations relating to providing a new regional plan, infrastructure protection, and social support to the local communities were progressed as a result of this invitation. This is about recognizing the importance of taking up invitations to influence the powerful parties in the conflict and not to shy away from the challenge of trying to shift the balance of power yet always remaining aware of the inherent risk of cooptation. Further, it was made possible by holding onto the relationship with Alcoa senior personnel and acting both with Alcoa and for the communities' interests at the same time in an open manner with both parties. In turn, the government of the day was able to follow the recommendations without being off side with Alcoa or the community, this being welcomed as they have double loyalties and legal obligations to both parties. Alcoa was enabled to hold the tension between its commercial interests and its duty of care to affected neighbouring communities without losing face or forgoing its strategic control over the situation. Here we see the value of a significant social work capacity of being able to analyse and work with power issues by holding onto relationships with all three stakeholder groups – the community, the corporation, and the government – and progressing matters of substance and mutual interest.

The influence of the research-based work at Wagerup near Yarloop was also evident in some of the recommendations arising from the Parliamentary Inquiry (Sharp, 2004). Here social workers contributed to the development of local knowledge of the situation which was really important to counterbalance unfounded claims and counter-claims. Other efforts by social workers in the research team to influence statutory obligations of the government centred on written submissions as part of the appeal process against Alcoa's plans for an expansion at its Wagerup refinery. These contributions allowing the local people to be heard represent important steps in enabling the least powerful to be listened to in the corridors of power. However, these examples should not be mistaken as strategies that in and of themselves can change the power imbalance towards more enduring favourable consideration of the local communities' socioeconomic and environmental sustainability. Nevertheless, they do show that power and ethics are inseparable and social justice efforts need to embrace this complexity in relationships in context, within specific historical situations, over time, with the people who are involved, and differently situated, in the controversy.

Post-structuralist notions of power (Ross, 2002b; Stanley and Wise, 1993) are consistent with this way of thinking about and responding to socioenvironmental issues of this order of impact and vested interests. Social workers need to be ready to work alongside the community, government, and corporation for the long haul, in multidimensional ways, using a broad range of (nonviolent) strategies and tactics, many of which will not be declared. For example, to the present time social workers from the original research team are actively involved behind-the-scenes with some of the community on the ongoing issues writing letters, providing support to community leaders, helping to protect community culture and history, writing for publication, and providing advice to other affected communities. Tellingly though, direct social work involvement with Alcoa has not endured, which sharply reduces the scope for relationship-based approaches in trying to change the unequal power dynamics underpinning the controversy.

Social work as contributions to efforts at dialogue

Social and environmental justice cannot be achieved without dialogue between the 'oppressed' and the 'oppressors' on matters of substance where the dominant party – the party being most advantaged by the status quo – is additionally legally or ethically held accountable by society. Ensuring that the legal obligations, ethical imperatives, and relational demands in the case study in question are all addressed is not the preserve of any one stakeholder group or intervention. What the research experience showed is the relational aspect needed to involve a three-way dialogue between the government, corporation, and community but this was incredibly hard to achieve and sustain over the long haul. In part, this was because of the contractual and outsider status of the researcher's relationship with Alcoa. But furthermore, Alcoa was operating in a legal manner (yet see the next point) and also believed it was behaving in an ethical manner. Some legal pressure was brought to bear on Alcoa when it was fined for breaches of its licensing requirements on various occasions (Community Alliance for Positive Solutions, 2011). However, these fines were regarded by locals as grossly inadequate relative to the harm done. Social workers need to actively embrace opportunities to influence legislative aspects of these types of issues. For example, part of the submission-writing process against Alcoa's plans to expand its operational capacity included an analysis of the limits of regulatory powers and recommendations on how to give greater strength to the precautionary principle (Drake, 2011) with regard to the issues identified in the case study. Adherence to the precautionary principle would give scope for the government not to support Alcoa's submission on the grounds of possible irrevocable harm to the environment in light of growing evidence of concerns by local people and a range of environmental experts. Bigger pro-development forces in the state government have meant little has changed on the basis of this micro level of intervention and point of law alone. However, Alcoa has been subject to the greatest number of conditions for its expansion plans ever required of a corporation in Australia (McGowan, 2006), meaning it has had to overcome more obstacles to achieve its economic objectives.

It is the case that social workers will not always be placed, either unilaterally or in collaboration with other parties, in a position to influence all the dimensions and actors in these kinds of controversies. These points notwithstanding, the use of social work knowledge and skills in the case study resulted in a concerted attempt with the community and Alcoa to negotiate a more equitable set of outcomes relating to the land purchases

Alcoa was undertaking. What was critical here was the timing of this attempt at dialogue: It was on Alcoa's invitation when it was reacting to strong threats to its credibility and, in fact, to its ability to operate its refinery at Wagerup. Here the legal and ethical imperatives that are the main leverages for securing more just and sustainable outcomes were intersected through the struggle over Alcoa's legal right to buy up a great deal of private land. Social workers supported local activists to raise this issue with Federal and State politicians but no basis could be found for illegal behaviour under the current legislation about foreign ownership of land. The lack of fairness in Alcoa's buy-up plan for adjacent private properties in Yarloop district was thoroughly scrutinized and required changes due to the evidence provided to the Parliamentary Inquiry by the research team.

Thus, timing when to intervene to ensure the best opportunity to influence the status quo of how corporations like Alcoa do their business is a key factor in socioenvironmental change efforts. The basis of the research contract with Alcoa was also crucial for gaining entry into the corporation's boardroom and key discussions about the issues. Aligning with other concerned stakeholders, including sitting members of parliament, in particular members of the Western Australian Greens party, was crucial for keeping the political and legal dimensions of the issue on the agenda. Further, another parallel focus was social work support of local leaders to resist involvement in government-led tripartite meetings aimed at assisting Alcoa's development interests. Over time, this local resistance has threatened the credibility of the tripartite process and resulted in the government's environmental protection agency working informally with the activists.

The research contract with Alcoa was crafted using social work skills of engaging conflicting parties, analysing the multilayered power dynamics, and applying socioenvironmental justice principles. Its purpose was to enable Alcoa to engage affected community members in a non-exploitative dialogue and genuine problem-solving partnership. It was based on the following warrants or agreements through which the research team asked Alcoa to:

1   Build a sincere relationship with the aggrieved parties who were disadvantaged and harmed by its actions.
2   Stay focused on relevant shared issues with willing attention to the effects of power imbalances.
3   Ensure substantive contributions to solving the problem between Alcoa (the dominant party) relative to the affected community (the non-dominant party) (Fox and Miller, 1995).

These warrants assumed that the more powerful party – Alcoa – would be more likely to break these agreements as it tried to exercise its authority and influence to maintain the status quo against the claims of the less powerful aggrieved community. In such unequal power situations, it is particularly important that social workers bear these power dynamics in mind so as to avoid becoming part of the problem through cooptation. It was assumed that naivety about the power dynamics involved would aggravate the problem in contention. When Alcoa started to default on willing attention to the substantive matters on the table in the social work led community dialogues, the research team decided to call the meetings to a halt. This dramatic decision had the effect of making clear what was happening rather than pushing on as if Alcoa were genuinely engaged in making real changes to its land management policy.

The case study experience showed that the community-based meetings with Alcoa and local residents over an 18-month period was a productive space for placing concerns 'on the table' and for Alcoa to have the opportunity to account for and change its behaviour. What the preceding comments show is that the meetings alone were not sufficient as a strategy since the corporation was acting on many fronts to protect its interests. How to gain full 'buy-in' from Alcoa's senior executive in Australia and the government to this grassroots, democratic, and power-alert approach, while still retaining their support, remains an unanswered question.

Emphasizing the 'social work' in CSR

Adopting social work principles and knowledge in the situation under discussion allowed attention to be given to the importance of emphasizing the *social* aspects of CSR when thinking about how to secure sustainable outcomes at Wagerup (Ross, 2009). The research was based on building trust, understanding, and respect between people involved in the conflict. It was thought that the relationships contained the possibility for doing things differently if the trust could be built and the power issues mediated by understanding, mutual respect, and collaborative problem solving. These are well honed skills for social workers. Post-structural notions of power recognize that unequal power relations are not only situated in the formal structures of society but also in the micro practices of the everyday relationships between people (Smith, 1990). The partnership approach (Tennyson and Wilde, 2000) and efforts to enable dialogue were premised on the value of the relationships between the corporation and community. While the relationships between key parties brought a keen appreciation of the persistent power dynamics and there were instances of genuine efforts to solve the problem, Alcoa's unfair land management practices ultimately triumphed. Alcoa now has its own buffer around its refinery at Wagerup. This unwelcome outcome for the community was in part because the trust established in some relationships at key points in the dialogue was lost and diluted by constant changes in the Alcoa personnel involved. Also there were undermining instances of key personnel in the government joining Alcoa or vice versa. Alcoa's most senior manager at the time of the research later took up the government-appointed post of The Chair of GESB Mutual Ltd., a

Western Australia government statutory authority, to oversee the state's biggest superannuation fund (Henry, 2008). Further, a key person in the government resigned his post and became a manager and spokesperson for Alcoa on matters to do with Yarloop. This served to feed some community members' perceptions that Alcoa and the government were 'in each other's pockets' and that they would act in every instance to maintain the status quo.

Thus, we come to the point of emphasizing the *social work* in efforts to enable CSR by multinational corporations to protect threatened communities and environments. Valuing relationships and attempting to effect socioenvironmental change through relationship-based strategies will continue to be important. However, to play on the idea of 'social work' here to make a point, learning from the case study, suggests that an equally strong emphasis needs to be given to the 'work' of social work, much of which may not be about fostering and supporting key relationships. That is, CSR is not a self-evident capacity that is readily embraced and upheld by mining corporations such as Alcoa World Alumina. It is the work of social work that has much to offer our understanding of the nature of struggles between people, place, and profit. There are extra-local and extra-relational aspects to the controversy that are not immediately amenable to interpersonal micro-skills and strategies. The work of social work, in turn, has to be multidimensional, and include indirect macro practice as well as localized direct efforts. It should involve forging broader alliances and networks, including formal representation around such matters by professional associations and other interest groups.

A mix of social work skills and knowledge is crucial to enabling a commitment to social justice and environmental sustainability in corporations *and* governments. Further, these capacities are not the sole preserve of professionally trained social workers. The sociologists, community artists, and social workers who comprised the research team from Edith Cowan University worked productively with a range of community leaders, activists, and lay people to leverage greater capacity to sustain the challenging dialogue with Alcoa during 2002 and 2003. This dovetailing with community members' capacities to protect their own interests, including the local environment, is crucial to avoid undermining local expertise and grassroots wisdom (Ife and Tesoriero, 2006).

In summary, the important social work skills and strategies employed in the case study that contributed to the efforts at dialogue to address the socioenvironmental issues at Wagerup are noted below. As the skill of critical analysis of power is central to all the others noted, a set of guiding questions are also presented.

Critical analysis of power issues and unequal relationship dynamics

The warrants framework presented earlier (Fox and Miller, 1995) shows a robust thinking strategy for monitoring how far the powerful party in the unequal situation is really committed to making changes that benefit the less powerful party. This model was employed alongside an adaptation of a set of 'value-rational' questions derived from Flyvbjerg's (2001) power-sensitive inquiry schema:

1   Where is sustainability going in the Wagerup situation?
2   Who gains, who loses, and by which mechanisms of power?
3   Is it desirable?
4   What should be done? (in Brueckner and Ross, 2010: 208).

In particular, the second question in the schema was constantly employed prior to any action or decision being taken by the research team. Brueckner and Ross (2010) provide a full response to Flyvbjerg's (2001) questions, which were used throughout the research, and allowed for constant re-positioning by the research team, and the adoption of new strategies in light of new understandings gained *in situ* as events unfolded.

Listening to the powerless

Prior to the research, the community felt unheard and resorted to national media releases (Mayman, 2002). The social work skills of advocacy for the marginalized resulted in the state government Minister's Council presentation (noted earlier), with Alcoa present, which placed community concerns on the table months prior to the Parliamentary Inquiry. This action allowed immediate actions by the government to provide infrastructure and planning support relating to threats to the viability of Yarloop as a result of Alcoa's commercial decisions.

Engaging powerful stakeholders

Alcoa sought help from the research team and this initiated the engagement of one of the powerful stakeholders. In turn, ready access to the state government was provided through association with Alcoa and via a specially convened Wagerup Working Party which the research team was permitted to attend. The engagement of the powerful stakeholders covered a two-year period and crucially the research team enabled the legitimacy of the community – members of the towns in the Yarloop district – to be at the table where important discussions and decisions were taken. The skills of diplomacy, negotiation, facilitation, representation, de-escalation of conflict, agenda setting, problem posing, problem solving, and creating spaces for the parties to meet and progress the issues were provided by the social work expertise in the research team.

Dialogue in pursuit of socially and environmentally just outcomes

The idea of dialogue used here relates to non-exploitative formal conversations between stakeholders. Most dialogue occurs through meetings and it is important that the parameters and purpose of these interactions are clear to all parties. While adherence to meeting rules act as safeguards against power abuses, flexibility is required. This was the most successful part of the research as a relatively safe and respectful space was created in an ongoing series of open public meetings where the agenda permitted often highly emotive resident input. It was important that neither party be allowed to be disrespectful or abusive to the other to ensure that residents and Alcoa personnel would continue to attend and have the tough conversations that did in fact happen. For example, the issue of whether the company would consider compensation for the socioenvironmental harm done to the area was highly sensitive and very unwelcome for Alcoa but it did occur. In addition to the social work skills noted above, an important activity in these meetings was constantly seeking and naming the common ground even as the differences were usually so large as to risk swamping any chance of the parties hearing one another, or reaching consensus. In tandem with the public meetings, the research team engaged in a range of de-briefings in which they supported company and community stakeholders and helped them reflect on, and make sense of, their interactions. The researchers' role was to maintain the integrity of the process and participants' goodwill for forthcoming meetings.

Ethical behaviour

Ethical behaviour involves accountability toward the less powerful stakeholders and their interests without antagonizing the powerful party. The main challenge for the research team was how to maintain its impartiality, independence, and integrity while acting for and on behalf of all the stakeholder groups involved: company, community, and government stakeholders. The research task was to develop local, experientially rich and collaboratively developed understandings that would assist the parties in their efforts to negotiate around their interconnected issues. The research team used an open and transparent approach, documented its activities, and shared its deliberations with all parties to improve awareness of their respective interests and differences. Alcoa's refusal to allow a key summary research report to be shared with the community in late 2003 marked the end of the research contract. Key members of the research team withdrew from the contract with Alcoa since the company abused its power and transgressed the key ethic of transparency.

Measuring success

The success or otherwise of the partnership was measured in terms of Alcoa's adherence to the warrants or agreements for engagement, which sought to equalize power between stakeholders. This is not necessarily how Alcoa would define success or think about the research. As already discussed, Alcoa's deviation from these warrants led to the breakdown of negotiations in the Yarloop community and led the researchers to terminate their contract with Alcoa. The research team's duty of care to the community, who continued to invest an enormous amount of time and energy in the meetings, outweighed Alcoa's interests. The decision to terminate the research contract was inevitable given Alcoa personnel's lack of commitment to advancing the main parts of the agreed recommendations to their land management policy.

Strategies to equalize power

Given the inherent power imbalances in this unjust socioenvironmental situation, it was important to develop strategies for respectful engagement. For a time, it seemed this was achieved in the public meetings. The researchers worked hard to maintain the goodwill and mutual respect between meetings but, ultimately, were unsuccessful and the reasons for this lay beyond the terms of the research contract. It became evident that the local Alcoa personnel with whom the researchers and community were working did not have the power to make the decisions necessary to fulfil the conditions and outcomes of their joint negotiations. The power lay with Alcoa's senior executive at the company's head office in Perth. Though the rural community of Yarloop was a mere two hours south of Perth, there was no direct contact with the company's senior executive and the Wagerup managers with whom they were negotiating, though well intentioned, were ultimately ineffective. It took a parliamentary inquiry to force Alcoa to engage in socially and environmentally just practices in the purchase of private properties to establish a buffer for its commercial interests.

Conclusion

Efforts directed towards emphasizing the socioenvironmental aspects of struggles around the human rights of people in local communities, corporate social responsibility, and pro-development government agendas necessarily bring matters of power abuse and privilege to the fore. This case study showed social work's normative, anti-oppressive stance and array of knowledge and skills provided no quick-fix answers. Much, though, can be done to advance social and environmental justice without necessarily fully solving problems. Social work can contribute to informed public debate about the irreconcilable interests between mining companies and their impacts on people and environments. They can align with local community-based activist groups working to protect local interests and social and environmental ecosystems against the damaging effects wrought by multinational mining companies, such as Alcoa. Social workers can engage with communities, harnessing their skills to those of environmental groups who share a commitment to social and environmental justice. Through these alliances, they might leverage political and financial resources and resist the damaging incursions of corporate expansion. Social workers can participate in corporate social responsibility programs to put environmentally sustainable and socially just practices in the mining industry firmly on the agenda. Though this case study presents an unsuccessful outcome in many respects, like the researchers involved, the people from the Yarloop community, some personnel from Alcoa Wagerup, and some state government officials and politicians made genuine attempts to respond to the multidimensional conflict but could, ultimately, not stand up to the power of this mining giant. The lesson to be learnt from this case study is that moral or ethical grounds – agreed warrants, transparency, and accountability, in this case, for example – are insufficient to counter dominant economic interests. Powerful alliances have to be formed with activist groups to withstand the power of mining corporates *vis-à-vis* community and environmental interests. Though socioenvironmentally committed people continue to pursue justice-informed and environmentally sustainable outcomes day by day, unless they harness their energy to organizations that share their interests and concerns and at the same time build productive relationships with the mining corporations, little will change.

References

Alcoa Australia. (2001/2002). *Alcoa Wagerup land management revised proposal.* Perth: Alcoa World Alumina.

Alcoa Australia. (2002). *Visions, values: Principles.* Retrieved September 11, 2002 from http://www.alcoa.com/australia/en/pdf/Community/2002_Sustainability. pdf.

Alcoa Australia. (2003). *Media reports on Wagerup expansion incorrect.* Alcoa letter. Booragoon: Alcoa World Alumina.

Alcoa Australia. (2008). *Sustainability 08: Unlocking the solutions to sustainability.* Perth, Western Australia: Alcoa World Alumina.

Australian Association of Social Workers (AASW). (2010). *Code of ethics.* Canberra: Australian Association of Social Workers.

Besthorn, F.H. (2002). Radical environmentalism and the ecological self. *Journal of Progressive Human Services, 13*(1), 53–72.

Brager, G., and Holloway, S. (1978). *Changing human service organizations: Politics and practice.* New York: Free Press.

Brueckner, M., and Ross, D. (2010). *Under corporate skies: A struggle between people, place and profit.* Fremantle: Fremantle Press.

Coates, J. (2003). *Ecology and social work.* Halifax, NS: Fernwood Press.

Community Alliance for Positive Solutions (CAPS). (2011). CAPS Newsletter, *Summer Issue 12.* http://www.caps6218.org.au/.

Crane, A., and Matten, D. (2010). *Business ethics: Managing corporate citizenship and sustainability in the age of globalization* (3rd ed.). Oxford: Oxford University Press.

Donoghue, A., and Cullen, M. (2007). Air emissions from Wagerup alumina refinery and community symptoms: An environmental case study. *Journal of Occupational and Environmental Medicine, 49*(9), 1027–1039.

Drake, G. (2011). *Precautionary principle: Mining perspective.* Retrieved July 15, 2011 from http://www.uow.edu.au/~sharonb/STS300/science/regulation/articles/artprinciple11.html.

Flannery, T. (2009). *Now or never: A sustainable future for Australia?* Melbourne: Black Inc.

Flint, J. (2005). It's unjust and a threat to our health. *The Sunday Times.* Nov 20, pp. 10–11.

Flyvbjerg, B. (2001). *Making social science matter: Why social inquiry fails and how it can succeed again.* Cambridge: Cambridge University Press.

Fox, C., and Miller, H. (1995). *Postmodern public administration: Toward discourse.* Thousand Oaks, CA: Sage.

Freire, P. (1970). *Pedagogy of the oppressed.* New York: Herder & Herder.

Global Social Agenda (2011). *Global agenda for social work and social development.* Retrieved July 11, 2011 from http://www.globalsocialagenda.org/.

Hawkins, C. (2010). Sustainability, human rights and environmental justice: Critical connections for contemporary social work. *Critical social work, 11*(3). Retrieved January 8, 2012 from http://www.uwindsor.ca/criticalsocialwork/the-nexus-of-sustainability-human-rights-and-environmental-justice-a-critical-connection-for-contemp.

Henry, L. (2008). *Inaugural GESB board announced.* Retrieved January 8, 2012 from http://www.gesb.com.au/cps/rde/xbcr/internet/media_20081002_gml_board_appointment.pdf.

Higgins, P. (2010). *Eradicating ecocide: Exposing the corporate and political practices destroying the planet and proposing the laws needed to eradicate ecocide.* London: Shepheard-Walwyn Publishers Ltd.

Holliday, C., Schmidheiny, S., and Watts, P. (2002). *Walking the talk: The business case for sustainable development.* Sheffield, UK: Greenleaf Publishing Limited.

Ife, J. (2008). *Human rights and social work: Towards rights-based practice.* New York: Cambridge.

Ife, J., and Tesoriero, F. (2006). *Community development: Community based alternatives in the age of globalism* (3rd ed.). Sydney: Pearson Education Australia.

International Federation of Social Workers (IFSW). (2011). *Ethics in Social Work, Statement of Principles.* Retrieved December 9, 2011 from http://www.ifsw.org/f38000032.html.

Leonard, P. (1997). *Postmodern welfare: Reconstructing an emancipatory project.* London: Sage.

MacDonald, C. (2011). *Alcoa and corporate social responsibility: Rhetoric vs reality.* Miller-McCune.com e-newsletter. Retrieved July 12, 2011 from http://www.caps6218.org.au/documents/Alcoa%20Rehetoric%20vs.%20Realty.pdf.

Mackenzie, C. (2004). Moral sanctions: Ethical norms as a solution to corporate governance problems. *The Journal of Corporate Citizenship, 15*, 49–61.

Mayman, J. (2002). The stink of uncle Al. *The Weekend Australian.* May 11 and 12, p. 19.

McDermott, Q. (2005). *Something in the air.* Four Corners, Canberra: Australian Broadcasting Commission.

McGowan, M. (2006). *Environmental approval for the Alcoa expansion: Statement by the Minister for the Environment.* Perth: Government of Western Australia.

McKibben, J., and Waters, J. (2010). *The importance of maintaining social licence to operate.* Retrieved July 11, 2011 from http://www.theajmonline.com.au/mining_news/news/2010/april/april-22-10/other-top-stories/the-importance-of-maintaining-2018social-licence-to-operate2019.

Mullaly, B. (1997). *Structural social work. Ideology, theory and practice.* Toronto, ON: Oxford University Press.

Porter, M., and Kramer, M. (2006). Strategy and society: The link between competitive advantage and corporate social responsibility. HBR Spotlight. *Harvard Business Review,* December, 1–14.

Ross, D. (2002a). *Yarloop at the crossroads: Naming the issues.* Bunbury, Western Australia: Centre for Social Research.

Ross, D. (2002b). *Enacting my theory and politics of an ethic of love in social work education.* Doctoral thesis. Bunbury, Western Australia: Edith Cowan University.

Ross, D. (2009). Emphasising the social in corporate social responsibility. In S.O. Idowu and Filho, L.W. (Eds). *Professional perspectives of corporate social responsibility.* Heidelberg: Springer.

Sharp, C. (2004). *Report for the standing committee on environment and public affairs in relation to the Alcoa refinery at Wagerup inquiry.* Perth: Government of Western Australia.

Smith, D. (1990). *The conceptual practices of power: A feminist sociology of knowledge.* Boston, MA: Northeastern University Press.

Stanley, L., and Wise, S. (1993). *Breaking out again: Feminist ontology and epistemology* (2nd ed.). London: Routledge.

Tennyson, R., and Wilde, L. (2000). *The guiding hand: Brokering partnerships for sustainable development.* Geneva: United Nations Office of Public Information.

Wagerup Medical Practitioner's Forum (2005). *Submission on ERMP: Wagerup refinery unit 3 expansion.* Perth: Wagerup Medical Practitioner's Forum.

Walker, J., and Howard, S. (2002). *Finding a way forward: How could voluntary action move mining towards sustainable development?* London: MMSD, Earthscan.

Young, I. (1990). *Justice and the politics of difference.* Princeton, NJ: Princeton University Press.

Part 3

Education

Challenging students to respond to environmental issues

11 Transforming the curriculum
Social work education and ecological consciousness

Peter Jones

> The human race is part of nature. We need to have this insight before we can have harmony between people (Thich Nhat Hahn, 2008: 36).

Virtually from its inception as a professional activity, social work has had an interest in the interactions between people and their environment. Indeed this interest has seen the emergence of a number of influential theoretical orientations and practice theories, including the 'person-in-environment' and ecological approaches (see, for example, Germain, 1979; Germain and Gitterman, 1980; Karls, 2002). However, within social work, environment and ecology have often been conceptualized as almost exclusively social domains, neglecting to take into account broader relationships between humans and the non-human world. For over a decade, a small number of writers have advanced the argument that a more fully developed, expanded ecological orientation was needed in social work (for example, Berger and Kelly, 1993; Besthorn, 2000; Coates, 2003a; Hoff and Polack, 1993; Park, 1996). While the evidence suggests that an expanded ecological orientation remains a marginalized perspective in social work, there are hopeful signs that the profession might be ready to begin shifting from its traditionally narrow view.

Social work education has, inevitably, mirrored this narrow conceptualization of the environment (Besthorn and Canda, 2002). In Australia, there is little evidence of attempts to integrate, in a meaningful, holistic manner, expanded ecological approaches into the social work curriculum, although there have been some laudable attempts at introducing some ecosocial content in a number of BSW and MSW programs. Similarly, an expanded ecological perspective, or indeed explorations of social work's interest in the relationship between humans and the non-human world, do not feature very strongly in most social work education and practice journals.

This lack of attention to environmental issues is problematic in the face of emerging evidence which suggests that climate change, and other dimensions of anthropogenic environmental damage, will become an important dynamic in social work practice. This is particularly the case as the social impacts of such change, and government policy responses to it, become clearer and more obvious. If future professionals are to be well equipped to deal with this changing landscape, then new ways of conceptualizing its relationship to the environment will need to become an integral part of social work education.

Social work and the ecological crisis

There can now be little debate about the profound effect of human activity on the global environment. The nature and extent of anthropogenic environmental damage, including climate change, has been well documented in many scientific reports and represents as close to a scientific consensus as it is possible to achieve (Beeton, Buckley, Jones, Morgan, Reichelt, and Trewin, 2006; Garnaut, 2011; Intergovernmental Panel on Climate Change, 2007). It is now clear that such environmental damage, in all of its dimensions, will have widespread and potentially devastating social impacts, particularly on those who are already disadvantaged (United Nations Environment Programme, 2007).

Despite this mounting evidence, social work as a profession has, in the main, been slow to recognize the centrality of issues pertaining to the natural environment as a determinant of human well-being. Indeed, it can be argued that the profession has generally reflected a binary approach to the human–nature relationship, seeing itself as primarily concerned with people and issues of social justice, while the environment and issues of environmental and ecological justice remain the concern of others, outside of the profession. Analyses of this situation often reflect on social work's position as a profession with its roots in modernity (Coates, 2003b). In spite of this, a small but significant body of literature has been developed within the profession arguing that social work should expand its existing 'social-ecological' orientation to take greater account of the non-human world. This body of literature has been reviewed and discussed in other places (see, for example, Jones, 2010; Molyneux, 2010; McKinnon, 2008) and includes a wide range of approaches to thinking about how the profession might engage with the environment.

Key to the thinking of many of these authors has been an explicit linking of the social and environmental in ways that demonstrate the interrelatedness of the concepts of social and environmental justice (for example, Hillman, 2002; Low and Gleeson, 2001). Environmental justice has, in this sense, emerged as an additional, related concern for the profession, usually as a result of recognition of the impact of environmental issues on human well-being. The particular focus for social work has been on the inequitable distribution of environmental costs (for example, pollution and toxic waste) on already disadvantaged communities (Rogge, 2008). Recognition of environmental justice as a significant concern for social work has been a welcome development, often expressed as the right to clean air, clean water, and a clean, safe environment. Indeed, it is through the increasing recognition of issues of environmental justice that the non-human world has really begun to enter into social work consciousness. However, there are powerful arguments that notions of environmental justice remain fundamentally anthropocentric and that a truly ecologically oriented social work will need to push its understanding of justice much further than the current accepted models. The issues at stake here are discussed in detail by Besthorn (see Chapter 1).

Social work that embraces an expanded ecological paradigm tends to refute the dualistic, binary thinking that has characterized previous thought on the human–nature relationship. The nature of the profession, which involves working with the most disadvantaged individuals, groups, and communities, means that, at the very least, social work will be called upon to ameliorate the effects of environmental crises. Such 'reactive' practice might include dealing with hunger and food security, supporting environmental refugees, managing the health consequences of climate change, or assisting low-income families to manage energy costs in a low carbon economy, among many other possibilities. In some areas, it is clear that social workers are already working with environmentally related social issues and this trend is likely to continue in the future (Alston, 2007; Rogge and Combs-Orme, 2003).

In addition to reactive practice, there will also be opportunities for more positive and proactive practice. Again, there are examples of such practice already in operation (Berger, 2006; Carrilio, 2007; Lane, 1997) and social work sits on the periphery of a global movement concerned with finding ways to address climate change and other negative environmental impacts of human activity. Positive environmental practice might take many forms, but could include working with individuals and families to adapt to new environmental realities, contributing to the development of ecologically sustainable communities, and making a contribution to wider political and social policy discussions and decisions.

If the inevitability of the consequences and challenges of the environmental crisis – and the increasing importance of such issues in the future – were accepted, then it is logical to ask what role social work as a profession wants, and needs, to play in this future. Perhaps, more importantly, are social work students receiving an education that will equip them with the values, knowledge, and skills to play an active role in addressing the consequences of environmental degradation? A sense of where the profession currently stands in this regard can be gleaned from even a cursory glance at the content of social work programs and at the articles relating to the environment appearing in social work education and practice journals.

Ecological content in Australian social work education

While a relatively crude tool, one way of beginning to get a sense of how social work education is engaging with the emerging environmental agenda is to examine the publicly available descriptions of course offerings. To this end, the websites of universities offering BSW programs in Australia were explored, searching for course and unit descriptions indicating content focusing specifically on environment, ecology, ecological justice, and sustainability. The limitations of such an approach are that not all content in a curriculum is adequately captured in unit descriptions nor do such descriptions always accurately label the content actually taught in specific units. However, as an initial impression such a review does say something about the inclusion of the environment in current curricula.

In Australia, 27 universities offer a BSW program. A small number of universities were identified that offer required or compulsory units with a specific and focused emphasis on environment, sustainability, and ecosocial issues. The University of the Sunshine Coast, for example, requires social work students to take a unit on *Environment, Technology and Sustainability*; the Royal Melbourne Institute of Technology requires *Sustainability: Society and Environment*; and James Cook University requires *Developmental Approaches to Eco-Social Justice*. Interestingly, at Flinders University, where the undergraduate program is a Bachelor of Social Work and Social Planning, a slightly more thorough inclusion of the environment can be discerned, with a number of required units, such as *Social Work/Social Planning and the Environment, Society and Space*, and *Cities as Human Environments* having a significant ecological orientation.

In the majority of BSW program descriptions, however, where issues of the environment or ecology are mentioned at all, they usually appear among a checklist of social or policy issues. The message conveyed is that the particular environmental issue listed is just one among many that might be of interest to social workers. In a number of programs, no mention at all of ecology or environment was discernible, except as those terms might be used in an exclusionary social sense. From this limited overview, it is clear that there are no BSW programs in Australia that could lay claim to being ecologically oriented, where a deep understanding of natural processes and humans' place in the natural world is the foundation for professional education.

A similar exercise with key journals from social work and social work education was also revealing for what it said about the level of the profession's interest and engagement in this area. The table of contents of seven journals – *Journal of Social Work Education*; *Social Work Education*; *Journal of Teaching in Social Work*; *Australian Social Work*; *British Journal of Social Work*; *European Journal of Social Work*; *Social Work* – were reviewed with the intent of identifying articles whose titles indicated that they were clearly concerned with the environment, ecology, ecological justice, or sustainability. Articles were excluded if their titles indicated an ecological or environmental interest but where this related to the narrower, 'social' understanding of these terms discussed above.

Since 2001, these seven journals had published a total of eight articles whose titles clearly indicated they were concerned with ecological issues.

Three appeared in *Australian Social Work* while one was identified in each of the other journals, with the exception of *Social Work Education*, where no articles were found. There were undoubtedly many more articles in all of these journals with some reference to the natural environment, ecology or issues of sustainability in, for example, discussions of Indigenous practice issues or work in drought-affected areas. However, it was telling that in these leading fora for social work thought so few authors had focused specifically on ecologically related topics. Outside of these establishment publications, there were other publications where the challenge of addressing issues of ecology had been taken up, such as the online journal *Critical Social Work* where issues of environment, ecology, and sustainability have been a theme over some years.

The inescapable conclusion is that Australian social work education's engagement with an expanded ecological perspective has been generally piecemeal and often peripheral. Given the strong arguments for greater attention to this area, it is worthwhile considering how changes in curricula might be approached to meet this end.

Pathways to ecological engagement

While an increased commitment to an ecological orientation will be essential in the future, there are many possible pathways to such change within social work education. These may be usefully grouped into three types: changes that: (1) focus on adding ecological content into the existing curriculum; (2) seek to 'embed' material on ecology and sustainability into the existing curriculum; and (3) endeavour to transform the entire curriculum to reflect a holistic ecological orientation.

The 'bolt-on' option

The first option for changing BSW offerings to reflect recognition of the environmental crisis, and the relationship of social work to this crisis, is the traditional curriculum content approach. Fundamentally, such an approach involves identifying an issue, skill, knowledge area, or practice approach that is currently not addressed and looking for places to insert such content into the existing curriculum. It is a content-driven approach and requires no change in pedagogy or shift in underlying values, beliefs, or ways of seeing the world. This process is, in effect, a response to the question 'what do students need to know?' and a recognition that the answer to this question may change or expand over time.

Such an approach could be used in relation to ecological issues, and indeed has been. When my colleague Robyn Lynn and I developed a stand-alone subject on socio-environmentalism for inclusion in the BSW program at James Cook University, it was in response to a perceived gap in this area (see Jones, 2008). For many years the subject stood as the only environmental component in the degree, effectively a 'bolt-on' solution. Where similar attempts to include ecological content in BSW programs can be identified, they are often of this nature, either subjects that have been introduced to address the gap or discrete material within subjects included to the same end.

Such methods can be effective ways of raising the profile of ecosocial issues and exposing students to new knowledge and ways of working. They are certainly much better than having no content included in the curriculum at all. There are also some serious limitations to this approach. The most obvious limitation is the crowding of the curriculum. While suggestions are often made, by academics, students, accrediting bodies, and the field for new content that should be included in the curriculum, seldom are suggestions made about what can be dropped. The result is an increasing amount of content that needs to be delivered in the same amount of time. More significantly, the bolt-on approach does nothing to change the fundamental ways of thinking about the relationship between social work and environmental issues. In many respects, it simply supports the status quo, both ideologically and pedagogically. Humans' relationship to the environment, and the implications of this relationship for social work, becomes simply another 'topic' to learn, one among a long list of content areas that can sometimes seem like items to be ticked off on the way through a degree.

Such a business-as-usual approach might be acceptable if it were believed that the existing curriculum and pedagogies employed in social work education had got it right. Given the discussion above, there seems little evidence to support this contention. But there is an argument to be made, following Coates' (2003b) critique of social work and modernity, that business as usual is actually part of the problem and, therefore, cannot really be the solution. If the genesis of the ecological crisis were, at least in part, related to the dualism, empiricism, rationality, and reductionism that characterizes modernity, then how would an approach to education firmly rooted in these dynamics help social workers find a way forward in addressing the environmental crisis?

In some respects this issue mirrors the debate (long since resolved) that existed within the field of environmental education: should students be educated *about* sustainability or *for* sustainability (see, for example, Martins, Mata, and Costa, 2006; Shephard, 2008, 2010). The first implies simply adding another content area to the curriculum, the second at least opens up the possibility of exploring new ways of doing things as well as new areas of knowledge. In some areas of higher education, generally outside of social work, such discussions have led to a re-thinking of what education is actually for as well as how it is practically done (Junyent and Geli de Ciurana, 2008; Lange, 2009; Orr, 1992). Taken to their logical conclusion, the arguments against bolt-on approaches to the ecological crisis suggest that what is really required is a more fundamental shift in the way social work education is conceptualized.

The 'embedding' option

The second pathway is employed when an issue or perspective is seen as possessing such fundamental importance that an attempt is made to ensure that the perspective permeates the curriculum. Embedding a perspective in this manner involves looking for the connections between the existing curriculum and the area of concern in each unit or component of a BSW program. An example of this approach can be seen in the BSW and MSW programs at James Cook University (JCU) in Australia. JCU's unique geographical location, coupled with a strong ideological commitment, has led to an attempt to embed Australian Indigenous perspectives into all core social work subjects within the program. On a unit-by-unit basis, this has meant exploring ways in which the traditional content might be linked to Indigenous perspectives (Gair, 2007; Gair and Pagliano, 2008).

The success of such an embedded approach is variable. At best, there is a new way of seeing the traditional content facilitated by the introduction of Indigenous perspectives. This has the potential to produce new and meaningful learning experiences for students. At its least effective, such an approach simply means adding in some Indigenous-focused reading material, or including a module on Indigenous perspectives within the existing unit schedule. In other words, there remains the risk of producing a 'bolt-on' solution, but in this case replicated in multiple individual units across the program.

There do not appear to be any clear examples of attempts to embed ecological or sustainability perspectives thoroughly within a BSW program in Australia. However, there are discussions of such approaches in other locations, such as Canada, and from other disciplines (see Kahn and Scher, 2002). There is significant potential under this approach to assist students to develop a deeper awareness of the importance of ecological issues for their profession and to gain a practical understanding of the ways such a perspective may manifest in practice. It is not, however, a fundamentally transformative approach.

The transformative option

The third option for shifting the focus of social work education towards a more ecologically informed and oriented approach is the most challenging and far-reaching. Rather than asking the question 'what do students need to know in order to practise social work', a transformative approach to social work education seeks first to discover the answer to a broader question, 'what do we need to know in order to survive on this fragile planet?' and only then asks the question 'how can such a deep, ecologically aware knowledge and value base inform and shape social work practice?' In many respects, such an approach turns the traditional thinking around social work education on its head. Rather than beginning with a list of topics and issues which a student should know in order to become a practitioner, an ecologically transformative approach would seek to develop deep understandings of the workings of the natural world (of which humans are inextricably a part) and to then explore the ways in which such an understanding might translate into social work practice. This shift in fundamental assumptions about what education should be about would, in practice, go further than an embedded approach and would be the antithesis of the bolt-on solution discussed above (see Chapter 1).

In such an approach, the purpose of education generally is to increase people's capacity to understand and contribute actively to a sustainable future. Such a goal can only be based on a deep and holistic understanding of humans' place in the natural world and a thorough critique and analysis of the ways in which human activity has impacted on this world (Harper, 2008). Professional education would then build on this holistic ecological foundation. The foundation could be seen as consisting of: a body of knowledge, about natural systems and humans' place within these systems; a critique of the existing situation that seeks to develop an understanding of what has gone wrong in the human–nature relationship; and a set of values that provide guidance for a way of living that reflects a deep ecological understanding and has the potential to take the profession forward to a sustainable future. It is at this stage that we would be in a position to return to the question 'how can such a deep, ecologically aware knowledge and value base inform and shape social work practice?'

Social work education would, in this scenario, be charged with exploring the ways in which deep ecological understandings might help social workers better understand, plan, and implement human systems. Educators would look to natural systems and a deeper understanding of key ecological concepts, such as relationship and interdependence, for guidance in many areas of social work education and practice: interpersonal communication, social policy, mental health, community development, values and ethics, reflexive practice, and so on. This process of looking to nature has been used extensively in other fields (Birkeland, 2002). An ecologically transformative approach to curriculum development privileges ecological understanding as the inevitable and necessary starting point for professional education.

Key dimensions of an expanded ecosocial approach

It is clear that an ecologically transformative approach to social work education would involve some significant shifts in the content and pedagogy of social work programs. Exactly what such a transformed program would look like is, at this stage, unclear and indeed it may be counterintuitive to overly prescribe such detail at this stage, thereby limiting the potential for organic development. Starting points for the development of such an approach, and some possibilities for changes in emphasis that might accompany such a shift, can, however, be identified. The key to developing a solid foundation for an ecologically transformed approach to social work education would be a focus on the understanding that students have of the natural world, its processes and systems, and the place that humans occupy within this world. This deep understanding has been referred to as the development of 'ecological literacy' (Orr, 1992), a concept that would sit at the heart of a transformed approach to education.

Ecoliteracy

As humans have become more technologically advanced and deeply alienated from nature, understandings of the natural world, its processes and systems, and our place in them, has declined or disappeared (Orr, 1992). A type of illiteracy has developed that leaves us unable to 'read' and understand the world around us, upon which our very existence depends. Ecological literacy refers to the capacity to understand nature's systems (Orr, 1992; Fleischer, 2011). To become ecologically literate is to relearn the processes of nature and our place in them. It is a process of reconnection that emphasizes the fact that human well-being, indeed existence, is predicated on the operation of such processes. Humans are not above or beyond the fundamentals of natural systems, but are rather entirely dependent upon them. The 'content' to be learned in becoming ecologically literate is relatively straightforward, including the centrality of the network as a form of organization, the cycling of matter through the web of life, and the sustaining of life through the flow of energy from the sun (Capra, 2005; Chiras, 2005). However, ecoliteracy also highlights the need for a new pedagogical approach to allow for deeper reconnection to the natural world (Chiras, 2005; Duailibi, 2006; Hill, Wilson, and Watson, 2004).

Indigenous ways of knowing

The development of ecological literacy would include not just an understanding of the operations of the non-human world, but also a critical analysis of the relationship of humans to this world and their impact upon it. Such a focus would highlight the importance of including Indigenous perspectives and ways of knowing as essential components of a transformed curriculum. A number of writers have explored the ways in which Indigenous understandings of, and connection to, place represent an important approach to ecological understanding and a necessary perspective in social work (Gray and Coates, 2010; Coates, Gray, and Hetherington, 2006; Woolhorton and Bennell, 2007). Indigenous perspectives often stand in stark contrast to Western, industrialized relationships with the non-human world and offer a worldview that highlights notions of reciprocity and connection to the land (Milroy and Milroy, 2008). As content, such knowledge becomes an important component of a transformative approach.

However, such knowledge also suggests new and different forms of pedagogy, shifting not only what is taught, but also the ways in which it might be taught (Townsend-Cross, 2011). Exploring these pedagogical possibilities in a manner that is inclusive and respectful of Indigenous Peoples would present another challenge for a transformed social work education.

Spirituality

An ecologically transformed social work education would also give more time to the exploration of spirituality and its role in shaping the human–nature relationship (Keefe, 2003; Zapf, 2005, 2008). Spirituality in this sense refers less to organized religious traditions and more to the broader sense of humans' place within something ineffably larger than ourselves. Ecologically, there are a number of ways in which this has been explored. Lovelock's (1979) Gaia Hypothesis, for example, sees humans as a small part of a larger organism, a complex self-sustaining and self-regulating system (Penton, 1993). Coates (2003b) has explored the importance of understanding cosmogenesis, the narrative of an unfolding universe, whose scope and scale puts human existence into some perspective, while Wilson's (1984) biophilia hypothesis suggests a biological basis for a deep, spiritual affinity with nature (Besthorn and Saleebey, 2003; Kellert, 2005; Lysack, 2009a). Of course, many Indigenous traditions also postulate a deeply spiritual approach to understanding the relationships of people to natural systems.

The significance of all or any of these ecospiritual understandings is that they provide another way of conceptualizing humans' place within a much larger, unfolding, and dynamic system. This is not simply a matter of new content that should be introduced into a program. Recognition of the spiritual dimensions of the human–nature relationship also suggests a range of different pedagogical approaches, including greater use of contemplative practices as pathways for learning (Lysack, 2009b, see Chapter 12). For students (and educators) exploring this dimension can serve to generate a sense of awe and indeed reverence for the larger whole and subsequently a deeper critical appreciation of human beings' place within it.

Criticality

While exploring ecological literacy, Indigenous ways of knowing, and ecospirituality as important dimensions of a transformed social work curriculum, it is important that some existing dimensions of traditional approaches to education be retained and emphasized as part of the construction of a new ecological foundation. Foremost among these is the centrality of a critical approach to education and, in particular, to the development of an understanding of humans' place in the natural world (O'Sullivan, 1999). It would be a mistake to see an ecologically oriented social work education as somehow 'softer', 'fuzzier', or less critically rigorous than existing approaches. Indeed, meticulous critical analysis would be essential in many areas of a transformed curriculum starting with developing an understanding of the genesis of the environmental crisis, through to analysing scientific data and exploring the impacts of government policies. Traditional issues of power and privilege would remain highly relevant for such a critical approach, as would concepts of human rights and social and environmental justice, but they would need to be reenvisioned from an ecocentric perspective to fashion a radical equalitarian ecological justice (see Chapter 1).

Congruence with existing approaches to curriculum

While the development of an ecologically transformed curriculum for social work education would represent a radical departure from current practices, it is also important to note that many elements of existing approaches to social work training remain relevant and would find a comfortable place within a transformed structure. There exists, in other words, significant levels of congruence between dimensions of existing approaches and what would be required of a transformed approach. This is an important realization as such congruence would allow continuity and ease the transitional process as changes were made towards a more ecologically oriented social work education.

Current emphases on, for example, interpersonal communication skills, social policy analysis, and the centrality of values and ethics would be retained in a transformed curriculum. In these and many other areas the difference would be that the teaching and exploration of this content would be informed by a deeper understanding of ecological principles and would include expanded notions of what would need to be addressed in a truly ecologically literate education. To take another example, community-based practice, or community development, appears in all Australian social work programs in one form or another. There are strong arguments for this to continue in an ecologically transformed approach. But within such an approach the notion of community would be explored from the foundation of a deeper understanding of the operation of dynamic natural systems (Steiner, 2002). The development of ecosocially sustainable community solutions would become the goal of community development practice as concepts of environmental and ecological justice altered existing anthropocentric values of social justice and human rights (see Chapter 14). Nature too has rights. Significant work has already been done in exploring these issues with community development (see, for example, Ife and Tesoriero, 2006; Wint, 2000) but in an ecologically oriented social work education such approaches would be central and integral rather than peripheral or marginal.

All social work programs place significant emphasis on the importance of humanistic values and ethics as part of the foundation for professional practice (Banks, 2005). A foundation of ecological literacy and critical ecological analysis would mean that discussions of values and ethics would need to take place within a fuller understanding of humans' place in the world, of the finite physical limits of the planet, and of the unequal distribution of ecological goods across and within societies. It would simply not be possible (or logical) in a transformed curriculum to discuss issues of ecological justice without consideration of ecocentric values (Attfield, 2003) or the consequences of human materialism and consumption for the natural world (Hamilton and Denniss, 2005). Discussions of ethical behaviour would need to include analyses of Western 'lifestyle choices' and the impact of these on the biosphere. In this way, students would get a sense of how such a transformed approach could accommodate an expanded ecological consciousness.

Ecology: A thematic lens for a transformed social work education

One of the criticisms that can be made of existing approaches to social work education and of the accreditation guidelines that shape them is that they tend to privilege practice content above concepts and theory. In other words, the prescribed curriculum within social work programs identifies a list of facts, topics, and skills students should understand and acquire in order to become professional practitioners. Writers, such as O'Sullivan (1999, 2002), have highlighted the deficiencies of contemporary models by describing what a radically, ecologically oriented approach to education might entail. The work of Erickson (2002) on curriculum design is useful in this respect. Erickson describes content, as it appears in traditional curriculum design, as usually representing a focus on lower-order thinking skills, a set of facts and topics to be consumed. While such knowledge is important, she argues that higher-order critical thinking skills should sit above and inform the content areas themselves. Effective curriculum should see content viewed through the overarching concepts that are integral to the goals of a program. Such a concept would represent a 'thematic lens' (Galloway, 2011) through which all subsequent content was viewed and understood. In a transformed social work curriculum, the relevant thematic lens would be the concept of ecology.

Sitting beneath this overarching thematic lens would be a set of key values and concepts critical to the development of an ecological understanding. There is enormous scope for discussion about what such key elements might be and there is no reason why significant variation might not occur between specific social work programs depending on an educational provider's particular interests and emphases. As an example, the key ecological values or concepts suggested by Coates (2003b) include the lessons to be learned from the story of cosmogenesis, such as 'all is one' – recognizing connectedness, interdependence, and self-organization; subjectivity – understanding that every part has intrinsic value and an important role in the evolution of itself and the whole; complexity – of an organic and dynamic universe where change is a constant, creative process; and boundaries – understanding sustainability and the finite nature of resources.

Kaza (2010) adopts a different approach in exploring a spiritual guide to ecological thought, identifying three key values: understanding energy; working with desire; and practising peace. Parkin (2010) argues for a knowledge base comprising ecocentric ethics and values; people and community; science and technology; and economics. An interesting choice might be to use the four pillars of the Earth Charter (United Nations Educational Scientific and Cultural Organization, 2004): respect and care of the community of life; ecological integrity; social and economic justice; and democracy, non-violence, and peace. These key concepts and values could provide the structure within which individual content areas might be examined. Taken together, the overarching thematic lens and key concepts would form the outline of the ecological foundation upon which specific social work content might be based. While the detailed content and pedagogical practices would, of course, require transformation and expansion, and would grow out of the deep, ecological understandings that flow from engagement with the foundation, it would be possible to see where many of the existing content areas of social work education might sit within such a transformed structure (see Figure 11.1).

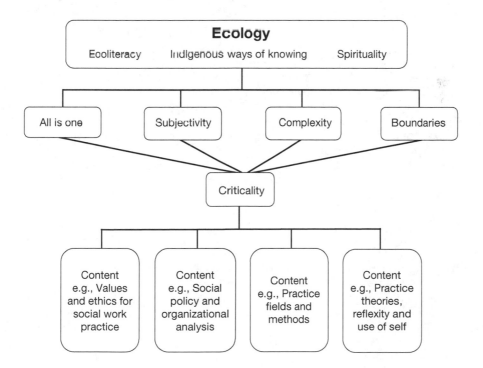

Figure 11.1 Ecologically oriented social work education

Conclusion

Given contemporary knowledge on the nature and extent of the ecological crisis, it is indisputable that the social work profession has a responsibility to respond to the social consequences of anthropogenic environmental damage. It can also be argued that, as a profession espousing human rights and social justice, social work has a responsibility to do more than simply ameliorate the consequences of such change, but should be part of the global movement to address environmental issues and steer humanity towards a sustainable future. Urgent attention must be paid to the way contemporary approaches to social work education fail to equip our students, future professional social workers, with the values, knowledge, and skills required in this challenging future.

To truly reorient social work in light of the environmental crisis would require a transformation of the very foundations of professional education and a rethinking of the purposes and goals of education itself. Using ecology as an overarching thematic lens, and ecological justice as a serious concern, social work education has an opportunity to identify key ecological concepts and ecocentric values that can act as the foundation from which the knowledge, values, and skills for professional practice might be developed. Key to such a foundation would be the establishment of ecological literacy as an essential component of all educational processes, and an integral aspect of social work education.

References

Alston, M. (2007). It's really not easy to get help: Services to drought-affected families. *Australian Social Work , 60*(4), 421–435.

Attfield, R. (2003). *Environmental ethics: An overview for the twenty-first century.* Cambridge: Polity Press.

Banks, S. (2005). The ethical practitioner in formation: Issues of courage, competence and commitment. *Social Work Education, 24*(5), 737–753.

Beeton, R., Buckley, K., Jones, G., Morgan, D., Reichelt, R., and Trewin, D. (2006). *Australia state of the environment 2006 – at a glance: Summary of the independent report to the Australian Government Minister for the Environment and Heritage.* Canberra: Department of the Environment and Heritage.

Berger, R. (2006). Using contact with nature, creativity and rituals as a therapeutic medium with children with learning difficulties: A case study. *Emotional and Behavioural Difficulties, 11*(2), 135–146.

Berger, R., and Kelly, J. (1993). Social work in the ecological crisis. *Social Work, 38,* 521–526.

Besthorn, F.H. (2000). Toward a deep-ecological social work: Its environmental, spiritual and political dimensions. *The Spirituality and Social Work Forum, 7*(2), 2–7.

Besthorn, F.H., and Canda, E. (2002). Revisioning environment: Deep ecology for education and teaching in social work. *Journal of Teaching in Social Work, 22*(1/2), 79–101.

Besthorn, F.H., and Saleebey, D. (2003) Nature, genetics and the biophilia connection: Exploring linkages with social work values and practice. *Advances in Social Work*, 4(1), 1–18.

Birkeland, J. (2002). *Ideas for sustainability.* London: Earthscan Publications.

Capra, F. (2005). Preface. In M. Stone and Barlow, Z. (Eds). *Ecological literacy: Educating our children for a sustainable world.* San Francisco: Sierra Club Books. xiii–xv.

Carrilio, T. (2007). Utilizing a social work perspective to enhance sustainable development efforts in Loreto, Mexico. *International Social Work*, 50(4), 528–538.

Chiras, D. (2005). *Ecokids: Raising children who care for the Earth.* Gabriola Island, BC: New Society Publishers.

Coates, J. (2003a). Exploring the roots of the environmental crisis: Opportunity for social transformation. *Critical Social Work*, 3(1), 44–66.

Coates, J. (2003b). *Ecology and social work: Toward a new paradigm.* Halifax, NS: Fernwood Publishing.

Coates, J., Gray, M., and Hetherington, T. (2006). An 'ecospiritual' perspective: Finally, a place for Indigenous approaches. *British Journal of Social Work*, 36(3), 381–399.

Duailibi, M. (2006). Ecological literacy: What are we talking about? *Convergence*, 39(4), 65–68.

Erickson, L. (2002). *Concept-based curriculum and instruction: Teaching beyond the facts.* Thousand Oaks, CA: Corwin Press.

Flcischer, S. (2011). Emerging beliefs frustrate ecological literacy and meaning-making for students. *Cultural Studies of Science Education*, 6, 235–241.

Gair, S. (2007). Pursuing Indigenous-inclusive curriculum in social work tertiary education: Feeling my way as a non-Indigenous educator. *Australian Journal of Indigenous Education*, 36, 49–55.

Gair, S., and Pagliano, P. (2008). 'Don't we already do that?' In search of an Indigenous and non-Indigenous academic symbiosis. *Journal of Australian Indigenous Issues*, 11(3), 3–18

Galloway, K. (2011). Refreshed in the tropics: Developing curriculum using a thematic lens. Paper delivered at Australasian Law Teachers' Association Conference, Brisbane, July 2–6.

Garnaut, R. (2011). *The Garnaut Review 2011: Australia in the Global Response to Climate Change.* Canberra: Cambridge.

Germain, C. (Ed.). (1979). *Social work practice: People and environments – An ecological perspective.* New York: Columbia University Press.

Germain, C., and Gitterman, A. (1980). *The life model of social work practice.* New York: Columbia University Press.

Gray, M., and Coates, J. (2010). 'Indigenization' and knowledge development: Extending the debate. *International Social Work*, 53, 613–627.

Hamilton, C., and Denniss, R. (2005). *Affluenza: When too much is never enough.* Sydney: Allen & Unwin.

Harper, C. (2008). *Environment and society: Human perspectives on environmental issues.* Upper Saddle River, NJ: Pearson Prentice Hall.

Hill, S., Wilson, S., and Watson, K. (2004). Learning ecology: A new approach to learning and transforming ecological consciousness. In E. O'Sullivan and Taylor, M. (Eds). *Learning toward an ecological consciousness: Selected transformative practices.* New York: Palgrave Macmillan. 47–64.

Hillman, M. (2002). Environmental justice: A crucial link between environmentalism and community development? *Community Development Journal, 37*(4), 349–360.

Hoff, M., and Polack, R. (1993). Social dimensions of the environmental crisis: Challenges for social work. *Social Work, 38*, 204–211.

Ife, J., and Tesoriero, F. (2006). *Community Development: Community-based alternatives in an age of globalisation.* Frenchs Forest, NSW: Pearson Education.

Intergovernmental Panel on Climate Change (IPCC). (2007). *Climate Change 2007: Synthesis Report. Contribution of Working Groups I, II and III to the Fourth Assessment Report of the Intergovernmental Panel on Climate Change* [Core Writing Team, Pachauri, R.K. and Reisinger, A. (Eds)]. Switzerland: Intergovernmental Panel on Climate Change.

Jones, P. (2008). Expanding the ecological consciousness of social work students: Education for sustainable practice. In *Sustainability in Higher Education: Directions for Change. Proceedings of the EDU-COM 2008 Conference.* Khon Kaen, Thailand: EDU-COM.

Jones, P. (2010). Responding to the ecological crisis: Transformative pathways for social work education. *Journal of Social Work Education, 46*(1), 67–84.

Junyent, M., and Geli de Ciurana, A. (2008). Education for sustainability in university studies: A model for reorienting the curriculum. *British Educational Research Journal, 34*(6), 763–782.

Kahn, M., and Scher, S. (2002). Infusing content on the physical environment into the BSW curriculum. *The Journal of Baccalaureate Social Work, 7*(2), 1–14.

Karls, J.M. (2002). Person-in-environment system: Its essence and applications. In A.R. Roberts and Greene, G.J. (Eds). *Social workers' desk reference.* New York: Oxford University Press. 194–198.

Kaza, S. (2010). *Mindfully green: A personal and spiritual guide to whole-earth thinking.* Sydney: Finch Publishing.

Keefe, T. (2003). The bio-psycho-social-spiritual origins of environmental justice. *Critical Social Work, 4*(1). Retrieved on July 22, 2011 from www.criticalsocial work.com/units/socialwork/critical.nsf/982f.

Kellert, S. (2005). The biological basis for human values of nature. In L. Kalof and Satterfield, T. (Eds). *The Earthscan reader in environmental values.* London: Earthscan. 131–150.

Lane, M. (1997). Community work, social work: Green and postmodern? *British Journal of Social Work, 27*(3), 319–341.

Lange, E. (2009). Fostering a learning sanctuary for transformation in sustainability education. In J. Mezirow, Taylor, E., and Associates (Eds). *Transformative learning in practice: Insights from community, workplace and higher education.* San Francisco, CA: Jossey Bass. 193–204.

Lovelock, J. (1979). *Gaia: A new look at life on Earth.* Oxford: Oxford University Press.

Low, N., and Gleeson, B. (2001). The challenge of ethical environmental governance. In N. Low and Gleeson, B. (Eds). *Governing for the environment: Global problems, ethics and democracy.* Basingstoke: Palgrave. 1–25.

Lysack, M. (2009a). Defending and protecting what we love: Biophilia and creating environmental citizenship. *Wild Lands Advocate, 17*(3), 14–16.

Lysack, M. (2009b). From environmental despair to the ecological self: Mindfulness and community action. In S. Hick (Ed.). *Mindfulness and social work.* Chicago, IL: Lyceum Press. 202–218.

Martins, A., Mata, T., and Costa, C. (2006). Education for sustainability: Challenges and trends. *Clean Technologies and Environmental Policy, 8*(1), 31–37.

McKinnon, J. (2008). Exploring the nexus between social work and the environment. *Australian Social Work, 61*(3), 256–268.

Milroy, G., and Milroy, J. (2008). Different ways of knowing: Trees are our families too. In S. Morgan, Tjalaminu, M., and Kwaymullina, B. (Eds). *Heartsick for country: Stories of love, spirit and creation.* Fremantle, WA: Fremantle Press. 21–42.

Molyneux, R. (2010). The practical realities of ecosocial work: A review of the literature. *Critical Social Work, 11*(2). Retrieved July 15, 2011 from http://www.uwindsor.ca/criticalsocialwork/the-practical-realities-of-ecosocial-work-a-review-of-the-literature.

Orr, D. (1992). *Ecological literacy: Education and the transition to a postmodern world.* Albany, NY: State University of New York Press.

O'Sullivan, E. (1999). *Transformative learning: Educational vision for the 21st century.* London: Zed Books.

O'Sullivan, E. (2002). The project and vision of transformative education: Integral trans- formative learning. In E. O'Sullivan, Morrell, A., and. O'Connor, M.A. (Eds). *Expanding the boundaries of transformative learning.* New York: Palgrave. 1–12

Park, K. (1996). The personal is ecological: Environmentalism of social work. *Social Work, 41,* 320–323.

Parkin, S. (2010). *The positive deviant: Sustainability leadership in a perverse world.* London: Earthscan.

Penton, K. (1993). Ideology, social work, and the Gaian connection. *Australian Social Work, 46*(4), 41–48.

Rogge, M. (2008). Environmental justice. In National Association of Social Workers (NASW), *Encyclopedia of Social Work.* New York: Oxford University Press. 136–139.

Rogge, M., and Combs-Orme, T. (2003). Protecting children from chemical exposure: Social work and U.S. social welfare policy. *Social Work, 48*(4), 439–450.

Shephard, K. (2008). Higher education for sustainability: Seeking affective learning outcomes. *International Journal of Sustainability in Higher Education, 9*(1), 87–98.

Shephard, K. (2010). Higher education's role in education for sustainability. *Australian Universities Review, 52*(1), 13–22.

Steiner, F. (2002). *Human ecology: Following nature's lead.* Washington: Island Press.

Thich Nhat Hahn (2008). *The world we have: A Buddhist approach to peace and ecology.* Berkeley, CA: Parallax Press.

Townsend-Cross, M. (2011). Indigenous education and Indigenous Studies in the Australian Academy: Assimilationism, critical pedagogy, dominant culture learners and Indigenous knowledges. In G.J.S. Dei (Ed.). *Indigenous philosophies and critical education.* New York: Peter Lang. 68–79.

United Nations Educational Scientific and Cultural Organization (UNESCO). (2004). *Records of the general conference, 32nd session, Paris, 29 September to 17 October, 2003.* Paris: UNESCO.

United Nations Environment Programme. (2007). *Global environment outlook: Environment for development (GEO4).* Retrieved on July 22, 2011 from http://www.unep. org/geo/geo4.

Wilson, E.O. (1984). *Biophilia.* Cambridge, MA: Harvard University Press.

Wint, E. (2000). Factors encouraging the growth of sustainable communities: A Jamaican study. *Journal of Sociology and Social Welfare, 27*(3), 119–133.

Woolhorton, S., and Bennell, D. (2007). Ecological literacy: Noongar way. *Every Child, 13*(4), 30–31.

Zapf, M.K. (2005). The spiritual dimension of person and environment: Perspectives from social work and traditional knowledge. *International Social Work, 48*(5), 633–642.

Zapf, M.K. (2008). Transforming social work's understanding of person and environment: Spirituality and 'common ground'. *Journal of Religion & Spirituality in Social Work: Social Thought, 27*(1–2), 171–181.

12 Emotion, ethics, and fostering committed environmental citizenship

Mishka Lysack

> [The] anxiety, loss of meaning and direction, and concern for the future that many people feel in modern society can be linked to the problems of modernity and environmental destruction (Coates, 2003: 134).

At first glance, this statement of ecosocial work scholar John Coates (2003) may appear to be a rather audacious, even reckless claim, overreaching its grasp in explaining the malaise permeating modern Western society. But Coates persists, and traces the implications of his insight into contemporary consciousness, proposing that addressing this malaise is a responsibility that falls to helping professions, especially social work. Coates (2003) writes:

> One task of social work and counselling professions will be to help people deal with their sense of anxiety and loss. While people may not be aware of the cause of these feelings, for many the distress will be rooted in trepidation about the present and the future.
>
> (p. 131)

Referring to what Buddhist teacher and environmental activist Joanna Macy (1990) calls the 'pivotal psychological reality of our time' (p. 56), Coates (2003) continues by asserting that the 'depth of the concern may be great as many people will be confronting that which provides their lives with meaning and ultimate answers' (p. 131).

While there may not be 'hard' empirical proof establishing the certainty of such a claim, there are certainly indications from other quarters that this intuition about the deepening unease in contemporary society is worthy of further consideration. Clearly, Coates (2003) is not alone in his suspicions, even though conclusions about the interrelationships between emotional well-being, material wealth, and ecological degradation vary. Ecological economist Anielski (2007) wrestles with the question, 'does consuming more of nature buy more happiness?', and concludes that research does indeed suggest that it is possible to 'achieve a higher quality of life with a smaller ecological footprint, based on a more moderate and frugal lifestyle' (pp. 222–223). In his book *Deep Economy*, McKibben (2007) outlines findings where 'research from many quarters has started to show that even when growth does make us wealthier, the greater wealth no longer makes us happier' (p. 2), a distressing finding when joined with 'our dawning understanding of our ecological peril and our psychological malaise' (p. 226).

But these pathways of inquiry do not equip us to explore the thorny issue as to the components of the emotional impacts of ecological decline. To be fair, McKibben (2007) does explore this issue in depth, especially in his earlier book *The End of Nature*. Even then, such explorations still do not quite lead to the 'holy grail' of how those emotional responses might contribute, or even be a critical element of the development of committed ecological citizenship. Such is the deeper concern of this chapter, one that is shared by all those involved in public education and movement building fostering the emergence of a resilient environmental advocacy to protect the planet.

The growing interest of the environmental NGO community in the critical role of emotion in the emergence of ecological awareness and environmental citizenship is especially striking, as it highlights the growing realization among ecological educators and environmental activists that information alone is insufficient to create the motivational wellsprings for sustained action and engagement on the part of ordinary citizens (Moser and Dilling, 2007). While the debate continues as to what specific elements contribute to the emergence of ecological engagement (Thomashow, 2002), educators now propose that affective images play a role in enhancing the likelihood of engagement in environmental action (Leiserowitz, 2007). In her research, climate change educator Moser (2007a) explores the risks of neglecting people's emotional responses to information regarding climate change impacts, while acknowledging that negative scare tactics using fear to motivate individuals do not promote the growth of commitment to effective environmental action.

Since the advent of Freud decades ago, it has been known that individuals and communities do not act primarily on the basis of fact or reason, but often on the basis of emotion, a fact that has not escaped the attention of those perfecting the science of propaganda and media manipulation begun in the Second World War and developed further in modern corporate society (Lakoff, 2004, 2009). Emotions by themselves do not promote prosocial behaviour, and in fact, have the capacity to be tethered to anti-social forces vectoring individuals to engage in destructive activity. However, as a powerful driver of human behaviour, emotional connection can also be foundational for building transformative social movements grounded in a moral vision and ethical perspective, such as the environmental or civil rights movements.

This chapter begins with an overview of the new ecological context in which humanity finds itself, facing serious threats from climate change and the sixth mega extinction of biodiversity. A growing number of scientists and environmental writers are concluding that humanity is either close to, or may have effectively 'crossed the line of no return', when it is no longer possible to turn these threats of climate change or the biodiversity mega extinction around. At the same time, these scientists also insist that there is much that humanity still can and must save. Environmental ethicist Hamilton (2010) is arresting in his directness in assessing the implications:

> Over the last five years, almost every advance to climate science has painted a more disturbing picture of the future. The reluctant conclusion of the most eminent climate scientists is that the world is now on a path to a very unpleasant future and it is too late to stop it. Behind the façade of scientific detachment, the climate scientists themselves now evince a mood of barely suppressed panic. No one is willing to say publicly what the climate science is telling us: that we can no longer prevent global warming that will this century bring about a radically transformed world that is much more hostile to the survival and flourishing of life.
>
> (pp. x–xi)

It is difficult to ascertain the specific impacts on the emotional life of individuals as humanity becomes aware of this historically unique and deeply threatening context of environmental decline and climate change. Such an inquiry exceeds the bounds of this chapter. However, it does need to be acknowledged that such effects are already being experienced by individuals, especially those who are working to protect the Earth, its climate, and its inhabitants, human and otherwise. What cannot be denied is that the increasing scale and severity of the impacts on life on Earth as the new inescapable context for human life moves the discussion deeply into the existential and ethical realm.

Following this exploration of the emerging context, the second section of the chapter surveys the writings of two ecological writers and advocates, Eban Goodstein and Bill McKibben, and examines the impacts of ecological decline on their emotional life, coalescing around this question: what are the emotional effects on environmental advocates, ecosocial workers, and public educators struggling against ecological decline, such as climate change and species extinction? From their writings, what are we able to discern regarding the elements and dynamics of their emotional responses to ecological degradation? Finally, the third focus of this chapter follows from this initial inquiry: how can emotional engagement play a role in the shift of ordinary individuals from being passive consumers to becoming committed environmental citizens? In what ways could environmental educators and ecosocial workers draw on this insight in order to enhance the emergence of deeper participation in environmental protection and advocacy? How could such insights contribute to an understanding of public engagement, providing tools for capacity-building for more intentional and sustained environmental advocacy among the public?

New environmental context: Serious climate change and mega extinction

Personal attachment and loss in the face of extinction

The theme of the human affection for the natural world, and a corresponding sense of grief and loss as people confront their complicity in the deterioration of the environment, is finding greater expression in recent ecological literature. One powerful literary expression of this emotional response to environmental decline may be found in Kathleen Dean Moore's writings (2010). She offers an eloquent evocation of her sadness and guilt in her observations of the degradation of the bioregion near her home. Moore (2010) invokes an intimately personal stance, holding her granddaughter and singing her to sleep in the outdoors, while watching the life of the ecological community around them: 'I held her close, weighing the chances of the birds and the butterflies. She fell asleep in my arms, unafraid. I will tell you, I was so afraid' (p. 392). Moore (2010) makes herself a compassionate witness to the death of other species, in this case, the death of the last salmon in the stream near her house:

> My husband and I were there when the last salmon died in the stream. When we came upon her in the creek, her flank was torn and moldy. She had already poured her rich, red life from her muscles into her hopeless eggs.
>
> (p. 392)

Moore (2010) attempted to help the last salmon, but to no avail, as:

> her jaws gaped, still trying to move water over her gills. Sometimes she tried to swim. But she bumped against rocks, spilling eggs onto the stones. Without reason she pushed her head into the air and gasped. We waded beside her until she died ... I buried my face in my hands.
>
> (p. 393)

Moore pours her grief into more than a mere moral exhortation or ethical imperative. She clothes her profound sense of loss in a spiritual longing so deep that she draws on an ancient Christian ritual to give voice to her loss as well as to her plea for hope: 'Ring the angelus for the salmon and the swallows ... Ring the bells for all of us who did not save the songs' (p. 392). In her poignant reflections, the recurring pattern of affection for the natural world can be seen, which then cedes into a deep sense of loss and grief as well as a guilt arising from how humans, as a species, are directly implicated in environmental deterioration through their fealty to the economic imperative of growth at all costs.

Mega extinction as an existential and moral crisis

For biologist E.O. Wilson (1999, 2002), the need for a robust environmental movement arises from his concerns about the assault of human activity on the biodiversity of the planet. Wilson (1999) insists that the Earth is presently entering a mega extinction, the sixth mega extinction that has occurred on the planet over a half billion years. While the other five mega extinctions (Ordovician, 440 million years ago; Devonian, 365 million; Permian, 245 million; Triassic, 210 million; and Cretaceous, 65 million) have been precipitated by natural occurrences, the present mega extinction, he argues, is being driven by human action. The tragedy of the current mega extinction of species is thrown into stark relief by Wilson's (1999) sense of wonder as he contemplates the ecological communities on the planet, and of each individual species as a survivor of history. Such is the:

> ultimate and cryptic truth of every kind of organism, large and small ... it *is* a miracle ... Every kind of organism has reached this moment in time by threading one needle after another, throwing up brilliant artifices to survive and reproduce against nearly impossible odds.
>
> (p. 345, emphasis in original)

But it is in their living relationship with each other that Wilson's (1999) wonder deepens further still, as he considers how organisms are 'all the more remarkable in combination ... a sample of the living force that runs the earth – and will continue to do so with or without us' (p. 345).

With this sense of awe of the wonder of biodiversity and its sheer tenacity in survival, Wilson (1999) reflects on the human-induced mega extinction that exceeds human rationality, entering the mystery of existential depth. He pours scorn on the trite responses of commentators who argue that extinction is a trivial matter that can be remedied by the course of biological development. Given the large-scale timelines that have been needed to recover from previous mega extinctions (for instance, the most recent mega extinction, Cretaceous, needed 20 million years for recovery of biodiversity health), Wilson (1999) replies that these large figures 'should give pause to anyone who believes that what *Homo sapiens* destroys, Nature will redeem. Maybe so, but not within any length of time that has meaning for contemporary humanity' (p. 31). Wilson's critical appraisal of these trivializing responses regarding humanity precipitating its extinction are echoed by ecosocial work scholars (Coates, 2003; Mary, 2008), who insist that it is 'reckless to believe that biodiversity can diminish without threatening our own survival as a species' (Coates, 2003: 36).

Ecological educator Thomashow (2002) suggests that facing the reality and meaning of the present mega extinction precipitated by human activity 'transcends ecological and political considerations and opens you up to all kinds of existential dilemmas. Anyone who studies global environmental change will eventually confront profound spiritual challenges – the contemplation of love and loss, life and death, creation and extinction' (p. 12). As humanity enters this confluence, disciplines such as social work will need to find ways of bridging the 'gaps among the environment, spirit, and science' (Mary, 2008: 89). Just as Leopold (1970) declared that for 'one species to mourn the death of another is a new thing under the sun' (p. 117), Wilson (1999) also ponders the inscrutable mystery of species extinction and the wistful absence of human witnesses as the last individual organism of a species dies. As a species slips out of existence, eternally, irrevocably, and irreplaceably, the extinction takes place usually without any human witness:

> Extinction is the most obscure and local of all biological processes. We don't see the last butterfly of its species snatched from the air by a bird or the last orchid of a certain kind killed by the collapse of its supporting tree in some distant mountain forest. We hear that a certain animal or plant is on the edge, perhaps already gone. We return to the last known locality to search, and when no individuals are encountered there ... we pronounce the species extinct. But hope lingers on ... but it is probably all fantasy.
>
> (Wilson, 1999: 255)

Other scientists have also explored the sense of loss and the emotional side of their scientific work, when scientists are witnesses to the extinction of a species (Ackerman, 1997; Stearns and Stearns, 1999).

Awareness of an impending mega extinction exacts a personal emotional toll that cannot merely be remediated through therapy, or tranquillized through medication in order to bring a person back to 'normal'. Living an emotional life in the crossfire of attachment and loss, affection and guilt is the 'new normal', rather like living in a 'world of wounds', as Leopold (1970) shrewdly points out. For environmental advocates, these emotionally complex states appear to be a critical part of their intense engagement, providing an affective dimension to their commitment to environmental advocacy. For ecosocial work academics, such as Mary (2008), a recognition of the sheer scale of the ecological problems necessitates a reconfiguration of the field of social work as a whole so that both social and environmental dimensions are integrated into a unified and more expansive profession oriented by a 'larger global imperative of planetary survival' (p. 1). Coates (2003) suggests that as individuals begin to realize the serious environmental crisis through 'critical analysis and personal reflection', they are 'freed to seek deeper meaning and purpose and discover the unifying force that connects all of life' (p. 101).

In Wilson's (1984) exposition of the motivational basis for ecological engagement that evolves into an ethical posture, he proposes that the 'goal is to join emotion with the rational analysis of emotion in order to create a deeper and more enduring conservation ethic' (p. 119). For Wilson, intellectual understanding needs to be integrated with an ongoing affective interaction with nature. But the coalescence of emotionality and rationality, including enlightened self-interest with respect to human health or a 'green economy', are not sufficient in themselves to produce a deep ethic capable of facing the challenge of mega extinction and the scale of the current ecological crisis:

> a healthful environment, the warmth of kinship, right-sounding moral strictures, sure-bet economic gain, and a stirring of nostalgia and sentiment are the chief components of the surface ethic. Together they are enough to make a compelling case to most people most of the time … But this is not nearly enough.
>
> (Wilson, 1984: 138)

So just what might be enough?

Emotion, ethics, and environmental action: Goodstein and McKibben

Goodstein: Politics and advocating for the environment

The themes of human emotional responses to environmental decline intermingling with joy from the natural world emerge in the work of two contemporary figures – Eban Goodstein and Bill McKibben – intriguing figures in their own right, uniting thoughtful reflection, sustained environmental advocacy, and innovative approaches to ecological public education, especially regarding climate change. Goodstein (1999, 2008) was an economics professor at Lewis and Clark College in Portland, Oregon, until recently becoming the Executive Director of the Bard Centre for Environmental Policy in New York State. While at Lewis and Clark, Goodstein was the leader of a series of three-day intensive educational workshops called the 'Green House Network' for community-based educators and organizers across the USA. Starting in 1999, over a period of merely three years, the Green House Network trained almost 250 activists in 30 states (Gelbspan, 2004; Goodstein, 2007), who themselves, in turn, organized 600 educational events in 30 states. After this, Goodstein (2007) became the director of *Focus the Nation*, which facilitated 1,900 teach-ins in universities and colleges across North America on January 31, 2008.

Goodstein's (2007) personal emotional response to the impacts of climate change on the environment spurred his desire to engage in building a morally based climate change movement. In *Fighting for Love in the Century of*

Extinction, he describes his emotions: his sadness in learning about the destruction of particular animal species (harp seals in this case); his hopelessness, numbness, depression, pain, loss, and failure, all heart-sinking reactions to scientific projections on the extent of species extinction as climate change accelerates. So deep was his love for nature, his biophilia (Wilson, 1984), his spiritual sense of life was 'facilitated through a deep love for creation' (p. 72). Like Wilson (1984), Goodstein (2007) maintains that the human 'biophilic' drive for affiliation with nature is expressed in strong emotions – joy and elation when experiences are positive, and depression and sadness when faced with loss of species and habitats in the natural world, whether real or anticipated (McKibben, 2006). Thence comes the drive to protect the environment as these emotions evolve into more nuanced emotional and volitional experiences, leading to a heightened sense of responsibility to care and advocate for the Earth. This is an *ethical* dimension which spurs action. The transition from an emotional response to ethical action is central to Goodstein's (2007) approach to fostering environmental citizenship: It 'is not merely sad that creatures are going extinct, it is wrong' (p. 84). Goodstein (2007) believed that a public moral language was needed for people 'to express feelings of either awe or anger' (p. 16). For Goodstein (2007), social movements grow from the embrace of a moral cause and evolve into public education and engagement to build a 'tide of moral sentiment' (p. 90) with a 'moral vision at the center pole' (p. 117).

McKibben: Advocacy as living gracefully on 'Eaarth'

Like Goodstein, Bill McKibben commands widespread recognition and acclamation, through his public profile and twelve books, including *Fight Global Warming Now* (McKibben *et al.*, 2007), a handbook on community-based environmental engagement co-written with six young activists and *Deep Economy*, McKibben's (2007) reflections on the emerging local economy and social order. His most recent book *Eaarth* (McKibben, 2010) explores the ways in which humanity must live on a fundamentally altered planet with climate change now in motion. Public figures as varied as Canadian author, Margaret Atwood and James Hansen, Director of the NASA Goddard Space Center, have pointed to McKibben's contemporary form of environmental activism in 350.org as one of the most successful expressions of global environmental engagement on climate change.

Across his body of work, McKibben explores the emotional impacts of environmental decline and accelerating climate change on his interior life. In *Eaarth,* McKibben (2010) meditates on the meaning of the changes evident in the weather and topography of his own home in Vermont. He felt an all-pervading sense of melancholy and loss (McKibben, 1989, 2006) then sadness 'turned into a sharper-edged fear' (McKibben, 2010: xii) as statistics on the relentless impacts of climate change continued to emerge. His creative reinvention of 'Earth' as 'Eaarth' is a powerful educative device to convey his compelling insight that the 'planet on which our civilization evolved no longer exists ... The earth that we knew – the only earth that we ever knew – is gone' (p. 27). Hence 'Eaarth represents the deepest of human failures. But we must still live on the world we've created – lightly, carefully, gracefully' (p. 212).

The foundation of McKibben's (2006) environmental advocacy is his emotional and relational bond with the natural world, and his ecological sensibility to the suffering of all species through environmental degradation. Like Goodstein (2007), he grounds his advocacy in his emotional response as a call to action. As the rhythm of nature and climate become more unstable, there is a shift from a comforting sense of the reliability of the cycles of the natural world to a growing environmental disequilibrium (see Lysack, 2007, 2010). In the Global South, ecological disequilibrium has deepened into environmental trauma with growing numbers of environmental and climate refugees responding to ecological deterioration arising from the policies of the Global North in its acquisition of resources to fulfil the rapacious appetite of the global economy (Lysack, 2008; McKibben, 2010).

For McKibben (2006), the initial sadness can give rise to a secondary series of emotional reactions, such as the denial of the reality, scale, and severity of environmental decline. His uncomfortable ambivalent relationship with nature engenders a sense of guilt as he fears attachment to that which he might lose. He believes resistance to engage with environmental action is more psychological than intellectual. This insight dovetails with climate change research showing that mere information is insufficient to engender committed environmental action and engagement (Moser, 2007b; Moser and Dilling, 2007).

Ecosocial work: Healing emotional responses to environmental decline

Emotional responses to ecological decline

Like McKibben and Goodstein, some ecosocial workers (Lysack, 2009a, 2009c, 2009d, 2010) have mapped the landscape of emotional responses to ecological degradation. In his groundbreaking *Ecology and Social Work*, Coates (2003) introduces the notion of first- and second-level emotional responses framed within a social justice perspective where the 'pervasiveness and magnitude of these problems and the widespread and unquestioned commitment of governments to technological solutions and market forces leaves many people feeling disempowered and immobilized' (p. 5). This induced powerlessness and helplessness, which discourages active engagement in solving the ecological crisis, is augmented by the realization that the collective decision-making power of governments and the global market economy are also aligned against decisive and timely action to intervene in environmental destruction. Coates (2003) observes a 'widespread indifference of the human community toward the eradication of species and habitats [reflecting] ... a lack of connectedness [and compassion] which permeates [modern society]' (p. 6). Its ultra-individualism cascades into a lack of empathy: with the 'emphasis placed on separateness and individual benefit, many people have lost their ability to be empathic and sensitive to the devastation and pain taking place' (p. 36). These emotional responses have a 'multiplier effect' leading to incapacitating and pervasive helplessness, rather than to a heightened sensitivity to ecological and social injustice and the desire to take effective environmental action.

Healing responses to ecological loss

Coates (2003) believes social work's neglect of environmental concerns results in a lack of clinical interventions to heal the emotional impacts of ecological losses. Fortunately, a small core of ecosocial workers is beginning to devise a social work response to the ecological crisis. For example, Mary (2008) sees social work's role in facilitating linkages between people's individual actions and the larger question of climate change and species mega extinction as integral to fostering environmental citizenship. The more people make connections between personal difficulties and global issues, 'the more they will see the interconnectedness between their own behaviors and consumer patterns and those of the larger global commons' (Mary, 2008: 177). Coates (2003) also stresses the importance of broadening concerns from the personal to the global through public education:

> [S]ocial empathy could be expanded to become global empathy, where the reality that a person experiences can be seen not only in the context of their immediate situation (such as abuse or poverty) but also in the context of global poverty and ecological destruction ... awareness ... [could be extended] toward a global consciousness within which a person can see how his/her situation is a position of privilege or is shared by many people around the world.
>
> (p. 101)

Other ecosocial workers, such as Besthorn (2004), have advanced their own educational models of empowerment that centre on challenging the disempowering effects of consumer culture on the ecological identity of ecosocial workers, and recovering alternative identities as advocates. Besthorn (2003) has also developed learning tools that ecosocial workers might use to deepen the connections between their social and environmental justice commitments and their skills in taking environmental action, integrating all of these dimensions into a unified professional identity as an ecosocial worker as a basis for resilient ecological advocacy.

Moral environmental reasoning, emotions, and ethics

To an extent still undervalued in culture, human existence depends on the human being's propensity to bond with nature. The work of key writers (Goodstein, 2007; McKibben, 2006, 2007, 2010; Wilson, 1984) reveals the emergence of an environmental ethical framework from the interplay of human emotional and intellectual responses to the growing ecological crisis (see Gray and Coates, 2011). For Wilson (1984), it is 'time to invent moral reasoning of a new and more powerful kind, to look at the very roots of motivation and understand why, in what circumstances and on which occasions, we cherish and protect life' (pp. 138–139). Wilson (1984) grounds this moral urge in 'the innate tendency to focus on life and lifelike processes ... We learn to distinguish life from the inanimate and move towards it like moths to a porch light' (p. 1). For Wilson (1984), this attraction to life is an intrinsic part of human nature, cascading into patterns of ordering social and cultural interactions. It is a heuristic device for understanding the role of the natural realm in shaping child and adolescent development (Kahn and Kellert, 2002; Kellert, 1997, 2002). In environmental education and advocacy, biophilia provides a generative metaphor for inquiry and practice in fields concerned with social change, community action, ecosocial work and public education (Besthorn and Saleebey, 2003; Lysack, 2009a, 2009b, 2009d, 2010). In ethics, biophilia explains the driving force behind contemporary activists and public educators (Goodstein, 2007; McKibben, 2006, 2007, 2010). How do these explorations into the emotional life of environmental advocates and into biophilia as a foundation for a deep conservation ethic overlap with research into engagement in public issues like climate change?

Implications for environmental advocacy

Research on education and public mobilization *vis-à-vis* climate change has shown that 'knowledge or information alone is not sufficient to produce behavioral change' (Moser, 2007b: 85–86). Rejecting the Enlightenment notion that humans act on the basis of rational self-interest, environmental advocates and educators focus on emotions as the force behind human rationality (Crompton, 2010; de Kirby, Morgan, Nordhaus, and Shellenberger, 2007). As Moser (2007a) notes, emotions are 'powerful motivators as well as de-motivators of action' (p. 69). Inner-focused or self-centred emotions such as fear, anxiety, guilt, and apathy incapacitate those gripped by these emotional states, while other-centred emotions (compassion) precipitate deeper engagement. Thus suggests Finley (2007): 'motivation to act comes from our caring' (p. 55). They are embedded in a frame of values, providing a 'moral compass' (Mary, 2008). In other words, human behaviour is determined by the way in which 'people perceive the material world and ... its relationship to their spiritual world of beliefs, values, and ethics drives human behavior' (Mary, 2008: 27). Hence educational and community-building activities – and the building of social change movements – capitalize on the human longing for a stronger sense of community. Environmental advocates seek to ground their activity on a 'moral sense of responsibility [transcending] … self-interest' (Moser, 2007b: 81). A critical task of the ecological educator is to foster an ethic of environmental responsibility by providing an 'engaging, morally compelling social vision' (ibid.: 82) and a hopeful vision for a positive future worth fighting for to animate and motivate individuals to become engaged in environmental advocacy. Climate change educators – and ecosocial workers – need to provide pathways for action inside a supportive set of relationships within a community of practice that embraces ecocentric values (Gray and Coates, 2011; Moser, 2007a).

Public educational campaigns strategically align personal values and emotional engagement. For example, *Common Cause*, a report written by Tom Crompton (2010) from the WWF-UK, affirms the 'mounting evidence that facts only play a partial role in shaping people's judgment. Emotion is often far more important … in particular, dominant cultural values, which are tied to emotion' (p. 8; see also Monbiot, 2010). Lakoff's (2009) study of voting behaviour shows that bias, prejudice, and emotion lead individual voters to 'vote against their obvious self-interest' (p. 8). Likewise psychologists Westen, Weinberger, and Bradley (2007) note that 'emotional pulls dominate judgment and decision-making in high-stakes, emotion-laden political situations, generally overriding even relatively strong cognitive restraints' (p. 691). Facts that are inconsistent with an individual's values merely 'bounce off' (Lakoff, 2004: 17). Hence copious data on climate science or declining biodiversity is neutralized by the psychological configurations of emotion and values.

Conclusion: Implications for social work

Drawing on these insights, environmental public educators have begun to develop templates for public education vectored towards deepening the engagement of individuals to make personal behavioural changes and increase their social and political involvement (Orr, 2004, 2009; Lysack, 2009b, 2009c, 2010; Macy, 1990, 1995; Seed and Macy, 2004; Meyer, 2007). Within social work, education is seen as an important vehicle through which social workers might forge a unified professional identity oriented to ecological advocacy (Besthorn, 2003, 2004; Coates, 2003). Social work educators could learn from environmental advocates and public campaigners to facilitate the movement of students' values and emotional responses towards an ecocentric worldview. But further than this, social workers could align themselves with environmental organizations to forge political and social change (see Chapter 6). Educational processes that promote environmental engagement are critically needed, if the struggle described by H.G. Wells as the race between education and catastrophe is to be won (in Orr, 2004). But the key question that humanity must answer is posed by Wilson (1984): "'Is it possible that humanity will love life enough to save it?'" (p. 145).

References

Ackerman, D. (1997). *The rarest of the rare*. New York: Random House.

Anielski, M. (2007). *The economics of happiness: Building genuine wealth*. Gabriola Island, BC: New Society Publishers.

Besthorn, F. (2003). Radical ecologisms: Insights for educating social workers in ecological activism and social justice. *Critical Social Work, 4*(1). Retrieved on March 19, 2007 from http://www.uwindsor.ca/criticalsocialwork/radical-ecologisms-insights-for-educating-social-workers-in-ecological-activism-and-social-justice.

Besthorn, F. (2004). Globalized consumer culture: Its implications for social justice and practice teaching in social work. *Journal of Practice Teaching in Health and Social Work, 5*(3), 20–39.

Besthorn, F., and Saleebey, D. (2003). Nature, genetics and the biophilia connection: Exploring linkages with social work values and practices. *Advances in Social Work, 4*(1), 1–18.

Coates, J. (2003). *Ecology and social work*. Halifax, NS: Fernwood Publishing.

Crompton, T. (2010). *Common cause: The case for working with our cultural values*. WWF, Oxfam, Friends of the Earth, CPRE, Climate Outreach Information Network. Retrieved on July 31, 2011 from http://assets.wwf.org.uk/downloads/common_cause_report.pdf.

de Kirby, K., Morgan, P., Nordhaus, T., and Shellenberger, M. (2007). Irrationality wants to be your friend. In J. Isham and Waage, S. (Eds). *Ignition: What you can do to fight global warming and spark a movement*. Washington, DC: Island Press. 59–72.

Finley, M.L. (2007). Shaping the movement. In J. Isham and Waage, S. (Eds). *Ignition: What you can do to fight global warming and spark a movement*. Washington, DC: Island Press. 33–56.

Gelbspan, R. (2004). *Boiling point*. New York: Basic Books.

Goodstein, E. (1999). *The trade-off myth: Fact and fiction about jobs and the environment*. Washington, DC: Island Press.

Goodstein, E. (2007). *Fighting for love in the century of extinction: How passion and politics can stop global warming*. Burlington, VT: University of Vermont Press.

Goodstein, E. (2008). *Economics and the environment*. Hoboken, NJ: John Wiley & Sons.

Gray, M., and Coates, J. (2011). Environmental ethics for social work: Social work's responsibility to the non-human world. *International Journal of Social Welfare, 21*, 1–9. Article first published online: 13 DEC 2011 | DOI: 10.1111/j.1468-2397.2011.00852.x.

Hamilton, C. (2010). *Requiem for a species: Why we resist the truth about climate change*. London: Earthscan.

Kahn, P., and Kellert, S. (Eds). (2002). *Children and nature*. Cambridge, MA: MIT Press.

Kellert, S. (1997). *Kinship to mastery: Biophilia in human evolution and development*. Washington, DC: Island Press.

Kellert, S. (2002). Experiencing nature: Affective, cognitive, and evaluative development in children. In P. Kahn and Kellert, S. (Eds). *Children and nature.* Cambridge, MA: MIT Press. 117–152.

Lakoff, G. (2004). *Don't think of an elephant! Know your values and frame the debate.* White River Junction, VT: Chelsea Green Publishing.

Lakoff, G. (2009). *The political mind: A cognitive scientist's guide to your brain and its politics.* London: Penguin.

Leiserowitz, A. (2007). Communicating the risks of global warming: American risk perceptions, affective images, and interpretative communities. In S. Moser and Dilling, L. (Eds). *Creating a climate for change: Communicating climate change and facilitating social change.* Cambridge: Cambridge University Press. 44–63.

Leopold, A. (1970). *A sand county almanac.* New York: Ballantine Books.

Lysack, M. (2007). Family therapy, the ecological self, and global warming. *Context, 91*, 9–11.

Lysack, M. (2008). Global warming as a moral issue: Ethics and economics of reducing carbon emissions. *Interdisciplinary Environmental Review, 10*(1&2), 95–109.

Lysack, M. (2009a). From environmental despair to the ecological self: Mindfulness and community action. In S. Hick (Ed.). *Mindfulness and Social Work.*   Chicago, IL: Lyceum Publications. 212–218.

Lysack, M. (2009b). The Teach-in on Global Warming Solutions and Vygotsky: Fostering ecological action and environmental citizenship. *McGill Journal of Education, 44*(1), 119–134.

Lysack, M. (2009c). Practices and skills for building social and ecological resiliency with individuals and communities. In S. Hick, Peters, H., Corner, T., and London, T. (Eds). *Structural social work in action: Examples from practice.* Toronto, ON: Canadian Scholars Press. 211–228.

Lysack, M. (2009d). Defending and protecting what we love: Biophilia and creating environmental citizenship. *Wild Lands Advocate, 17*(3), 14–16.

Lysack, M. (2010). Environmental decline, loss, and biophilia: Fostering commitment in environmental citizenship. *Critical Social Work, 11*(3). Retrieved on February 12, 2012 from http://www.uwindsor.ca/criticalsocialwork/2010-volume-11-no-3.

Macy, J. (1990). The greening of the self. In A. Badiner (Ed.). *Dharma Gaia: A harvest of essays in Buddhism and ecology.* Berkeley, CA: Parallax Press. 53–63.

Macy, J. (1995). Working through environmental despair. In T. Roszak, Gomes, M., and Kanner, A. (Eds). *Ecopsychology: Restoring the earth, healing the mind.* San Francisco: Sierra Club Books. 240–259.

Mary, N. (2008). *Social work in a sustainable world.* Chicago, IL: Lyceum Books.

McKibben, B. (1989). *The end of nature.* New York: Random House.

McKibben, B. (2006). *The end of nature* (2nd ed.). New York: Random House Trade Paperbacks.

McKibben, B. (2007). *Deep economy: The wealth of communities and the durable future.* New York: Henry Holt and Company.

McKibben, B. (2010). *Eaarth: Making a life on a tough new planet.* Toronto, ON: Alfred Knopf Canada.

McKibben, B., Aroneanu, P., Bates, W., Boeve, M., Henn, J., Osborn, J., and Warnow, J. (2007). *Fight global warming now: A handbook for taking action in your community.* New York: Times Books, Henry Holt and Company.

Meyer, D. (2007). Building social movements. In S. Moser and Dilling, L. (Eds). *Creating a climate for change: Communicating climate change and facilitating social change.* Cambridge: Cambridge University Press. 451–461.

Monbiot, G. (2010). The values of everything. *The Guardian,* October 11, 2010. Retrieved on August 3, 2011 from http://www.monbiot.com/2010/10/11/the-values-of-everything/.

Moore, K.D. (2010). The call to forgiveness at the end of the day. In K. Dean Moore and Nelson, M. (Eds). *Moral ground: Ethical action for a planet in peril.* San Antonio, TX: Trinity University Press. 390–393.

Moser, S. (2007a). More bad news: The risk of neglecting emotional responses to climate change information. In S. Moser and Dilling, L. (Eds). *Creating a climate for change: Communicating climate change and facilitating social change.* Cambridge: Cambridge University Press. 64–80.

Moser, S. (2007b). Communication strategies. In J. Isham and Waage, S. (Eds). *Ignition: What you can do to fight global warming and spark a movement.* Washington, DC: Island Press. 73–93.

Moser, S., and Dilling, L. (Eds). (2007). *Creating a climate for change: Communicating climate change and facilitating social change.* Cambridge: Cambridge University Press.

Orr, D. (2004). *Earth in mind: On education, environment, and the human prospect* (10th anniversary ed.). Washington, DC: Island Press.

Orr, D. (2009). *Down to the wire: Confronting climate collapse.* Oxford: Oxford University Press.

Seed, J., and Macy, J. (2004). Gaia meditations. In R.S. Gottlieb (ed.). *This Sacred Earth: Religion, nature, environment* (2nd ed.). New York: Routledge. pp, 552–553

Stearns, B.P., and Stearns, S. (1999). *Watching, from the edge of extinction.* New Haven, CT: Yale University Press.

Thomashow, M. (2002). *Bringing the biosphere home: Learning to perceive global environmental change.* Cambridge, MA: MIT Press.

Westen, D., Weinberger, J., and Bradley, R. (2007). Motivation, decision making, and consciousness: From psychodynamics to subliminal priming and emotional constraint satisfaction. In P.D. Zelazo and Moscovitch, M. (Eds). *Cambridge handbook of consciousness.* Cambridge: Cambridge University Press. 671–700.

Wilson, E. O. (1984). *Biophilia.* Cambridge, MA: Harvard University Press.

Wilson, E. O. (1999). *The diversity of life.* New York: W.W. Norton & Company.

Wilson, E. O. (2002). *The future of life.* New York: Vintage Books.

13 Social work education on the environment in contemporary curricula in the USA

*R. Anna Hayward, Shari E. Miller,
and Terry V. Shaw*

> Our task must be to free ourselves ... by widening our circle of compassion
> to embrace all living creatures and the whole of nature and its beauty
> (Albert Einstein, in Eves, 1977).

Trends in social work employment in the United States have continued to focus the profession in the areas of health and social assistance (Bureau of Labor Statistics (BLS), 2011), securing professional social workers' roles in micro-level, direct practice arenas. Despite an increased public interest in sustainability and environmental issues, the thrust of social work education and practice continues to be directed toward individual-level processes and agency-based practice settings. A viable congruence between social work values and environmental and ecological justice has been noted (see Chapter 1). However, the educational and practice experiences of most social workers do not reflect values outside of an individualistic or humanistic focus. Two recent US studies suggest social work students and practitioners express interest in and commitment to environmental issues (Shaw, 2011; Shaw, Miller, and Hayward, 2008) and leaders in the field point to the convergence of social work and environmental concerns (Besthorn and Canda, 2002; Besthorn and Saleebey, 2003; Coates, 2003; Coates, Gray, and Hetherington, 2006; Gray and Coates, 2011; Rogge, 1993). Efforts to infuse the social work curriculum with an understanding of environmental and ecological justice are a key step in expanding the social work profession's role in the environmental arena but typical practice settings in the USA may not offer social workers opportunities to practise in an ecologically conscious way. This chapter explores employment prospects for social workers in the USA, social workers' attitudes and beliefs toward the environment, and potential areas for infusing environmental issues and concerns into social work education and the most social worker dense practice arenas.

Social work employment trends and outlook in the USA

Twenty-eight years ago, Rubin and Johnson's (1984) study on social work students' practice preferences found that, upon entry into social work education, 86 per cent said they wanted to become private practitioners at some point in their careers and held 'little or no commitment to social work's mission' (p. 13). In a follow-up study two years later, Rubin, Johnson, and DeWeaver (1986) reported that the percentage of students who wanted to enter private practice upon entry into their MSW programs had decreased from 86 per cent to 73 per cent upon graduation from their MSW programs, while those preferring a social care orientation, which is 'characterized by a focus on institutionally-based services and community-based alternatives to institutional care' (ibid.: 99) had increased during their education. Rubin *et al.* (1986) attributed this change in part to the professional socializing influences of their MSW education. In a national survey, Abell and McDonell (1990) found that most entry-level MSW students preferred direct practice activities with individuals, families, and children (see also Aviram and Katan, 1991; Butler, 1990). However, unlike earlier studies (Rubin and Johnson, 1984; Rubin *et al.*, 1986), the students reported a commitment to working with the disadvantaged as one of the reasons they had chosen a career in social work. However, Specht and Courtney's (1994) influential *Unfaithful Angels* proclaimed the shift toward private practice and psychotherapy away from public sector work addressing pressing social problems showed that social work had abandoned its social mission. Since then, a growing body of research has questioned whether or not social workers have abandoned their social mission in their chosen fields of practice, practice roles, and populations of focus. Findings from this body of literature are mixed, with some studies agreeing with Specht and Courtney's (1994) diagnosis of the profession showing students wanted to be clinically trained (Weiss, Gal, and Cnaan, 2004) with others not sharing their concerns (Abell and McDonell, 1990; Bogo, Michalski, Raphael, and Roberts, 1995; Butler, 1990; Limb and Organista, 2003, 2006; Miller, 2008; Perry, 2001). Divergent findings regarding students' interest in pursuing private practice are particularly relevant to discussions on an expanded environmental justice or ecological focus for social work because they attest social workers' commitment to social justice and may be indicative of internal forces within the profession towards broader social and environmental concerns.

More recently, Dulmus, Bass, and Bunch (2005) sought to determine how social work practitioners viewed their professional mission with 66 per cent of respondents favouring clinical work with individuals, families, and groups, followed by 13 per cent who selected social justice. Miller's (2008) study on the professional socialization of social workers sought to determine whether undergraduate and graduate students and MSW-qualified practitioners (n=489) identified strongly with the profession's values and social mission. Findings indicated that the respondents had a strong professional identity and idealistic orientation. However, consistent with the earlier studies cited above, most expressed a strong preference for direct practice with individuals and families in agency-based mental health, family, and children's services despite the fact that nearly 75 per cent said they had entered the profession to help the disadvantaged.

In short, repeated studies have found that social work students and practitioners have an overwhelming interest in direct agency-based practice, which accords with Ginsberg's (2005) synopsis of the future of US social work. Ginsberg (2005) pointed to employment trends suggesting further increases in social workers employed in direct practice in metropolitan areas in the fields of aging, school-based services, and substance-abuse treatment.

The US National Association of Social Workers' (NASW) 2004 workforce survey similarly suggested a continued demand for social workers across the USA and identified over 254,000 social workers holding a state licence[1] (NASW, 2006). A random sample of 10,000 licensed social workers identified mental health (37 per cent), child welfare (13 per cent), health (13 per cent), and aging (9 per cent) as the most dominant areas of practice, with the most common social work role involving direct services to clients (96 per cent). Only 25 per cent held employment positions in federal, state, or local governments (NASW, 2006).

Five years later, the US Bureau of Labor Statistics' (BLS, 2011) reflected the culmination of many of the trends Ginsberg (2005) had predicted. In 2009, 54 per cent of social workers were employed in the healthcare and social assistance industries, while only 31 per cent worked for city, state, or federal government. A trend that continued to show projected growth was social work with the aging population where jobs tend to focus on individual and family work to assist with quality of life and medical case management. The BLS (2011) estimated that there were about 620,000 social workers, of whom 46 per cent were employed in child, family, and school practice, 22 per cent in medical and public health, 21 per cent in mental health and substance abuse, and 11 per cent in other sectors. Further, while the 2004 BLS report discussed by Ginsberg (2005) pointed to increases in services in metropolitan areas, the 2009 report projected more work in rural settings.

These practice settings, especially those within large county and state bureaucracies, may not lend themselves to the integration of environmental social work. Social workers who work in direct services need to meet accountability demands and those who work in hospital settings or with the aging population may not see a clear link between their day-to-day work and environmental issues and concerns. In any event, social work's traditional mission is grounded in humanistic, democratic, and Judeo-Christian values,

---

1   Licensure and education requirements for work under the title 'social worker' vary by State in the USA.

and personal and social issues and problems (Gibelman, 1999), with an exclusive focus on the person-in-*social* environment. Placing ecological consciousness in the extant epistemology and ontology of social work represents a fundamental challenge, though some suggest it is possible to fold a different definition of environment into social work practice that goes beyond the social and constructed human environment to extend to the natural, ecological environment (Besthorn, 1997; Coates, 2003; Mary, 2008; Miller, Hayward, and Shaw, 2011; Zapf, 2009). These authors suggest that an ecologically conscious ethos can be infused into social work practice across the continuum from micro to macro practice by building on and expanding a continued commitment to social justice to include environmental and ecological justice and, in so doing, expand the profession's mission (Miller *et al.*, 2011). Hence despite predictions on social work's employment market trajectory, these authors suggest innovative environmentally-mindful ecosocial approaches are possible. Rather than indicate that social workers have abandoned their social mission and despite the factors influencing these shifts, including the demands of the human services market (Perry, 2001), social work education (Miller, 2008; Rubin *et al.*, 1986), differing perspectives on social justice, and how and where it fits into social work practice (Miller, 2011; Solas, 2008), these authors believe it is imperative for the profession to engage in transformative environmental practice.

NASW policy statement regarding the environment

As social work slowly continues to determine its place in addressing the global ecological crisis, the National Association of Social Workers (NASW) – a professional organization for licensed social workers in the USA that mostly comprises those employed in direct services (NASW, 2006) – has issued a series of policy statements on the environment. In 2003, its statement read:

> People share a common need for and a right to a fair share of the Earth's resources, including a clean, safe, and healthy environment. Today, human beings are at risk of life-threatening consequences, including many health problems, from environmental degradation. The consequences of environmental neglect and harm will continue for generations to come. Environmental exploitation violates the principle of social justice and is a direct violation of the NASW *Code of Ethics.*
>
> (NASW, 2003: 120)

This policy statement offers a starting place for an expanded understanding of the environment for social workers, claims to support environmental laws that protect humans and the planet, and advocates for populations adversely affected by environmental impacts.

Social workers' attitudes and beliefs towards environmental issues

Shortly after the publication of NASW's (2003) environmental policy statement, two independently conducted surveys sought to understand the attitudes and beliefs of social work students in Maryland (Miller and Hayward, 2006) and social work professionals in California (Shaw, 2006).

During the 2005–2006 academic year, 800 foundation and advanced Master of Social Work (MSW) students in a school of social work were asked to complete a survey distributed to their mailboxes; 159 surveys were returned, a response rate of 20 per cent. In the same year, a mailed survey was sent to a randomly selected sample of 1,000 NASW members in California. Both surveys included the New Environmental Paradigm Scale (NEPS), which is used to measure attitudes towards the environment. It has been used to compare: (i) the environmental attitudes of environmental organizations to the general population (Dunlap and Van Liere, 1978; LaTrobe and Acott, 2000), (ii) farmers to the general population (Albrecht, Gordon, Hoiberg, and Nowack, 1982), (iii) hunters to non-hunters (Tarrant, Bright, and Cordell, 1997), and (iv) changes in the general population's attitudes to the environment between 1978 and 1990 (Dunlap, Van Liere, Mertig, and Jones, 2000). The prior Ecological Paradigm Scale (EPS) was found to have internal consistency reliability (cronbach alpha=0.81) (Dunlap and Van Liere, 1978) while the revised NEPS was found to have slightly higher internal consistency reliability (cronbach alpha=0.83) (Dunlap *et al.*, 2000), predictive validity in the studies comparing the general population to an environmentally conscious group (Albrecht *et al.*, 1982; Dunlap and Van Liere, 1978; LaTrobe and Acott, 2000), and construct validity with other measures of environmental attitudes (Dunlap *et al.*, 2000; Tarrant *et al.*, 1997). The NEPS comprises 15 questions designed to gauge respondents' environmental worldview and is scored across five different dimensions of environmental attitude:

1   limits to growth (including the impact of modern industry and the Earth's ability to absorb population and industrial growth)
2   anti-anthropocentrism (including human interference with natural processes)
3   fragility of nature (including humans' rights and responsibilities in modifying the natural environment)
4   rejection of exceptionalism (including the equal rights of plants and animals with humans), and
5   possibility of an ecological crisis (including the delicate balance of nature).

The response rate for the mailed NASW survey was 39 per cent and, as reported earlier, 20 per cent for the student survey. The students were mainly enrolled in the clinical track (57 per cent) with only 11 per cent

Table 13.1 New Environmental Paradigm (NEP) scores of survey participants

Dimension	Student Survey (Mean)	NASW Survey (Mean)	General Population*
Limits to growth	08.88	11.07	–
Anti-anthropocentrism	10.13	12.19	–
Fragility of nature	11.45	11.19	–
Rejection of exceptionalism	11.62	11.76	–
Possibility of an ecological crisis	12.33	10.14	–
Total Score	52.15	56.20	**56.20
	N=159	N=373	

*   General population of Washington residents (Dunlap *et al.*, 2000).
** Only overall scores available for this study.

following a macro or community practice focus and 21 per cent undecided (often students do not decide on a concentration until the end of their first year). The distribution by race and gender of 87 per cent female and 76 per cent white Caucasian was representative of the institution – a large State University program – where the research was conducted. Results suggested that MSW students and NASW members had similar scores in comparison with studies of the general population (see Table 13.1).

NASW members expressed similar levels of concern with the environment as compared to participants in studies of the general population, with MSW students scoring slightly lower than both. The relatively high scores in all groups could be attributed to the response rate in both studies: perhaps those individuals who already had an interest in environmental issues were more likely to complete the survey in the first place. It could also be that the scale captures issues in the hypothetical and asks only about attitudes and beliefs, not about specific actions.

Miller and Hayward's (2006) study of MSW students also sought students' attitudes toward the integration of environmental issues in social work and their exposure to content on environmental issues in the MSW curriculum at their institution. Eighty-eight per cent either strongly agreed (50 per cent) or agreed (38 per cent) that environmental issues were important for social work, and 88 per cent also strongly agreed (43 per cent) or agreed (45 per cent) that environmental issues were an important aspect of social justice. When asked whether or not content on environmental issues should be included in the MSW curriculum, 64 per cent agreed or strongly agreed. Despite students' apparent interest in environmental issues, only 8 per cent reported there was enough content in the MSW curriculum and 24 per cent reported being exposed to some content during their MSW education. Similarly, 68 per cent of the NASW respondents stated that their social work education did not include discussions of the natural environment and 90 per cent believed that it should. In addition, Shaw's (2011) survey of NASW members asked respondents about their knowledge of the NASW's (2003) policy statement on the environment. As noted previously, the NASW issued this statement to articulate its stance on issues related to the environment, and environmental justice in particular. The majority of respondents (68 per cent) stated that they did not know whether or not the NASW had a statement on the natural environment and 21 per cent (incorrectly) indicated that it did not while 11 per cent correctly responded that it did. This suggests that this statement is not well known or the NASW has a minimal impact on the profession in day-to-day practice.

Social work education

On the basis of these findings, Shaw *et al.* (2008) and Shaw (2011) concluded that primacy should be given to finding where ecological concerns might fit into the social work MSW curriculum. In 2008, the Council on Social Work Education (CSWE) introduced revised Educational Policy and Accreditation Standards (EPAS) for all CSWE-accredited social work programs in the USA. These standards guide social work educators to focus on the development of professional competencies. The EPAS (CSWE, 2008) indicated that:

> the purpose of the social work profession is to promote human and community well-being. Guided by a person and environment construct, a global perspective, respect for human diversity, and knowledge based on scientific inquiry, social work's purpose is actualized through its quest for social and economic justice, the prevention of conditions that limit human rights, the elimination of poverty, and the enhancement of the quality of life for all persons.
>
> (p. 1)

In 2010, CSWE accredited baccalaureate and masters level social work programs in 527 institutions serving over 53,000 students in the USA. With a focus on a global person-in-environment perspective, CSWE advocates that social work education should foster a quest for socioeconomic justice and enhancement of the quality of life for all citizens. An expanded emphasis on the environment and related environmental justice concerns aligns with this call, and provides opportunities for innovative educational approaches that begin to *ecologize* the notion of environment for social work.

Opportunities for integration in field and practice settings

Jones (2010) speaks to the need to overhaul the Australian social work curriculum in order to shift to a transformative social work education approach (see Chapter 11). He believes the focus needs to be on educating social workers so they might more deeply understand and contribute to the development of a sustainable future. He argues against add-on approaches that paste bits of eco-relevant content onto the already packed social work curriculum, or approaches that attempt to embed eco-relevant content within the existing curriculum. Only a radically transformed curriculum could support the philosophical shifts necessary to make a place for a naturalistically defined environment in social work (Jones, 2010).

A possible starting point for this transformation is the infusion of a service-learning component across the social work curriculum. Service-learning has been defined in a variety of ways, but one unifying feature of most definitions is the notion that there is balance and reciprocity between the service and the learning, and that the structure of the learning and service benefit both the student and the involved community partner(s): 'Service learning not only enhances students' knowledge ... but also requires that they apply that knowledge to the practice of addressing social problems in collaboration with community partners' (Phillips, 2007: 4). Drawing on the philosophy of John Dewey and building on by Paolo Freire's critical pedagogy, underlying service-learning is the idea that learning does not emerge through the service experience alone, but through the necessary integration of experience with reflection (Deans, 1999). Service-learning, while it shares some similarities to field education in social work, differs in a particularly elemental way because of its focus on service: 'While strong intentions to benefit the recipients of the service are evident, the focus of field education programs tend to be on maximizing the student's learning of a field of study' (Furco, 2003: 14). Service-learning programs however are designed specifically to benefit the student providing the service and the community partner receiving the service, equitably, and through collaboration; the emphasis is shared equally between the learning engendered and the service performed (Furco, 2003).

The University of Georgia provides an example of a service-learning course focused on eco-consciousness within social work practice (Miller, 2011). It includes a hefty interdisciplinary service component that places students in after-school programs for children in Kindergarten (approximately five years old) through to fifth grade (approximately 10 years old) located in on-site food gardens. This one-semester elective course (approximately 15 weeks) is designed for undergraduate (BSW) and graduate (MSW) social work students. BSW students are eligible to enrol in the course during their final year of study (during which they are also engaged in a year-long field internship) to satisfy a required elective, and MSW students can enrol in the course at any point in their studies. Students who choose to enrol in the course work with others from the horticulture and food and nutrition majors to create twice-weekly programming for children focused on their relationship to nature, sustainability, where food comes from, nutrition and well-being, sustainable involvement of parents and community, with an emphasis on food security in a sustainable environment (Miller, 2011). Outside of the service-learning site, social work students are asked to reflect upon and challenge their values and assumptions, to read about and expand their understanding of the environment, nature, and ecology, and to locate its relevance to social work. Service-learning of this nature can be incorporated into social work courses, even though it is not part of core content. Service-learning opportunities by design require instructors to rethink their courses (and potentially the entire curriculum) and redesign them to accommodate the newly defined environment in support of a transformative approach, as Jones (2010) suggests. They draw on the experiential and reflective learning components central to effective social work education (see Chapter 11).

While there have been recent pockets of efforts to infuse a broader understanding of environment and a shift away from a focus on the individual in social work curricula, especially in Human Behaviour and the Social Environment (HBSE) courses (see for example Van Wormer and Besthorn, 2011), which are core to most BSW and MSW programs, these efforts have been scattered and vary widely across the broad array of US social work programs (Mary, 2008). Outside of the classroom, service-learning projects, transdisciplinary approaches, and non-traditional field placements offer alternative methods for transforming social work education to an ecosocial model for students who express interest, as a starting point, in pursuing an environmental or ecological justice-focused practice. Students can be placed in agencies and nongovernmental organizations focused on sustainability and environmentally or ecologically just work.

'Tom', a student at the University of Georgia, School of Social Work, for example, has completed his foundation year field placement with a local organization focused on sustainable land use. For his second year concentration on community and organizational practice, he will work in an elementary school setting to develop a multifaceted school gardening program with a focus on grassroots community organizing and the development of a therapeutic garden program for students diagnosed with behavioural disorders. Not only do these field placements diverge from the typical social work field education placement model, they also place central emphasis on a sustainable relationship to land. They also, by design, serve to merge a potentially artificial divide between direct (micro) and indirect (macro) practice. Educational opportunities such as these set the stage for shifting social work's relationship to its environment and broadening its practice roles (Heinsch, 2011). A shift away from the micro–macro divide in education and practice serves to take some of the artificial out of a purely social construction of environment, and expand to a holistic construction of the natural environment. As some social work educators move toward a more integrative social work curriculum that directly addresses our place in a global ecosystem and promotes social workers' roles in addressing local, national, and global environmental concerns, students such as Tom push to pursue ecosocial justice in their local communities. Hopefully, future social work students like Tom with an acute awareness of environmental concerns will demand that the curriculum focus on ecosocial practice.

However, despite efforts by educators and students alike, broader market forces continue to demand employment in direct practice, particularly in individual mental health and state and local governmental services, which do not immediately create supportive work environments for the integration of environmental practice for social workers entering the profession to engage in ecosocial practice. Changes in the day-to-day working lives of the majority of professional social workers may be slow to emerge, but through fundamental shifts in the purpose and delivery of social work education and demands *on* the market by social work students and new professionals in the field, these workplaces may adapt to provide a receptive environment for ecosocial practice.

Conclusion

In direct service-practice settings in the USA, the integration of ecosocial practice is rare but not unknown. The use of forest experiences or 'Nature Therapy' for children and especially for adolescents holds promise as intervention for psychosocial and mental health concerns (Berger and McLeod, 2006; Milligan and Bingley, 2007; Shin *et al.*, 2010). These interventions do not simply focus on clinical issues but also reconnect individuals to their natural environment. With such a large percentage of social workers employed in mental health (BLS, 2004), integrating these and other ecotherapies into social workers' repertoire might allow the integration of environmental issues into direct practice work. Heinsch (2011) further suggests ways to integrate the natural environment into office settings by the use of photographs and sounds of nature, plants, and animal companions. Community food groups, while often operated outside the purview of social work practice, also offer opportunities to integrate community organizing and development with sustainable land development, nutrition, and education (Heinsch, 2011). Edible schoolyard programs are another example that can be developed even in the confines of a large state-run institution in the public school system (Briggs, 2005; Stone, 2005). These programs combine a focus on ecological education with the immediate nutrition needs of children and offer a model of integrated individual, community, and environmental intervention but, up until now, have not involved social workers.

Social work's agility as a profession and within its own professional culture offers some hope in the face of a labour market that, on first glance, creates obstacles for ecosocial practice. As the public interest shifts and policymakers respond to these shifts, ecosocial work becomes increasingly likely. Change tends to happen incrementally, and the very existence of this volume itself (along with the growing ecosocial work literature that has preceded it) speaks to the progress social work has made on this front. There is still a great deal of work to be done. Much of the ecosocial work literature emanates from the academic realm. This is a reasonable starting point. If the literature is robust enough to support curriculum change and students continue to take up the mantle and advocate for ecologically just practice experiences, it is likely that changes will begin to reach further into the practice arena.

References

Abell, N., and McDonell, J.R. (1990). Preparing for practice: Motivations, expectations and aspirations of the MSW Class of 1990. *Journal of Social Work Education, 26*(1), 57–64.

Albrecht, D., Gordon, B., Hoiberg, E., and Nowak, P. (1982). The new environmental paradigm scale, *Journal of Environmental Education, 13*(3), 39–43.

Aviram, U., and Katan, J. (1991). Professional preferences of social workers: Prestige scales of populations, services and methods in social work. *International Social Work, 34,* 37–55.

Berger, R.M., and McLeod, J. (2006). Incorporating nature into therapy: A framework for practice. *Journal of Systemic Therapies, 25*(2), 80–94.

Besthorn, F.H. (1997). *Reconceptualizing social work's person-in-environment perspective: Explorations in radical environmental thought.* Unpublished doctoral dissertation, University of Kansas, Lawrence.

Besthorn, F.H., and Canda, E.R. (2002). Revisioning environment: Deep ecology for education and teaching in social work. *Journal of Teaching in Social Work, 22,* 79–101.

Besthorn, F.H., and Saleebey, D. (2003). Nature, genetics, and the biophilia connection: Exploring linkages with social work values and practice. *Advances in Social Work, 4*(1), 1–18.

Bogo, M., Michalski, J., Raphael, D., and Roberts, R. (1995). Practice interests and self-identification among social work students: Changes over the course of graduate social work education. *Journal of Social Work Education, 31*(2), 228–246.

Briggs, M. (2005). Rethinking school lunch. In M.K. Stone and Barlow, Z. (Eds). *Ecological literacy: Educating our children for a sustainable world.* San Francisco: Sierra Club Books. 241–249.

Bureau of Labor Statistics, U.S. Department of Labor (2011). Social Workers. *Occupational Outlook Handbook, 2010–11 Edition.* Retrieved on November 5, 2011 from http://www.bls.gov/oco/ocos060.htm.

Butler, A.C. (1990). A reevaluation of social work students' career interests. *Journal of Social Work Education, 26*(1), 45–56.

Coates, J. (2003). *Ecology and social work: Toward a new paradigm.* Halifax, NS: Fernwood Publishing.

Coates, J., Gray, M., and Hetherington, T. (2006). An 'ecospiritual' perspective: Finally, a place for indigenous approaches. *British Journal of Social Work, 36,* 381–399.

Council on Social Work Education (CSWE) (2008). *Educational Policy and Accreditation Standards.* Alexandria, VA: CSWE.

Deans, T. (1999). Service-learning in two keys: Paulo Freire's critical pedagogy in relation to John Dewey's pragmatism. *Michigan Journal of Community Service Learning, 6,* 15–29.

Dulmus, C.N., Bass, L.L., and Bunch, S.G. (2005). Perspectives on the mission of the social work profession: A random survey of NASW members. *Advances in Social Work, 6*(2), 231–239.

Dunlap, R.E., and Van Liere, K.D. (1978). A proposed measuring instrument and preliminary results: The 'new environmental paradigm'. *Journal of Environmental Education, 10*(1), 10–19.

Dunlap, R.R., Van Liere, K.D., Mertig, A.G., and Jones, R.E. (2000). Measuring endorsement of the new ecological paradigm: A revised NEP scale. *Journal of Social Issues, 56*(3), 425–442.

Eves, H.W. (1977). *Albert Einstein, letter dated 1950, Mathematical circles adieu: A fourth collection of mathematical stories and anecdotes.* Boston, MA: Prindle, Weber and Schmidt.

Furco, A. (2003). Service-learning: A balanced approach to experiential education. In S. Jones (Ed.). *Introduction to service-learning toolkit. Readings and resources for faculty* (2nd ed.). Providence, RI: Campus Compact, Brown University. 11–14.

Gibelman, M. (1999). The search for identity: Defining social work – past, present, future. *Social Work, 44*(4), 298–310.

Ginsberg, L. (2005). The future of social work as a profession. *Advances in Social Work, 6*(1), 7–17.

Gray, M., and Coates, J. (Eds). (2011). Environmental social work. Special Issue, *International Journal of Social Welfare, 21*, 1–9. Article first published online: 13 DEC 2011 | DOI: 10.1111/j.1468-2397.2011.00852.x.

Heinsch, M. (2011). Getting down to earth: Finding a place for nature in social work practice. *International Journal of Social Welfare,* Special Issue on Environmental Social Work. Article first published online: 13 DEC 2011. DOI:10.1111/j.1468-2397.2011.00860.x.

Jones, P. (2010). Responding to the ecological crisis: Transformative pathways for social work education. *Journal of Social Work Education, 46*(1), 67–84.

LaTrobe, H.L., and Acott, T.G. (2000). A modified NEP/DSP Environmental attitudes scale. *The Journal of Environmental Education, 32*(1), 12–20.

Limb, G.E., and Organista, K.C. (2003). Comparisons between Caucasian students, students of color, and American Indian students on their views on social work's traditional mission, career motivations, and practice preferences. *Journal of Social Work Education, 39*, 91–109.

Limb, G.E., and Organista, K.C. (2006). Change between entry and graduation in MSW student views on social work's traditional mission, career motivations, and practice preferences: Caucasian, student of color, and American Indian group comparisons. *Journal of Social Work Education, 42*(2), 269–290.

Mary, N. (2008). *Social work in a sustainable world.* Chicago, IL: Lyceum Books.

Miller, S.E. (2008). *Becoming a social worker: Factors that predict socialization to the profession and differences between groups* (Doctoral dissertation). Retrieved on December 15, 2011 from ProQuest Dissertations and Theses (3323589).

Miller, S.E. (2010). A conceptual framework for the professional socialization of social workers. *Journal of Human Behavior in the Social Environment, 20*, 924–938.

Miller, S.E. (2011). Community engagement from the ground up: An interdisciplinary school garden initiative. Paper presented at the *Council on Social Work Education, 57th Annual Program Meeting: Increasing Access: Confronting Disparity and Inequality.* Atlanta, Georgia, October 30.

Miller, S.E., and Hayward, R.A. (2006). *Knowledge of and attitudes toward environmental issues among social work students.* Unpublished raw data. Stony Brook University School of Social Welfare.

Miller, S.E., Hayward, A., and Shaw, T.V. (2011). Environmental shifts for social work: A principles approach. *International Journal of Social Welfare,* Special Issue on Environmental Social Work. Article first published online: 13DEC2011 DOI: 10.1111/j.1468-2397.2011.00848.x.

Milligan, C., and Bingley, A.F. (2007). Restorative places or scary spaces? The impact of woodland on the mental well-being of young adults. *Health & Place, 13,* 799–811.

National Association of Social Workers (NASW). (2003). Environmental policy. *Social Work Speaks.* Washington, DC: NASW Press. 116–123.

National Association of Social Workers (NASW). (2006). *Licensed social workers in the United States, 2004.* The NASW Center for Workforce Studies, Washington, DC. Retrieved January 20, 2012 from http://workforce.socialworkers.org/studies/fullStudy0806.pdf.

Perry, R. (2001). The classification, intercorrelation, and dynamic nature of MSW student practice preferences. *Journal of Social Work Education, 37,* 523–542.

Phillips, A. (2007). Service learning and social work education: A natural but tenuous connection. In M. Nadel, Majewski, V., and Sullivan-Cosetti, M. (Eds). *Social work and service learning: Partnerships for social justice.* Lanham, MD: Rowan & Littlefield. 3–19.

Rogge, M.E. (1993). Social work, disenfranchised communities, and the natural environment: Field education opportunities. *Journal of Social Work Education, 29,* 111–120.

Rubin, A., and Johnson, P.J. (1984). Direct practice interests of entering MSW students. *Journal of Education for Social Work, 20*(2), 5–16.

Rubin, A., Johnson, P.J., and DeWeaver, K.L. (1986). Direct practice interests of MSW students: Changes from entry to graduation. *Journal of Social Work Education, 22*(2), 98–108.

Shaw, T.V. (2006). *Social workers' knowledge and attitudes toward the ecological environment* (doctoral dissertation). Retrieved on January 20, 2011 from ProQuest Dissertation and Theses (3254075).

Shaw, T. (2011). Is social work a green profession? An examination of environmental beliefs. *Journal of Social Work.* Published online before print June 2, 2011, doi:10.1177/1468017311407555.

Shaw, T., Miller, S., and Hayward, R.A. (2008). Social work knowledge and attitudes toward the natural environment. Paper presented at the *Council on Social Work Education, 54th Annual Program Meeting: Social Work Policy and Practice: Linking Theory, Methods and Skill.* Philadelphia, PA, November 2.

Shin, W.S., Yeoun, P.S., Yoo, R.W., and Shin, C.S. (2010). Forest experience and psychological health benefits: The state of the art and future prospect in Korea. *Environmental Health and Preventive Medicine, 15*(1), 38–47.

Solas, J. (2008). What kind of social justice does social work seek? *International Social Work, 51*(6), 813–822.

Specht, H., and Courtney, M.E. (1994). *Unfaithful angels: How social work has abandoned its mission.* New York: The Free Press.

Stone, M.K. (2005). Sustainability – A new item on the lunch menu. The slow school: An idea whose time has come? In M.K. Stone and Barlow, Z. (Eds). *Ecological literacy: Educating our children for a sustainable world*. San Francisco, CA: Sierra Club Books. 227–240.

Tarrant, M.A., Bright, A.D., and Cordell, H.K. (1997). Attitudes toward wildlife species protection: Assessing moderating and mediating effects in the value-attitude relationship. *Human Dimensions of Wildlife, 2*(2), 1–20.

Van Wormer, K., and Besthorn, F. (2011). *Human behavior and the social environment: Groups. Communities and organizations* (2nd ed.). New York: Oxford University Press.

Weiss, I., Gal, J., and Cnaan, R.A. (2004). Social work education as professional socialization: A study of the impact of social work education upon students' professional preferences. *Journal of Social Service Research, 31*, 13–31.

Zapf, M.K. (2009). *Social work and the environment: Understanding people and place*. Toronto, ON: Canadian Scholars Press.

14 Environmental sustainability

Educating social workers for interdisciplinary practice

Cathryne L. Schmitz, Tom Matyók,
Channelle D. James, and Lacey M. Sloan

> In a few decades, the relationship between the environment, resources and conflict may seem almost as obvious as the connection we see today between human rights, democracy and peace (Wangari Maathai).

The relationship between social justice, environmental sustainability, and positive peace has been well established by theorists who highlight the need for multidisciplinary community-level responses to conflicts resulting from environmental issues and concerns. Schmitz, Matyók, Sloan, and James (2011) argue that many of the issues of poverty, injustice, and quality of life are connected to the health of the physical environment and its long-term sustainability. Increasingly, social workers, with their commitment to social justice, are called upon to recognize the relationship between social work, the environment, and human well-being (Coates, 2003).

The quality of the biophysical environment – the water, air, food, and living spaces – is pivotal for human existence. While the interdependence of these resources is critical, there have been historical attempts to separate human experience from concerns for the health of the biophysical environment, creating a dichotomy in practice and theory (Barry, 2010). This contributes to thinking of questions addressing environmental issues as separate from other living concerns and manufactures a limited understanding of sustainability (see Chapter 3). Globalization exacerbates the problem contributing to increased conflict between diverse communities around the world (Agyeman and Carmin, 2011).

In this chapter, an interdisciplinary approach to teaching environmental sustainability is examined from a community perspective, mindful of the part national and global issues play in informing this analysis. The approach is based on the belief that an understanding of environmental sustainability, positive peace (the presence of justice and absence of cultural, structural, and direct violence), and community-invested economic models are crucial to the long-term health of the biophysical environment and human survival within it. The course introduced herein focuses on the relationship between community, conflict, peace, economic systems, and environmental sustainability. Students are exposed to complexity (or complex systems) theory and the ecosystems perspective as a framework for assessing the relationships intertwined across social justice, community, environmental sustainability, and positive peace.

A framework for understanding the impact of development and widespread conflict within human communities, along with the turmoil created at the hands of humans, often without awareness, provided a lens for reflecting on human responsibility for global ecological degradation. The model was based on a critical pedagogical approach informed by the values of social and environmental justice (see Chapter 1) in which the 'oppressed must be their own example in the struggle for their redemption' (Freire, 1970: 54). This, too, is the focus of community development, which requires people, individually and collectively, to take responsibility for creating the type of world in which they want to live. Thus a theoretical framework was needed to establish a connection between human action and environmental sustainability, one in which issues of morality and justice are engaged (Lysack, 2008, 2010).

Teaching sustainability

'Sustainability challenges – such as global climate change, biodiversity loss, poverty, and patterned social inequalities, to name just a few – are real-life problems with fuzzy boundaries, complexly interconnected components, unspecified parameters, missing information, conflicting societal values, and no single solution' (Myers and Beringer, 2010: 53). As a result of this increased complexity, and the nature of problems faced regarding sustainability, new and innovative pedagogies are required, pedagogies that focus on collaboration, not exclusion. In order to understand the complex relationship between community and environmental sustainability, social workers need to learn to work in fluid and changing environments within interdisciplinary spaces and as part of multidisciplinary teams. The teaching of environmental sustainability, as discussed in this chapter, was developed through the lens of community response, a sound knowledge of theory, and practice in a multidisciplinary context.

According to the United States Environmental Protection Agency (EPA), sustainability 'creates and maintains the conditions under which humans and nature can exist in productive harmony, that permit fulfilling the social, economic and other requirements of present and future generations' (n.d., p. 1). This 'requires far more ... than the cheap, shallow, and superficial measures commonly taken under the guise of sustainability' (Carroll, 2004: 2). Rather, environmental sustainability is a discourse that explores 'the relationship among economic development, environmental quality, and social equity' (Rogers, Jalal, and Boyd, 2008: 42).

Students learn that working in community contexts to ensure environmental sustainability requires a multidisciplinary response. Hence they are taught how to work in multidisciplinary teams at the community level. To this end, realistic experiences are provided to help them explore the multiple interconnected factors involved in meaningful and sustainable community change. The tensions of working within multidisciplinary teams are recreated in the classroom as students evaluate the value of holistic community engagement.

Interdisciplinary education provides multiple lenses through which to assess, engage with, and remediate the issues constituting the focus of this course. The interdisciplinary areas on which the course draws include social work, peace studies, economics, and the natural sciences. Each of these disciplines brings 'insightful observations about the dynamics of environmental sustainability and its impact on individual decision-making, public policy formation, and economic development [within local communities]' (Schmitz, Stinson, and James, 2010: 84). In focusing on sustainability, these disciplines are trying to discern a way to deal with environmental problems so as to protect the Earth for future generations (Smith, 2011). The study of environmental sustainability, therefore, represents 'a nexus for many disciplines seeking to examine issues of resource allocation, poverty, social justice, and globalization' (Schmitz *et al.*, 2010: 84). Drawing on their respective disciplines, the faculty educated one another on the interconnections between biodiversity, economics, conflict, and sustainable community development. This professional development approach was a precursor to the team development and the crossing of disciplinary boundaries for students.

Theoretical framework

It is increasingly recognized that social development theorists and practitioners have to understand that environmental sustainability rests on a healthy biosphere capable of sustaining diverse life forms, including humans. The biophysical environment is the context within which human social, economic, and political systems operate (Schmitz *et al.*, 2011). Figure 14.1 reflects these overlapping relationships.

Social, political, and economic human systems are embedded in the ecological (biophysical) environment (Schmitz *et al.*, 2011) and human growth that does not consider the multiple dimensions of environmental health is problematic and threatens all forms of life on the planet. This is the complexity through which the professional development of social workers – often charged with addressing critical, and frequently contradictory, issues comprising the social fabric of communities and relationships – must be viewed. Having a theoretical lens provides for critical analysis and supports the development of holistic practice models.

Complex systems theory provides a frame for analysing the web of interdependent relationships and the inherent complexity of human–environment transactions (Peterson, Allen, and Holling, 2010; Smith,

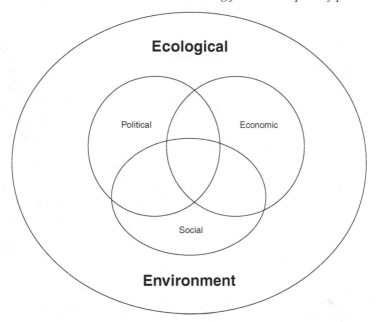

Figure 14.1 Human systems within the ecological environment (Schmitz *et al.*, 2011). Reproduced with permission

2011). Complex systems (and chaos) theory helps learners to frame analysis of the myriad interdependent relationships inherent in human–environment transactions (Gleick, 2008; Kay, 2008; Kiel and Elliott, 2004; Peterson *et al.*, 2010; Smith, 2011). Through awareness of complex systems theory, and the intricacies and interconnections between systems (ecosystems perspective), human responsibility for achieving environmental sustainability becomes the focus of analysis, knowledge creation, and the development of professional practice.

An ecosystems perspective, derived from complex systems theory, establishes the biophysical environment as part of a chaotic universe where 'the outcomes of changing variable interactions cannot be known' (Kiel and Elliott, 2004: 6). The ecosystems perspective further informs effective practice in complex community environments (see Waltner-Toews, Kay, and Lister, 2008). It also enhances understanding that there are no longer any ecosystems unaffected by humans (Berkes and Davidson-Hunt, 2008). Hence, a thorough examination of the evolution of human communities requires an understanding of the way in which ecosystems interact reciprocally to sustain life and the environment (McCright and Clark, 2006). This focus supports the development of the skills for critical analysis in complex environments.

Establishing the structure

Three main ideas guided course development. The first involved establishing how issues impacting on local communities, such as poverty, ineffective social systems, violent conflict, and inadequate models for economic development, are connected to global concerns of environmental sustainability. The second centred on understanding the role of community development, the transformative potential of conflict, and alternative economic models in bringing about progressive change. The third was the importance of teaching environmental sustainability from an inter-disciplinary perspective in a context where dialogue across disciplines was incorporated. Interdisciplinary practice for environmental sustainability can involve practitioners from a range of disciplines, including social work, community development, peace studies, business and economics, engineering, health, education, and multiple natural sciences.

The field of environmental studies is most established in the natural sciences, moderately developed in business and economics, and has great potential for expansion in many of the social sciences. Although there is a long history of investigating the impact of specific toxic substances on human health, the impact of human social systems within the environment and on sustainability is an interaction that is only beginning to be explored. Fields such as social work and peace studies have a large body of knowledge about creating change, community and relationship building, networking and collaboration, group work and team building, and development that can make significant contributions to environmental sustainability efforts. Each discipline involved in the development of this course (social work, peace studies, business, and economics) brings a degree of clarifying focus to the theory, knowledge, and skill interchange (see Table 14.1).

As social workers enter the field of environmental practice, they bring their commitment to issues of social and economic justice, community and organizational change, and policies and politics (Coates, 2003; Marlow and van Rooyen, 2001; Mary, 2008; Ungar, 2002; Zapf, 2009). Social workers come to the field of environmental practice with the skills and knowledge to work as change agents, community builders, political advocates, and educators. These skills are transferable to environmental practice when the contextual focus is expanded to include how the environment is central to sustaining every other system of concern in a global society. The nature of social work is one in which understanding sustainability is critical in producing acceptable environmental outcomes for human lives.

Social workers can enter the field of environmental practice at multiple levels. Barlow (2001) emphasized the link between free trade, social justice, environmental sustainability, and social programs. Understanding this interconnection highlights the potential for social workers to enter with their skills as group workers, team leaders, networkers, organizational consultants, community organizers, and change advocates. Social work

Table 14.1 Disciplinary links to environmental issues

Discipline	Core principles or theory	Knowledge	Skills and application
Social work	Collaboration Diversity Empowerment Social and economic justice	*Micro*: Person-in-environment and biopsychosocial *Meso*: Organizational practice *Macro*: Community development, multicultural engagement, and policy practice *Mega*: Social change	Advocacy Alliance building Communication Community-based practice Group work and team building Networking Problem solving
Peace and conflict studies	Human needs centred Humanistic conflict management Inclusive Non-violence Respect for diversity Social justice	*Micro:* Cultural fluency *Meso*: Organizational conflict *Macro*: Civic engagement, sustainable public policy development *Mega*: Global knowledge-base and transformative change	Consensus building Elicitive conflict resolution practices Joint problem-solving skills in mediation, facilitation, negotiation, and training
Economics	Externalities Democratic and living economy Limited natural resources Supply and demand curves	*Meso*: Economic development and business models *Macro*: Taxation and economic policies	*Micro*: Enterprise development Microfinance Social entrepreneurship

engagement moves from the micro to the macro as reflected in the developing environmental literature. In 2005, Coates drew attention specifically to the role of social work in responding to the growing environmental crisis. Borrell, Lane, and Fraser (2010) emphasized the need to integrate environmental issues into social work, highlighting overlapping financial, social, and environmental issues, while Durie (2010) reflected on the connection of the local, regional, and global spheres in responding to natural disasters. Lysack (2008) stressed the links between violent conflict, environmental decline, and what he called 'ecosocial' stress.

In addition to the knowledge and skills for engaging in change at the micro to macro levels, the field of peace and conflict studies is unique in tackling conditions of peace and ways of creating and replicating positive peace throughout society. A positive peace requires the presence of justice and the absence of cultural, structural, and direct violence. It is a field of scholarship and practice that begins from investigating what is absent in conflict situations that prevents peace from breaking out. From two different starting points, scholars and practitioners in the field seek to study conditions of peace, strategies for constructing and advancing increasing levels of justice, and ways to use the creative energy of conflict as a base for transformative change. A primary role of conflict and peace studies' practitioners and educators working in multidisciplinary teams is to engage in, and educate about, nonviolent conflict transformation, which involves moving conflictual community interactions to a *healthier* condition, one that reduces cultural, structural, and direct violence. Conflicts, in essence, are not really resolved, they are simply transformed.

Social work and peace studies practitioners bring the knowledge and skills for assessing the potential access points for precipitating community change. Community exists along a continuum anchored at one end by democratic, civic engagement – social inclusion – and, at the other, by disengagement or social exclusion. Communities can exclude in order to define themselves. Here, when we speak of community, we are instead referring to the engagement of citizens in the civic process and of local communities in grassroots community development. This form of community is open to dialogue and consensual decision making. All members of the community have a voice and should be given a chance to speak (Bantas, 2010).

The role of business and economics enters at three levels. At the most basic level, tax policies and regulatory requirements can be tools for imposing the economic cost of externalities on firms that create a negative public impact. Concepts like externalities (Scitovsky, 1954) are explored in connection with environmental protection (Baumol and Oates, 1971) in order to determine the real cost to the community as a result of processes that create profit inside the organization. In this context, students recognize that resources are finite and their use can have a significant impact on the whole community, locally and globally. At another level, business and economic theory exposes students to models for development at the local community level that are inclusive and empowering. The focus helps students understand potential efficiencies present in the marketplace for social good (Bornstein, 2007; Hawken, 2010). Social entrepreneurship, microfinance, and enterprise development are key models introduced. Last, at a macro level, models for *living* economics, economies committed to community renewal, are taught (Fickey, 2011).

Multidisciplinary approach

In order for students to develop the knowledge and skills needed to work effectively in multidisciplinary settings on issues related to environmental sustainability, they needed to recognize and understand complex global issues, such as poverty, economic stagnation, and political strife. To this end, students explored issues relating to environmental degradation, such as water usage, groundwater contamination, and air and water pollution, and, in parallel, they explored models of sustainability drawing on the work of Coates (2003), Hawken (2010), Mary (2008), and Orr (2011) with their clearly constructed critiques of the relationship between human development, democratic civic engagement and community building, justice economics, and sustainability. Other core models included Korten (2005, 2010), Shiva (2005), and Schumacher's (1989) models for *living* democracies with *living* economies, which assume a commitment to environmental citizenship, community, compassion, relationship, and equality. Gamble and Weil (2010) provided the framework for engaging in models of community practice anchored from the local to the global. These models, rather than focusing only on fixing symptoms, claim to respond to systemic issues by providing for the possibility of transformation toward economic self-reliance at the community level (Korten, 1996). Because economic oppression, environmental decline, and structural and interpersonal violence are linked, meaningful change must address these issues simultaneously.

Over the course of the semester, students from a diverse range of disciplines worked within multidisciplinary teams to study the work of those who had engaged with the global–local dialectic, such as Coates (2003, 2005), Mary (2008), Orr (2011), Shiva (2005), and Zapf (2009). Students most often came from biology, peace studies, engineering, business and economics, and social work. The goal was to discern the potential for transformative change through the advancement of civic engagement, democratic community building, just development, and social work centred in the biophysical environment. The United Nations' Millennium Development Goals (World Commission, 1987) were used to frame the global context. A *case study approach* and interactive learning methods, such as group discussion, community engagement, and team building, were used as students examined:

1   *Global and local issues.* Students explored the root causes of the problems experienced by local communities through studying the Millennium Development Goals (World Commission, 1987). Readings and experiential activities facilitated student exploration of these issues in their own communities along with their connections to the wider community. Because sustainability issues play out in global, unbounded spaces, students were encouraged to view their actions from the perspective of global actors. Teams explored historical and contemporary issues relating to the environment and structural violence, economic disparities, health inequalities, oppression, and injustice.

2   *Community engagement.* Some students engaged directly with communities while others conducted theoretical analyses. The instructors encouraged students to take a critical view of community as a context

for positive change with the potential to move beyond division, control, and exclusion. Through a series of debates and readings from critical visionaries and theorists, such as bell hooks (2009, 2010), Coates (2003, 2005), Mary (2008), Shiva (2005), Maathai (2010), Hawken (2010), Schumacher (1989), and Orr (2011), students began to question their notions of individual behaviour and community relationships. Students were introduced to a range of community-building methods, such as organizing, development, social action, and coalition building. This engagement allowed students to better understand the roots of sustainability issues in economic justice, global health initiatives, population shifts, and migration patterns, and to gain the confidence to participate in community work (Rosing and Hofman, 2010). Students were encouraged to examine potential roles for supporting positive change at the community level through critical reflection, journalling, small group discussions, and analysis of their team building and group development process.

The course brings knowledge from multiple disciplines to prepare students to work in multidisciplinary teams where they link individuals and communities to the environment. This individual–community relationship was established as core to balancing community responsibility with personal interests (Johnson and Scicchitano, 2009). An outcome of the class was to prepare students for work within chaotic and ill-defined contexts. Rather than providing students with cookbook responses, faculty sought to help students develop their ability to be comfortable with chaos and complexity as interdisciplinary solutions emerged (McGibbon and McPherson, 2011). Students were encouraged to take the knowledge and skills from their disciplines as a base for innovative recreation and the conceptualization of transformative models for change. They were urged to grow beyond their professional boundaries and engage in analysis across disciplinary lines (Mendoza and Matyók, 2012 in press).

Multidisciplinary teams and the case study approach

Case studies were used to engage students in the issues being explored in the classroom. To make the cases come alive, community change agents were sometimes invited as guest speakers to address critical concerns and identify the mechanisms they had used for transformative change towards sustainability in their communities. The use of case studies provided multidisciplinary student teams an opportunity to appreciate the interconnections between issues. Students moved away from prescriptive vertical approaches, which have the tendency to impose solutions from above (the top-down expert model). Rather, they were encouraged to engage in conflict transformation using an elicitive horizontal approach (Lederach, 1995), engaging actors as co-equals in their own liberation.

The case study learning method provided an opportunity to identify the patterns of conflict and the programmed behaviours that keep conflicts intact. Learners were propelled into situations that required them to use past and newly acquired knowledge to create innovative change strategies. Through this process, students were provided with the opportunity to analyse, evaluate, and judge in a safe environment. Conflicts were framed as patterned behaviours directed against individual and collective goals, with the potential for a disruption at any level to create a ripple of change. Analysis was introduced as an intervention, based on the assumption that what they analyse they change. The case study approach enhanced student learning by disrupting the tendency to disconnect what is happening on the local level from what occurs on the global level. The use of cases gave students an opportunity to apply ethical decision-making processes and reflect on the social impacts of their choices in relation to environmental issues and their global implications, deep historical roots, future ramifications, and social, economic, and political dimensions. Students completed independent research, produced a paper or presentation, and offered a debate on a current occurrence happening in their community or in society (McWilliams and Nahavandi, 2006).

Through case study analysis, teams assessed critical aspects of social problems and the various social, economic, and political components. In this way, attention was focused on analysis and problem solving that respected but moved beyond personal experience and local knowledge. Students avoided the tendency to become bogged down in the details of specific events, which drew their focus away from engaging in higher-order reasoning about the complexity of the issues. Participating in this reflective practice allowed students to develop their critical thinking skills, which did not simply occur, but rather needed to be nurtured. Students learned to engage in metacognitive actions, thinking about their thinking, not just how to follow rules (Sandel, 2009).

The Analysis of Violence Worksheet (see Figure 14.2) provided a tool for organizing a process of investigating an existing condition. The worksheets were introduced as a framework for analysis, not as templates offering a solution. The attitudes, behaviours, and contradictions toward the concern being explored (such as resource use and community health) were analysed at the mega, macro, meso, and micro levels. Attitudes such as hatred, distrust, and apathy, behaviours including physical and verbal violence, and contradictory goals that block and stymie in conflict situations were explored (Santa Barbara, Dubee, and Galtung, 2009). Using this tool, students explored the fluidity of the structure as characteristics at each level of analysis move freely across the dimensions. The worksheets guided analysis and encouraged students to see conflict in multiple dimensions, simultaneously.

Patterns were analysed with identification of interventions at all levels of a system and social structure. Interventions impacted on conflict at multiple

Level of analysis (of violence)	Attitudes	Behaviours	Contradictions
Mega – global			
Macro – community or policy			
Meso – organizational			
Micro – family and neighbourhood			

Figure 14.2 Analysis of Violence Worksheet

locations simultaneously, establishing new crises and conflict response patterns. The matrix introduced here also assisted students in framing their analysis of events. Through this process, they developed an appreciation of the nuances of conflict and its potential for disruption and transformation.

Cases such as water use and misuse have clear links locally and globally. A cursory review of multiple news media sites suggested the growing dominance of water-related concerns. It is now suggested that the world may be running out of water (Behr, 2010), that wetlands are disappearing (Weeks, 2010), and that the biodiversity of our oceans is collapsing (Woodard, 2010). Coastal communities around the globe are hugely impacted by water-related issues (see Mathbor, 2008 for coastal development discussion). This is an issue that impacts on communities in which social workers can engage at local and global levels. The complexity of water issues demands that social work students develop a holistic view of interrelated human actions that manifest themselves in environmental issues and crises. Case studies like this provided a means by which students were able to engage in the investigation of ongoing conflicts and their impact on community issues, such as water supplies and food security.

Water conflicts

Using case studies focusing on water concerns was something students could grasp in relating the local and the global. Students might be asked to analyse the water conflicts that arise when corporations buy the rights to water a local community needs for survival. Or, they might be asked to examine coastal issues, which affect resource use, environmental pollution, and community well-being. Georgia, on the East Coast of the United States of America (USA), provided a framework for multiple case studies used in our classrooms. Students identified manifestations of water conflicts from the interpersonal to the global recognizing the attitudes, behaviours, and contradictions involved. For example, the Altamaha River Basin on the Georgia coast was used as it is one of the largest breeding grounds for shell and fin-fish on the East Coast of the USA, and accounts for 18 per cent of the fresh water flowing into the South Atlantic. It is 'one of the highest quality and most expansive estuarine and salt marsh systems in the world' (The Nature Conservancy, n.d.). Land use changes and water withdrawals, coupled with water run-off upriver, threaten the health of the coast's biodiversity. The economic health of coastal communities also relies on tourism, and sport and commercial fishing, all connected to the condition of the river – positive and negative. In fact, tourism is the second-largest industry in Georgia, and the largest economic generator along the coast (Georgia Department of Economic Development, 2011). In 2004 tourism generated US $1.7 billion for the 10 coastal counties. Students were asked to create models for development that were socially and economically just and attended to the unique biodiversity found along the coast.

Through their research using the Analysis of Violence model, students began to understand the multiple layers of structural and direct violence. Students gained an understanding of how cultural, structural, and direct violence moves horizontally and vertically within and across the four levels of analysis: micro, macro, meso, and mega. Individually and in groups, students conducted a case analysis to determine what attitudes, behaviours, and contradictions were present at each level of analysis. Because of the flexibility and potential inherent in the model, teams could focus on any level as primary while analysing the impact across all four levels. Each student filled in the form from the perspective of their discipline. In coming together as an interdisciplinary team, they shared and integrated information as viewed through multiple lenses. Students were introduced to perspective taking (viewing situations/circumstances from multiple angles) and the importance of analysing conflicts from diverse viewpoints.

At the micro level, teams explored attitudes such as trust or distrust at the family and neighbourhood levels. Particularly salient were issues of trust among those engaged in commercial fishing in the local area. Students then explored related behaviours and contradictions, for example, the contradiction between distrust of their peers and their need to depend on them. At the meso level, they could proceed to organizational culture and distrust of the formal systems. At the macro level attitudes toward government policies were investigated to understand how laws, rules, and regulations impact individual fishing boats. An example here was the conflict between environmentalists and commercial fishers regarding the use of turtle exclusionary devices. And, at the mega level, environmental policy, global economic competition, and international conventions had the opportunity to be explored. Identifying the conditions present at each level then became the foundation for recommended solutions. Solutions were developed that addressed each condition at each level ensuring a unity of effort. Solutions complemented each other and ensured focused effort.

Presentation and debate helped students achieve a better understanding of the global reach of local issues. For instance, students became aware of how industrial shrimp farming in Asia affects local shrimp boats and processing facilities along the Atlantic coast. Commercial shrimping on the Atlantic coast is in a state of decline impacted by commercial shrimp farming practices, global economics, and environmental decline. Analysis that moved across interacting local and global concerns created a broader and more in-depth understanding. The multidisciplinary teams constructed in the course focused cross-disciplinary expertise that was useful in addressing diverse situations relating to East Coast water supply *vis-à-vis* industrial shrimp farming. In these cases, students not only had an opportunity to understand theory in action, but also were encouraged to develop skills in planning, resource allocation, civic engagement, and community development. Economic models explored included microfinance, enterprise development, and social entrepreneurship. Some proposals included developing commercial shrimping coops. The coops would pool resources in order to reduce operating costs such as boat insurance and fuel. Another proposal suggested creation of a city-operated dock for unloading and processing catches. This approach would place a local bond issue on the ballot to fund the project and merge commercial and governmental interests. Students suggested marketing locally caught shrimp as a boutique item, and the development of an internet marketing plan to expand the customer base. One group discussed developing a plan for *aquaculture tourism* that would open working shrimp boats to individuals who want to experience a week at sea doing commercial fishing.

Disaster relief in Haiti

In another case assignment, teams explored the work of multidisciplinary response teams in Haiti to provide a grassroots response that tended to be more effective than official relief efforts. Students were asked to consider the aftermath of the earthquake in Haiti and to design appropriate responses that delve deeply into the social, economic, and environmental issues. In this case Numana, a nonprofit organization, was positioned to address the needs of those experiencing hunger (for more information see Numana, 2011), thus teaching students an approach to disaster management from the meso level. Numana used a grassroots community approach to offer an effective redevelopment process in Haiti (Ballard-Reisch, 2011). The Numana process connected local volunteer organizations in the United States with trusted relief organizations in Haiti. Organizations that had already developed strong reputations for their relief work maintained over decades were able to provide strategic information on how food and materials are most likely to be effectively distributed to the residents of Haiti, and to address cultural concerns and the spread of rumours that interfered with the relief process. The organizers of Numana used this information throughout their whole process from food packaging to food delivery. Without this critical information, it is highly likely that donations would be wasted, or not reach those most in need of food and supplies. Students examined how Numana approached recovery efforts to address community concerns that supplies are distributed equitably and effectively to the whole community, and that children in particular would not be harmed in the process. Children were of particular concern because of rumours circulating that they were being traded for bags of food provided. Because Numana relied in part on the volunteer work of college students, our students had the opportunity to imagine how they might personally respond as members of disaster response teams (Mathbor, 2007; Pawar, 2008, see Chapter 15). In choosing a contemporary and global concern, students were connected to prominent issues. While the case study highlighted micro- and meso-level response, through the use of the Analysis of Violence Worksheet, teams of students analysed the macro and mega context. This learner-centred pedagogical approach (Myers and Beringer, 2010) provided the foundation upon which students were able to develop concern for their relationship to the environment and the local community and envisage community-based solutions and responses to the human and environmental devastation wrought by natural disasters.

Community gardening as a lens to sustainable agriculture

A concrete example of the transformative nature of the course was the community garden project assigned during one semester of the course. The garden was a symbol of community engagement around a concern for sustainable local agriculture that served as a context for learning about food security as a local and global issue (Phillips, 2009; Polack, Wood, and Bradley, 2008). With community gardens scattered across Greensboro – a mid-sized city situated within a metropolitan area surrounded by more rural communities struggling with agriculture-based economies – a local environmental organization wanted to raise awareness of the gardens and related economic and social issues. The students were asked to identify and explore possible issues arising for communities around food security. They were taught about Kretzmann and McKnight's (1993) approach to assets-based community development, pivotal to which is assets mapping. This enabled students to consider local community conditions and concerns through building on available strengths and resources and human and social capital. Through this process, students were able to understand the relationship between poverty and food security, and community gardening as a possible strategy to address this concern at the local level. Students from social work, peace studies, the natural sciences, and business brought to bear prior course work as they developed a business model that would help to better organize the community garden system in their local communities. The students developed a social entrepreneurship model with a multidimensional focus on social, economic, and environmental factors. This model recognized the role of community gardens in enhancing community solidarity, food security, and economic well-being while growing vegetables using environmentally friendly methods, such as biodegradable waste recycling (see Chapter 6). From a peace studies perspective, students also considered how conflict might arise around community gardening and how it might be dealt with. Community gardens are constantly under threat from local developers and conflicts between business economic interests often threaten the security and livelihoods of local communities. Using a team-building approach, students explored strategies of networking, advocacy, political action, and community development. They also considered the importance of leadership when exploring related issues such as nutrition and resource availability.

Beyond local engagement activities, community gardens are an ideal vehicle through which to teach students about the relationship between local and global environmental concerns. Poverty and food security affect huge numbers of people in the Global South and an increasing number of urban communities in the developed North. It has moved closer to home following the global financial crisis so the issue was topical for students. By using the Analysis of Violence model, students gained an awareness of how international aid and food policy affects people at the micro level and how this connects to the meso aid organization level, and mega global development level. Students entered the project with a linear view of what they could do with the community garden. However, after their research and discussions with community partners and local residents, they recognized the complex nature of food security and the influence of policy locally and globally. Their cross-disciplinary knowledge enabled them to develop a deeper understanding of food security and the influence of neoliberal development policy which encouraged local community self-reliance, social entrepreneurship, micro-enterprise, and cooperative development. Student and community members benefited from this symbiotic learning with the course culminating in student presentations to local community partners.

Environmental degradation in the midst of war

Some teams were more mega focused. The ongoing conditions of violence and chaos in the failed state of Somalia provided a case study at the mega level. The violence of war, environmental destruction, and crippling poverty provided the opportunity for analysis of these interconnected concerns followed by the creation of mechanisms with the potential to disrupt the destruction (see Lederach and Lederach, 2011 for history and context). Students learned lessons from the changes demanded by the women of Liberia (see Disney and Reticker, 2008). The use of the change action in Liberia as an exemplar has the added advantage of centring a social worker as a lead social change agent. The women of Liberia, in demanding a voice in the decision-making process, created the space for whole community civic engagement and opened a path to democracy. Using this example, they designed models for creating opportunities for civic engagement at every level, including the creation of grassroots civic engagement. In doing so, a disruption to the conflict and power structure was established. Conflict has relational and transformative characteristics. It did not matter at what level the conflict pattern was disrupted. In disturbing the patterns, room was created for the introduction of new patterns that could be replicated throughout the social context.

Conclusion and implications for social work practice

The authors used a multidisciplinary course to help students learn how to work in multidisciplinary teams to confront environmental problems at the local, national, and international level. Teaching sustainability involved introducing students to forms of analysis and interaction with local communities situated in a global context. The process was strengthened through the use of reflective decision making. The interdisciplinary framework has the potential to address the complexity inherent in the work of multidisciplinary teams with the goal of sustainable transformation in a global context. The interconnection between environmental concerns and issues of peace, war, and economic violence was highlighted within the context of a transformative learning environment.

Issues overlap and so do response systems. The ecological (or biophysical) environment is interactively impacted by the tightly connected human social, economic, and political systems. The tension at the intersection of these systems with the ecological environment often produces conflict, yet conflict can be viewed as creative energy. Collaborative interchange across disciplines can support the context for discourse designed to enhance understanding and the reciprocal creation of knowledge. As students and faculty from multiple disciplines share their knowledge, new spaces can be created for knowledge building (Schmitz *et al.*, 2010).

By using real-world case studies, students gained an in-depth awareness of networked interconnections, multilevel conflicts, and costs involved for humans and the environment. Concerns with water as a resource, disaster recovery, war, food security, and poverty were made real, removed from the isolation of the antiseptic classroom. Students were challenged to investigate the political, economic, and social dimensions involved at the micro, meso, macro, and mega levels of analysis. The complexity of human interaction across systems and within the environmental context created points of tension and conflict. Having this multidimensional framework for analysing conflict was useful. Recognizing the holistic and networked nature of conflict suggested that complex practice could be initiated at any level and impact all other levels, simultaneously.

With faculty and students from diverse academic fields, students were exposed to multiple perspectives regarding problem solving. Pedagogically, projects were designed to support the development of collaborative analysis and knowledge building. Through the action of people from diverse disciplines with varied interests, experiences, and knowledge, students came to critically examine local and global social, economic, and political systems from a multidimensional perspective. They explored individual and community sustainability, evaluated issues of diversity and justice, and generated collaborative change models. It is suggested that this strategy for education enabled our students to become active players in the world around them, working for a truly sustainable future.

References

Agyeman, J., and Carmin J, (2011). Introduction: Environmental injustice beyond borders. In J. Carmin and Agyeman, J. (Eds). *Environmental inequalities beyond borders: Local perspectives on global injustices.* Cambridge, MA: The MIT Press. 1–15.

Ballard-Reisch, D. (2011). Feminist reflections on food aid: The case of Numana in Haiti. *Women & Language, 34*(1), 53–62.

Bantas, H. (2010). *Jürgen Habermas and deliberative democracy.* Melbourne: Smashwords.

Barlow, M. (2001). *The free trade area of the Americas and the threat to social programs, environmental sustainability and social justice in Canada and the Americas.* The Council of Canadians. Retrieved on December 18, 2011 from http://www.ratical.org/co-globalize/MBonFTAA.html.

Barry, C. (2010). The environment/society disconnect: An overview of a concept tetrad of environment. *Journal of Environmental Education, 41*(2), 116.

Baumol, W., and Oates, W. (1971). The use of standards and prices for protection of the environment. *The Swedish Journal of Economics, 73*(1), 42–54.

Behr, P. (2010). Looming water crisis: Is the world running out of water? In *Issues for debate in environmental management: Selections from CQ researcher,* 323–352. Thousand Oaks, CA: Sage.

Berkes, F., and Davidson-Hunt, I.J. (2008). The cultural basis for an ecosystem approach: Sharing across systems of knowledge. In D. Waltner-Toews, Kay, J.J., and Lister, N.-M.E. (Eds). *The ecosystem approach. Complexity, uncertainty, and managing for sustainability.* New York: Columbia University Press. 109–124.

Bornstein, D. (2007). *How to change the world: Social entrepreneurs and the power of new ideas.* New York: Oxford University Press.

Borrell, J., Lane, S., and Fraser, S. (2010). Integrating environmental issues into social work practice: Lessons learnt from domestic energy auditing. *Australian Social Work, 63*(3), 315–328.

Carroll, J. (2004). *Sustainability and spirituality.* New York: State University of New York Press.

Coates, J. (2003). *Ecology and social work: Toward a new paradigm.* Halifax, NS: Fernwood Publishing.

Coates, J. (2005). The environmental crisis: Implications for social work. *Journal of Progressive Human Services, 16*(1), 25–49.

Disney, A.E. (Producer), and Reticker, G. (Director) (2008). *Pray the devil back to hell.* USA: Forks.

Durie, M. (2010). Global transitions: Implications for a regional social work agenda. *Journal of Indigenous Voices in Social Work, 1*(12), 1–9.

Fickey, A. (2011). 'The focus has to be on helping people make a living': Exploring diverse economies and alternative economic spaces. *Geography Compass, 5*(5), 237–248.

Freire, P. (1970). *Pedagogy of the oppressed.* New York: Continuum.

Gamble, D.N., and Weil, M. (2010). *Community practice skills: Local to global perspectives.* New York: Columbia University Press.

Georgia Department of Economic Development. (2011). *Georgia at a Glance.* Retrieved on January 9, 2011 from http://www.georgia.org/GeorgiaIndustries/Tourism/Pages/IndustryResearch.aspx.

Gleick, J. (2008). *Chaos: Making a new science.* New York: Penguin.

Hawken, P. (2010). *The ecology of commerce: A declaration of sustainability* (revised edition). New York: Harper.

hooks, b. (2009). *Belonging: A culture of place.* New York: Routledge

hooks, b. (2010). *Black on Earth: African American ecoliterary traditions.* Athens, GA: University of Georgia Press.

Johnson, R.J., and Scicchitano, M.J. (2009). Willing and able: Explaining individuals' engagement in environmental policy making. *Journal of Environmental Planning and Management, 52* (6), 833–846.

Kay, J.J. (2008). An introduction to systems thinking. In D. Waltner-Toews, Kay, J.J., and Lister, N.E. (Eds). *The ecosystem approach: Complexity, uncertainty, and managing for sustainability.* New York: Columbia University Press. 3–13.

Kiel, L., and Elliott, E. (2004). *Chaos theory in the social sciences: Foundations and applications.* Ann Arbor, MI: University of Michigan Press.

Korten, D. (1996). *Sustainable development: Conventional versus emergent alternative wisdom.* New York: The People Centered Development Forum.

Korten, D. (2005). *The great turning: From empire to earth community.* Bloomingfield, CT: Kumarian Press.

Korten, D. (2010). *Agenda for a new economy: From phantom wealth to real wealth* (2nd ed.), San Francisco: Berrett Kochler.

Kretzmann, J.P., and McKnight, J.L. (1993). *Building communities from the inside out: A path toward finding and mobilizing a community's assets.* Chicago, IL: ACTA publications.

Lederach, J.P. (1995). *Preparing for peace: Conflict transformation across cultures.* Syracuse, NY: Syracuse University Press.

Lederach, J.P., and Lederach, A. J. (2011). *When blood and bones cry out.* New York: Oxford University Press.

Lysack, M. (2008). Global warming as a moral issue: Ethics and economics of reducing carbon emissions. *Interdisciplinary Environmental Review, 10*(1/2), 95–109.

Lysack, M. (2010). Environmental decline and climate change: Fostering social and environmental justice on a warming planet. In N.J. Negi and Furman, R. (Eds). *Transnational social work practice.* New York: Columbia University Press. 52–75.

Maathai, W. (2010). *Replenishing the Earth: Spiritual values for healing ourselves and the world.* New York: Doubleday.

Maathai, W. (n.d.). *Meet the Laureates: Wangari Maathai.* Nobel Women's Initiative. Retrieved February 21, 2012 from http://nobelwomensinitiative.org/meet-the-laureates/wangari-maathai/.

Marlow, C., and van Rooyen, C. (2001). How green is the environment in social work? *International Social Work, 44*(2), 241–254.

Mary, N. L. (2008). *Social work in a sustainable world.* Chicago: Lyceum.

Mathbor, G.M. (2007). Enhancement of community preparedness for natural disasters: The role of social work in building social capital for sustainable disaster relief and management. *International Social Work, 50*(3), 357–369.

Mathbor, G.M. (2008). *Effective community participation in coastal development.* Chicago, IL: Lyceum Press.

McCright, A.M., and Clark, T.N. (2006). Place: Where community and environment meet. In A.M. McCright and Clark, T.N. (Eds). *Community and ecology: Dynamics of place, sustainability, and politics (Research in urban policy, Volume 10).* San Diego, CA: Emerald Group Publishing Limited. 17–19.

McGibbon, E., and McPherson, C. (2011). Applying intersectionality and complexity theory to address the social determinants of women's health. *Women's Health & Urban Life, 10*(1), 59–86.

McWilliams, V., and Nahavandi, A. (2006). Using live cases to teach ethics. *Journal of Business Ethics, 67* (4), 421–433.

Mendoza, H.R., and Matyók, T. (2012 in press). We are not alone: When the number of exceptions to a rule exceeds its usefulness as a construct, it is time for a change. In T. Poldma (Ed.). *Meanings of design: Social, cultural and philosophical essays about people, spaces and interior environments.* New York: Fairchild.

Myers, O.R., and Beringer, A. (2010). Sustainability in higher education: Psychological research for effective pedagogy. *Canadian Journal of Higher Education, 40*(2), 51–77.

Numana (2011). Numana: saving the starving. Downloaded February 10, 2012 from http://numanainc.com/index.php

Orr, D.W. (2011). *Down to the wire: Confronting climate collapse.* Washington, DC: Island Press.

Pawar, M. (2008). Interventions in disasters. *Asia Pacific Journal of Social Work and Development, 18*(2), 72–83.

Peterson, G., Allen, C.R., and Holling, C.S. (2010). Ecological resilience, biodiversity and scale. In L. Gunderson, Allen, C.R., and Holling, C.S. (Eds). *Foundations of ecological resilience.* New York: Island Press. 167–193.

Phillips, R. (2009). Food security and women's health: A feminist perspective for international social work. *International Social Work, 52*(4), 485–498.

Polack, R., Wood, S., and Bradley, E. (2008). Fossil fuels and food security: Analysis and recommendations for community organizers. *Journal of Community Practice, 16*(3), 359–375.

Rogers, P.P., Jalal, K.F., and Boyd, J.A. (2008). *An introduction to sustainable development.* London: Earthscan.

Rosing, H., and Hofman, N.G. (2010). Notes from the field: Service learning and the development of multidisciplinary community-based research initiatives. *Journal of Community Practice, 18* (2/3), 213–232.

Sandel, M. (2009). *Justice: What's the right thing to do?* New York: Farrar, Straus and Giroux.

Santa Barbara, J., Dubee, F., and Galtung, J. (2009). *Peace business: Humans and nature above markets and capital.* Oslo, Norway: Kolofon Press.

Schmitz, C.L., Stinson, C.H., and James, C.D. (2010). Reclaiming community: Multidisciplinary approaches to environmental sustainability. *Critical Social Work, 11*(3), 83–95. http://www.uwindsor.ca/criticalsocialwork/2010-volume-11-no-3.

Schmitz, C.L., Matyók, T., Sloan, L., and James, C.D. (2011). The relationship between social work and environmental sustainability: Implications for interdisciplinary practice. *International Journal of Social Welfare, 21.* Article first published online: 13 DEC 2011 DOI: 10.1111/j.1468-2397.2011.00855.x

Schumacher, E.F. (1989 [1973]). *Small is beautiful: Economics as if people mattered.* New York: Harper & Row.

Scitovsky, T. (1954). Two concepts of external economies. *Journal of Political Economy, 62*(2), 143–151.

Shiva, V. (2005). *Earth democracy: Justice, sustainability, and peace.* Cambridge, MA: South End Press.

Smith, T. (2011). Using critical systems thinking to foster an integrated approach to sustainability: A proposal for development practitioners. *Environment, Development & Sustainability, 13,* 1–17.

The Nature Conservancy. (n.d.). *Georgia Altamaha River Basin.* Retrieved on January 9, 2011 from http://www.nature.org/ourinitiatives/regions/northamerica/unitedstates/georgia/placesweprotect/altamaha-river.xml.

Ungar, M. (2002). A deeper, more social ecological social work practice. *Social Service Review, 76* (3), 480–499.

United States Environmental Protection Agency (n.d.). *What is sustainability?* Retrieved on December 8, 2011 from http://epa.gov/sustainability/basicinfo.htm.

Waltner-Toews, D., Kay, J.J., and Lister, N.E. (2008). *The ecosystem approach: Complexity, uncertainty, and managing for sustainability.* New York: Columbia University Press.

Weeks, J. (2010). Protecting wetlands: Is the government doing enough? In *Issues for debate in environmental management: Selections from CQ researcher.* Thousand Oaks, CA: Sage. 299–352.

Woodard, C. (2010). Oceans in crisis: Can the loss of ocean biodiversity be halted? In *Issues for debate in environmental management: Selections from CQ researcher.* Thousand Oaks, CA: Sage. 353–380.

World Commission on Environment and Development. (1987). *Our common future.* New York: Oxford University Press.

Zapf, M.K. (2009). *Social work and the environment: Understanding people and place.* Ontario: Canadian Scholars' Press.

15 Social work education for disaster relief work

Lena Dominelli

> We thought that the students had come to help with donations. But they had only come to gather information.[1]

Disasters, whether 'natural' or (hu)man-made, feature prominently in contemporary life and, moreover, it seems, with increasing frequency. Hence, though social workers have been supporting disaster survivors through the United Nations (UN) humanitarian aid program since the end of the Second World War in Europe, recently there has been a spate of literature on social work in the aftermath of disasters. For example, Desai (2007) at the TATA Institute has written on social work involvement in disaster relief in India since 1947 and a special edition of *International Social Work* on disaster interventions was published in May 2007. These interventions include the provision of emergency medicines, food, water, clothing, and shelter, and, during the recovery phases, efforts to reunite families, enhance resilience, and help people rebuild their lives. Long-term interventions include community reconstruction and the development of mitigation and preventive strategies to avoid future catastrophes.

Much of the social work literature on disasters, however, ignores the physical environment (Jones, 2010), focusing instead on what social workers do or should do, for example, in a number of manuals published through the UN and humanitarian agencies, such as the Red Cross (see www.ifrc. org) or the US Federal Emergency Management Agency (FEMA) (see www. fema.gov). The social work literature linking disasters, care for the physical environment, and social justice builds on notions of the person-in-the-social-environment articulated by Bronfenbrenner (1978), redefines

---

1 Sri Lankan villager, talking about the 2004 Indian Ocean Tsunami and replying to the question about the social work students who had gone to their village to help within two weeks of the tsunami. Note, this interview took place in January 2009 and the students were from Sri Lanka and another overseas country – 'Internationalising Institutional and Professional Practices Project' funded by the Economic and Social Sciences Research Council (2009–2012).

environment to include the physical, spiritual, and social (Rogge and Combs-Orme, 2003; Van Wormer and Besthorn, 2011). Also, a cursory search of social work curricula on the web, using the key words of 'disaster interventions', 'environmental justice', and 'social justice', shows that most social work courses do not cover practice in disaster situations and there is little social work research on this topic, though some, like Zakour (1996), called for such initiatives some time ago.

Despite a growing number of proponents of environmental and social justice based practice (Besthorn and Canda, 2002; Coates, 2003; Coates, Gray, and Hetherington, 2006; Dominelli, 2011, 2012a; Hoff and McNutt, 1994; Rogge, 1994; Soliman and Rogge, 2002; Sherraden and Fox, 1997; Zakour, 1996), social work's voice is virtually invisible in disaster discussions because most interventions in catastrophic circumstances are undertaken under practically oriented, national and international humanitarian-aid agencies, particularly the Red Cross and Red Crescent societies. Given that social work sees humanitarian work as part of its practice terrain, and its professional mission is to enhance peoples' well-being at the individual, group, and community levels, this is a surprising omission and leads to questions as to whether contemporary curricula are 'fit for purpose'.

This chapter argues that this can be rectified and suggests that the remit for disaster interventions ought to be broad and holistic and draw upon the social work values of social justice and human rights; equitable distribution of power and resources; respect for persons-in-their-environment redefined to include the physical, spiritual, and socioeconomic environments, while being contextualized within families, communities, cultural traditions, and historical conjunctures. As demonstrated below, embedding social work practice in protecting these environments calls for:

- treating these as entities requiring attention and care in their own right; integrating disaster interventions that impact upon the environment broadly defined into social work curricula;
- having social workers move into new knowledge areas, including working across disciplinary boundaries to engage with physical scientists to share information about earthquakes, landslides, flooding, tsunamis, and volcanoes that is useful at the practice level;
- becoming locality specific, culturally relevant, and environmentally aware, especially about issues of environmental degradation and the exploitation of resources with a disregard of the consequences on the earth's peoples, flora, and fauna; and
- working with local residents to encourage collective solutions to environmental problems and the coproduction of new knowledge that addresses their concerns based on residents, experts, practitioners, and policymakers working together.

'Natural' disasters, exacerbated through (hu)man action, alter the living environment

Social workers can play various roles in undertaking social-ecological disaster work, such as promoting the health of people and planet Earth when responding to environmental disasters and preventing the exploitation of people and their surroundings, as well as of other sentient beings inhabiting these places with them. Rooting disaster interventions within a human rights and social and environmental justice frameworks enable practitioners to act as: *educators*, giving out information about how to access relief aid and avoid diseases like cholera and gastro-intestinal diseases that can follow a disaster, e.g., as occurred in Haiti; *therapists* helping people to deal with the emotional consequences of disaster; or *innovators*, involved in developing coalitions to lobby for the enactment of a Universal Declaration of Environmental Rights for People, the Biosphere and the Material Environment (Dominelli, 2010). For practitioners to implement this remit, a 'social-ecological system does not only need to have the potential or capacity to cope and adapt but the *resources, skills, power, and willingness to realize this capacity* into real actions' (Moser, 2008: 14, original emphasis).

Disasters, whether 'natural' or (hu)man-made, have considerable implications for the physical environment and all life forms. Disasters alter the physical environment in ways that can be extremely beneficial or highly destructive. Their effects can be compounded by human interaction within and upon this altered environment. People, plants, and animals are not separate from the physical environment, but embedded within it. Human activity, e.g. agricultural production, has shaped what is considered the 'natural' environment by encouraging domesticated animals to graze fields, bringing previously unfarmed lands under arable production. Human settlements, farming and hunting practices also contributed to the extinction of particular species, e.g. the bear and wolf in England; the dodo bird in Mauritius. These activities make it difficult to draw distinct separations between 'natural' and (hu)man-made disasters, although it can be useful to do so when developing preventative and mitigation plans because different entities can be targeted depending on the cause of the disaster.

Disasters are usually perceived as 'natural' events occasioned by natural forces that upset the stability of the surroundings in which people live, e.g. earthquakes, tornadoes, hurricanes, flooding, tsunamis, and volcanoes. While some elements of these hazards are beyond the realm of human intervention, it is becoming increasingly clear that human actions have aggravated the havoc and extent of damage endured by marginalized groups living in poor communities affected by these (Rogge and Darkwa, 1996). A good example is the impact of Hurricane Katrina in the 9th Ward of New Orleans where African-Americans were the most severely affected and the relief offered was seriously inadequate, despite the disaster occurring in one of the richest countries in the world (Pyles, 2007). How can poor countries like Haiti recover from earthquakes or Ethiopia and Somalia from drought without an equitable sharing of the earth's resources including clean water? Even where environmental disasters are shaped, in part, by climate change, one of the most hotly contested arenas in the disaster field, the role nature and people play in producing poor outcomes for those with the least resources, is considerable (Dessler and Parsons, 2006). The dispute around such claims centres on whether 'man' or 'nature' plays the greater role in the resulting destruction of people, livelihoods, and physical environments.

Physical environments provide one of the essential settings for life on Earth. People are of the earth, not out of it. As a life-giving source, earth should be cared for and respected by all those who use its bounty to ensure it is not exploited for the benefit of the few and its use is protected for future generations. Caring for those living in the present and the future is a key tenet of environmental justice and underpins notions of sustainability that are holistic and inclusive (Brundtland Report, 1987). Indigenous people talk about this relationship and the responsibilities associated with it as part of the spiritual connection between human beings, the material environment, and other living things (Coates *et al.*, 2006). This circle of connectivity can be considered in secular terms as having usufruct rights, that is, only the right to use the earth's resources without leaving a footprint that destroys these resources for others (see Figure 15.1). Damaging this

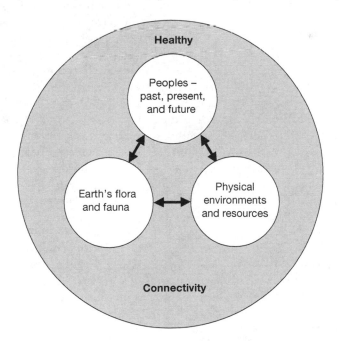

Figure 15.1 Circle of connectivity between peoples and their environments

connectivity through exploitative human actions, such as those practised by companies that dump toxic substances into the air, soil, and water, pollute food chains, and are indifferent to the plight of poor, marginalized communities on their doorsteps (Hanson, 2009) or inadequately built infrastructures, such as levées that break and cause extensive flooding as occurred in New Orleans during Hurricane Katrina (Curtis, Li, Marx, Mills, and Pine, 2011; Greenough, 2008; Pyles, 2007), exacerbates the damage caused to people and the physical terrain they inhabit

(Hu)man-made disasters include pollution of the earth's water, lands, and air to produce devastating environmental degradation, poor human health, the extinction of flora and fauna, and global climate change. Intractable levels of poverty provide the largest (hu)man-made disaster for human beings and degrade poor people's physical and built environment most (Dominelli, 2010). Poverty masks a taboo in emergency discussions because a conspiracy of silence makes invisible the need to transform exploitative economic relations that subject the needs of people and the biosphere to economic imperatives. For example, many homes in the Chilean earthquake of 2010 were destroyed because poor people could not afford to construct buildings that met existing building codes.

Armed conflicts over finite resources involving land, water, minerals, and oil (Buhaug, Gleditsch, and Thiesen, 2008) and violence against women and children are increasing globally (United Nations Division for the Advancement of Women (UNDAW), 2000). These produce deaths, mass migrations, substantial human suffering, and environmental degradation. Less commented upon in the literature is the cost these conflicts impose upon the environment by contributing to carbon emissions. Tons of exploded firepower and plumes of smoke rising into the air cause pollution and ill-health. Thousands of hectares of land have become uninhabitable because they have been mined or littered with cluster bombs.

Environmental degradation, industrial pollution, and 'natural' or (hu) man-made disasters can destroy a locale either through sudden, cataclysmic events that produce short-sharp shocks or those with long-term, gradual, and insidious cumulative effects. Short-term responses to shocks draw upon existing coping capacities, while sustained or longer-term responses depend on people's adaptive capacity. The potential of a particular response rests on a combination of coping and adaptive capacities (Gallopin, 2006; Moser, 2008). Social workers require knowledge that enables them to intervene at the pre-disaster, recovery, and reconstruction stages if they are to help protect, sustain, and rehabilitate the physical environment, people's livelihoods, and health of people, plants and animals. Their activities include working with multidisciplinary response teams to develop preventive and emergency services in case disaster strikes; reduce the number of deaths and casualties among people, animals, and plants; assess people's needs within the context of promoting a healthy and sustainable physical environment and biosphere; enhance resilience in the social, physical, and built environments; and enable disaster survivors to flourish in the future. While resilience implies a capacity to return to a previous state, sometimes this is impossible because the damage is severe and irreparable, as when a family's home is covered by volcanic lava and ash, as occurred in Montserrat. Kasperson, Kasperson, and Turner (1995) call this *environmental criticality*, which they define as 'a situation in which the extent and/or rate of environmental degradation preclude the continuation of current human-use systems or levels of human-well-being, given feasible adaptations and societal capabilities to respond' (p. 25). In such circumstances, social workers can intervene to help people dealing with grief and loss to consider alternative solutions and then move on. This necessitates the development of a psychosocial perspective and the ability to conduct multidimensional needs assessments, often undertaken jointly with other agencies to avoid individuals having to retell painful stories to a stream of helping professionals. Hence interagency coordination and interprofessional liaison is essential, especially in locating suitable alternative housing and places in which to live. Understanding human nature and exploring survivors' worries, hopes, and aspirations in their new surroundings are also important. Reminiscence narratives or memory work (Završek, 2008) might help people make the transition from their pre-disaster to post-disaster situation.

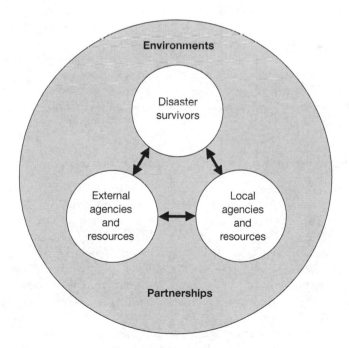

Figure 15.2 Disaster Intervention Chart

Social and environmental justice underpin social work interventions in disaster situations

Western practitioners intervening in non-Western countries have to exercise care to ensure they do not impose their assumptions, particularly those relating to age, gender, ethnicity, disability, class, caste, or religion, upon non-Western others. Learning how to use appropriate terminology and a local language or work with skilful interpreters and create locality-specific and culturally relevant services is essential to empowering forms of practice. However, this would be impossible to achieve without an egalitarian partnership being formed between local residents and external actors providing assistance in disaster situations. 'Natural' disasters are catastrophes that require resources from beyond the locality to promote restoration and resilience (Perez and Thompson, 1994) and so it is crucial that externally led interventions are not disempowering. Some disasters that are caused by (hu)man activity, such as the destruction of indigenous peoples' way of life through colonialism, are better addressed through the mobilization of local actors who can promote their own resilience and sustainable responses. Industrial pollution, though externally caused, is likely to require external resources and expertise to deal with the magnitude of the disaster, as in Bhopal (D'Silva, 2006). Knowing what local resources, facilities, and outreach activities are available and how these might be accessed will be invaluable in creating culturally appropriate local provisions. Co-produced problem-focused responses are likely to be locally empowering. Forming empowering partnerships, with local people in control, enables practitioners to play a brokerage role that facilitates residents' access to resources and external expertise. They may also advocate for a socially just world that is based on upholding the human, social, and environmental rights of all peoples and the realization of an equitable distribution of power, services, and aid, and learn the skills necessary for putting their aspirations to practice.

Social work curriculum for disaster interventions

Disaster interventions are complex, but social work educators teach students how to handle problematic situations and their generic skills can be transferred from other areas of practice into disaster arenas. Specific teaching can ensure that social workers have the capacity to undertake a variety of roles, including those of facilitator, coordinator, community organizer (of people and systems), mobilizer of resources, negotiator or broker between communities and regional and national levels of government, mediator between conflicting interests and groups, consultant to government and other agencies, and advocate for and supporters of people's rights and entitlements at national and international levels, including through the United Nations and International Court of Human

Rights. Engaging practitioners in environmental issues in the broad sense identified above through the curriculum will be a major challenge for social work educators and practitioners throughout their professional careers. According to McKinnon (2008), the 'university curriculum and continuing professional development program for social workers [has to] ... raise these issues and consider processes for sustaining reflexive and relevant social systems alongside mediating economic and ecological factors' (p. 10).

Existing curricula provide pedagogic bases on which social workers can draw. For example, the value base of anti-oppressive, socially and environmentally just, and empowering practice is useful in engaging with local residents in environmentally degraded areas, including those suffering from 'environmental racism' whereby pollutants are dumped in marginalized neighbourhoods (Rogge, 1994), poor African-American communities (Bullard, 2000), and low-income households with children (Rogge and Combs-Orme, 2003), and through large-scale hydro projects that undermine Indigenous People's lives by destroying the biosphere in tropical rainforests (Liebenthal, 2005), such as those owned by the Mapuche tribes in Chile (Carruthers and Rodriguez, 2009). Covering Indigenous perspectives in the curriculum can help students understand connections between people and their living environments (Grande, 2004).

An awareness of discrimination and oppression is insufficient if it excludes recognition of ensuing power dynamics being played out differently among diverse groups and locations. Women and children are particularly adversely affected, and their voices are seldom heard either in pre-disaster planning or in post-disaster reconstruction (Alston, 2002; Dominelli, 2012c; Pittaway, Bartolemei, and Rees, 2007; Seballos, Tanner, and Gallegos, 2011). Social justice has been an important feature of empowering social work for several decades (Dominelli, 1997) as has environmental justice (Coates *et al.*, 2006; Rogge, 1994; Ungar, 2002; see Chapter 1). Some authors have argued that Indigenous knowledge and spirituality add new dimensions to mainstream ecological concerns that focus largely on social and material considerations (Coates *et al.*, 2006; Rosenhek, 2006; Zapf, 2005). McKinnon (2008) notes:

> The links between social justice and environmental justice, and social and ecological sustainability, are topics that need to be firmly entrenched in the social work curriculum to enable the transition to social work as a profession that effectively interprets and enacts its environmental responsibilities.
>
> (p. 4)

In neoliberal, industrialized societies, social and environmental justice are interlinked with economic justice. The absence of economic justice in environments destroyed by industrial pollutants and natural disasters undermines the potential for social workers to realize social and environmental justice, and requires urgent attention in the academy and in the field (Rogge, 1994; Rogge and Darkwa, 1996). Consequently, economic questions about paid employment and workplace organization and their impact upon people's social status and income levels become important aspects of practice in environmental disasters and other catastrophic situations. Achieving economic justice is extremely problematic in an age of austerity, where public policy and public expenditure cuts affect poor people more than rich people, and social workers do not have direct access to the necessary resources or the political power to implement needs-led assessments. However, social workers can be taught how to advocate and lobby for policy changes to transform economic relations and reorient these in more egalitarian and environmentally friendly directions. They can also become involved in alliances that draw attention to the plight of poor people in disaster situations, manage the processes of change in communities (Maquire and Cartwright, 2008) and learn the skills for doing so in their courses.

Accessing the wide range of expertise necessary for operationalizing social, economic, and environmental justice does not mean social workers have to be experts in every discipline that impacts upon their work but learning how to work with the experts that do in ways that empower people is crucial. With regards to economic justice, McKinnon (2008) claims:

> [t]his is not to say that social workers are economists, they are not, but social workers do need to have an understanding of the ways in which economic factors affect the lived reality of the people with whom they work.
>
> (p. 10)

She also argues that social workers do not have to be environmental scientists either to engage in environmental issues and the same could be said about other disciplines that cover knowledge relevant to interventions in natural and (hu)man-made disasters. These include local and indigenous knowledges (Mercer, Kelman, Taranis, and Suchet Pearson, 2010) and that from disciplines like sociology, social policy, psychology, politics, economics, seismology, vulcanology, mathematics, chemistry, engineering, and climate change, complexity, environmental, and earth sciences. Of course, it is not possible for one social worker to learn the knowledge encompassed by all of these fields. However, recognizing the impact that degraded environments have on the lives of service users is indispensable (Dominelli, 1997). Learning how to work in interdisciplinary teams and knowing how to coordinate activities and facilitate working between them are important aspects for inclusion in the social work curriculum. Additionally, those practising in disaster situations are challenged to address their own needs for self-care to avoid burnout even though this injunction is poorly adhered to (Cronin, Ryan, and Brier, 2007).

Developing a curriculum for disaster interventions focusing on environmental and social justice draws on knowledge from various systems and presupposes action. Cash, Wilson, Alcock, Dickson, Eckley, Guston, Jager, and Mitchell's (2003) knowledge-action system has three components: *Credibility* refers to the scientific adequacy of expert technical evidence; *salience* to the relevance of information given to decision makers; and *legitimacy* to stakeholder involvement in the production of information and knowledge, the validation of their values, having their beliefs respected, and fair treatment of their views and interests, if disagreements arise. Social workers can use these principles to rethink the link between universal and particular dimensions of practice following disasters, and be mindful of the particular context and time in which they take place. The wide variety of disasters to be covered in social work curricula implies that, while there are certain problems that are relevant across the entire range of catastrophic events, there will also be considerable differences between them. Thus, guidelines for practice will have to engage with both similarities and differences in types of environmental disaster and avoid the attraction of one response to fit all scenarios because it may be highly inappropriate in many situations (Ramon, 2008). To promote environmental justice, the curriculum has to include respect for the physical environment and a positive duty to care for it. Additionally, group work that pays attention to the specific context in which external aid is given can provide useful techniques for enabling people to move on. Such approaches helped children survivors of the 2004 Tsunami in Sri Lanka to learn to trust the sea again (Dominelli, 2012b). Self-help groups comprising local and overseas volunteers also cleared debris and made the clean-up less arduous.

To intervene effectively in hazardous situations, social workers need a considerable array of locality-specific and culturally relevant knowledge. They need to: (1) understand the nature of the disaster, its causes, and associated secondary hazards; (2) know the spatial contours or geographic particularities of each disaster; (3) understand the social, cultural, economic, political, and historical contexts of the locality in which the disaster has occurred; and (4) appreciate the physical environment as an end in itself as well as the context in which they live. Social workers' generic knowledge, including practice theories, methods, and communication, interviewing, coordinating, organizational, group work, community, and social development skills, along with their understanding of human relationships and interactions and social and material systems and structures, should make them well-equipped to intervene in disaster situations. Additionally, there are key concepts that social workers have to understand and contextualize, and whose relevance to a particular culture and society they have to determine, including risk, vulnerability, adaptation, and resilience. Moser (2008) suggests that practitioners have considerable knowledge about these concepts, although they have to tailor them appropriately for disaster interventions:

Resilience is scale, context, and disturbance specific. Thus it is not merely an inherent characteristic of a given social-ecological system but rather an emergent property that arises from the interaction of the system, its environment, and the forces that act on both.

(p. 6)

Adger (2006) suggests that vulnerability refers to a susceptibility to harm in the context of a disturbance or stress, and that there are three dimensions that affect the degree of vulnerability: *exposure* to shock; *sensitivity* (or resistance) to stress; and *capacity* to react and adapt. Swift and Callahan (2010) believe that social workers consider risk as 'part of everyday life … most closely associated with fear and the efforts that people make to increase their security and safety' (p. 6). Moreover, they advise that incorporating notions of social justice in practitioners' understanding of risk is essential for good practice that transcends the 'tick box' mentality to assessment processes.

Social workers can become involved in assessing the immediate aftermath of disaster situations and developing plans for meeting basic needs involving the distribution of aid, as well as reuniting families and participating in long-term development. Dominelli (2011, 2012a) focuses on key processes that can assist social workers in carrying out their tasks during disaster interventions, including preventive or mitigation activities during the pre-disaster, recovery, and reconstruction stages. These include the following:

1 *Consciousness-raising* to highlight the interdependencies between people and planet Earth by discussing scenarios that might mitigate the hazards causing concern and promote an equitable and sustainable world.
2 *Advocating and lobbying* for equal access to green technologies and an equitable sharing of the earth's resources locally, nationally, and internationally.
3 *Mobilizing* communities to devise strategies for forms of development that promote solidarity and sustainability while caring for other people, and the earth's flora, fauna, and mineral resources.
4 *Dialoguing* with residents, policymakers, and the media to transform policies at the local, national, and international levels into more life-enhancing ones that the planet can sustain.
5 *Developing* curricula that cover disasters ranging from poverty to climate change and promote interventions that build individual and community resilience, capabilities, and sustainability among people and the biosphere (Dominelli, 2011, 2012a).

Each of these activities involves specific skills covered by existing social work curricula, albeit in generic terms. However, they need to be rethought for their relevance in particular disaster situations and contexts where responses to shock might be short term and focus on the coping capacities of individuals and communities or longer term and draw upon adaptive capacities or a combination of both. Kasperson, Kasperson, and Turner (1995) define *environmental* criticality as the extent to which environmental degradation precludes 'the continuation of current levels of human consumption and human-well-being' (p. 25), feasible adaptations, and the development of societal capabilities to respond to environmental degradation. Understanding when this critical point has been reached and how it can be avoided becomes an important ecological consideration to be covered in a social work curriculum for disaster interventions. It is also the point at which critical reflection can facilitate dialogue that leads to understanding how to formulate supportive actions that empower local residents (Jones, 2010).

In order to demonstrate how these generic skills and knowledge come together, a case example is provided of a social work intervention following a flood, bearing in mind that social workers often have to respond to emergency situations with little directly applicable training. In the UK, the Cabinet Office oversees the implementation of the Civil Contingencies Act (2004), the key piece of legislation outlining the duties provided by the Emergency Services. The local authorities are responsible for the safety and well-being of people during a disaster. The police and fire services play the leading roles at the beginning of the disaster, especially in evacuating people. Each area also has a local Emergency Response Team and an Action Plan that would have been developed long before a disaster occurred. This would have identified local resources that could be used when it did. General modelling techniques and scenario training used in mock exercises are not always easy to adapt to local circumstances.

Social workers become involved once people are moved to a place of safety to distribute water, food, clothing, and medicine; find temporary shelters and later permanent housing (or arrange the return home); and reunite families. Disaster legislation and procedures exist in other countries and knowledge of these is essential in planning responses appropriate to a specific locality. Being prepared suggests social workers should be aware of the legislation and emergency action plans for the particular area in which they are working, know how to access these, and discuss them with local residents and colleagues at their workplace before they are implemented. Such preparedness becomes even more important in the context of the increasing frequency of extreme weather events that can initiate a drought if hot and dry, freezing cold, or flooding if wet. People are likely to die in all these circumstances unless good mitigation and adaptation strategies are in place and their resilience is enhanced (United Nations International Strategy for Disaster Reduction (UNISDR), 2005). Social workers can help local people work with emergency planners to develop these, while ensuring that local people's participation is meaningfully and empowering (Buckingham and Percy, 1999).

Case example

A social work team in Beachside, an ethnically mixed community with a significant proportion of young and older people, including a range of (dis)abilities among them, was faced with a devastating flood following torrential rains that damaged the transportation and communication infrastructures, water, power, and other utilities and 90 per cent of its buildings (commercial, public, and residential). Beachside was in one of the poorest areas in the country and had limited resources to recover without the help of external jurisdictions. Two people in the population of 4,000 were killed. As it was holiday time, there were more women than men at Beachside. The death rate was uncertain with several people missing and the hotel registers unavailable. The primary school, which was hosting holiday activities, was seriously affected and one of the dead was a young child who could not swim. Parents were distraught that several missing children were supposed to have been at the school. The other death involved an older woman who was walking along the coastal promenade and was buried under a landslide triggered by rain and huge ocean waves that undermined the integrity of the cliffs.

The community centre, on a slightly higher slope, was one of the few buildings that remained usable and provided the social work team with an emergency office where people could come for help in accessing needed resources, including medicines, food, water, clothing, and temporary shelter; getting information about the disaster, missing relatives and friends; seeking support in reuniting with missing family members; and receiving counselling. The social workers also liaised with other agencies, including the Red Cross and a number of volunteers to assist survivors and ensure that all those that needed it were housed in temporary accommodation. The weather at the time of the flood was very cold and predicted to get colder. This increased the pressure on social workers to ensure that people were quickly rehoused. The government also declared Beachside a national disaster area and asked for other parts of the country to go to its assistance. This action brought additional resources, including finances, materials, equipment, and personnel into the rescue and recovery effort at Beachside.

An emergency meeting for the Beachside disaster which involved a range of stakeholders with an interest in Beachside, including representatives from the police and fire services, the local authority, education, social services, the business community, and residents was held in a city 100 miles away. Its aims were to: consider how well the existing emergency plans were being implemented; identify gaps in provisions, and determine how these could be filled, as well as learn lessons for the future. A social worker and a community worker from Beachside attended this meeting. While they felt confident in raising practical questions about people's immediate needs and other social work concerns, they felt bypassed when strategic matters were discussed, even though they tried to intervene and draw attention to, what seemed to them, obvious points. The meeting also highlighted for them the remoteness of those charged with creating the emergency plans they were discussing and how little real input community residents had in the process. This, they thought, should be changed, and they raised the issue of those affected by such disasters having greater input into the future plans that were being discussed to ensure that the plans that were being devised could resonate more with people's real needs.

During this emergency response meeting, those present were informed that a number of individuals and several overseas civil society organizations were coming to help. Nobody knew why they were coming, what they planned to do, where they were going, to whom they would be accountable, or the skills or resources they would bring. The social worker in the emergency response meeting was concerned about this development and raised several questions about whether they would be placing additional strain on already stretched resources, who was authorizing these unknown individuals and groups to enter the area, and the risks vulnerable groups would encounter as a result of their entry. Unfortunately, no one at the meeting could answer these questions which highlighted the lack of capacity in controlling those who could enter the area and ensure that their activities were consistent with what assistance was needed. Whether or not they were the ones local people needed was best left for others to consider, one of the politicians argued.

This case study reveals the complexities that have to be addressed during disaster interventions. Social workers can and do play important roles, often asking questions that others do not, and advocating on behalf of stricken communities. However, their own position at the decision-making tables tends to be one of supporting others rather than taking the initiative in determining what has to be done. This can lead to frustration and feelings of disempowerment that are not easily resolved.

Conclusion

Social workers are involved in disaster interventions in a variety of roles. Most of their activities are related to meeting people's basic emergency needs, providing psychosocial support and assisting long-term reconstruction endeavours. Social workers are not usually consulted about the impact of the malfunction of the built infrastructure upon health and social care delivery during disaster situations, nor are they automatically brought in as having expertise to contribute to decisions about the impact of human activity on the physical environment. The Deep Ecology movement in social work and green social workers have sought to change this state of affairs by arguing that social workers have important insights into protecting the physical environment and mobilizing people to defend their interests in maintaining healthy, sustainable communities and the geographical space in which these are located in order to ensure that environmental and social justice is realized by poor, marginalized communities that bear the brunt of degraded physical environments and their deleterious implications for their health and livelihoods.

The mainstream social work curriculum generally does not address environmental degradation and its impact on practice. Although this can make it unfit for purpose, some would argue that the curriculum is so overcrowded it cannot cover more terrain. While there is an issue about how much material can be considered in a given period of time, this is an inadequate response to the problem. Environmental considerations are embedded in sustaining all aspects of social life – from the food that is eaten to the fuel used for a variety of purposes, including heating and constructing the buildings in which people conduct their lives. The demands these make upon the earth's physical resources and other sentient beings are damaging the very basis of life, and precipitating 'natural' and (hu)man-made disasters that are increasing in frequency and damage caused. Their impact on poor people is much worse than on rich people and their effect on the earth's flora and fauna is significant enough to cause the extinction of many plant and animal species. Neglecting this state of affairs raises considerable moral and ethical questions for practitioners to address.

This chapter has argued that an ethical and moral social work practice fit for the twenty-first century cannot ignore the social and physical environmental problems that people's demands for a decent standard of living impose upon the earth. If people are to care about and for others, share the earth's resources equitably, and cause minimum damage to the biosphere, social workers have little option but to respond to the environmental crises shaping life, whether human, animal, or plant. Moreover, the social exclusion, social injustice, and marginalization which already exist in society are intensified in disaster situations and compounded by environmental degradation caused by destroyed built infrastructures, including housing, power, transportation, communication systems, and toxic rubble. Contemporary practitioners have an ethical and moral responsibility to future generations of people, plants, and animals. This places holistic sustainability at the core of curricula endorsing non-exploitative social and human development.

Disasters alter physical and geographic environments by seriously polluting and changing irrevocably the features of existing landscapes as occurred in Sichuan, China when landslides created lakes where none existed before. Working in these situations is complicated and calls for social workers with skills in navigating complexity, interacting with experts from many fields, and empowering local residents. Acquiring professional competence to intervene in such situations demands an extensive curriculum that cannot treat the environment in any of its forms as an 'add on' to an overcrowded curriculum or to be covered in one short course. While short, intensive courses on the subject might be useful tasters for beginners and students on undergraduate programs to see if this aspect of social work practice is for them, it is better to offer a specialist degree program at Masters level to enable students to learn about and explore effectively the range of materials, situations, complexities, and uncertainties of practice that could be encountered in the field.

References

Adger, W.N. (2006). Vulnerability. *Global Environmental Change, 16*(3), 268–281.

Alston, M. (2002). From local to global: Making social policy more effective for rural community capacity building. *Australian Social Work, 55*(3), 214–226.

Besthorn, F.H., and Canda, E.R. (2002). Revisioning environment: Deep ecology for education and teaching in social work. *Journal of Teaching in Social Work, 22*(1/2), 79–181.

Bronfenbrenner, U. (1978). *The ecology of human development: Experiments by nature and design.* Cambridge, MA: Harvard University Press.

Brundtland, G.H. (1987). *Our common future: Report of the World Commission on Environment and Development.* New York: Oxford University Press.

Buckingham, S., and Percy, S. (1999). *Constructing local environmental agendas: People, places and participation.* London: Routledge.

Buhaug, H., Gleditsch, N., and Thiesen, O. (2008). *Climate change and the implications for armed conflict.* Washington, DC: World Bank.

Bullard, R. (2000). *Dumping in Dixie: Race, class, and environmental quality* (3rd ed.). Boulder, CO: Westview Press.

Carruthers, D., and Rodriguez, P. (2009). Mapuche protest, environmental conflict and social movement linkage in Chile. *Third World Quarterly, 30*(4), 743–760.

Cash, D.W., Wilson, G., Alcock, F., Dickson, N., Eckley, N., Guston, D., Jager, J., and Mitchell, R. (2003). Knowledge systems for sustainable development. *PNAS, 100*(14), 8086–8091.

Civil Contingencies Act. (2004). Retrieved October 29, 2011 from http://www.legislation.gov.uk/ukpga/2004/36/contents.

Coates, J. (2003). *Ecology and social work: Towards a new paradigm.* Halifax, NS: Fernwood Press.

Coates, J., Gray, M., and Hetherington, T. (2006). An 'ecospiritual' perspective: Finally, a place for Indigenous approaches. *British Journal of Social Work, 36*(3), 381–399.

Cronin, M., Ryan, D., and Brier, D. (2007). Support for staff working in disaster situations: A social work perspective. *International Social Work, 50*(3), 370–382.

Curtis, A., Li, B., Marx, B., Mills, J., and Pine, J. (2011). A multiple additive regression tree analysis of three exposure measures during Hurricane Katrina. *Disasters, 35*(1), 19–35.

D'Silva, T (2006). *The black box of Bhopal: A closer look at the world's deadliest industrial disaster.* Victoria, BC: Trafford Publishing.

Desai, A. (2007). Disaster and social work responses. In L. Dominelli (Ed.). *Revitalising communities in a globalising world.* Aldershot, Hants: Ashgate. 297–314.

Dessler, A., and Parsons, E. (2006). *The science and politics of climate change: A guide to the debate.* Cambridge: Cambridge University Press.

Dominelli, L (1997). *Sociology for social workers.* London: Macmillan.

Dominelli, L. (2010). *Social work in a globalising world.* Cambridge: Polity Press.

Dominelli, L. (2011). Climate change: Social workers' roles and contributions to policy debates and practice interventions. *International Journal of Social Welfare*, *20*(4), 430–438.

Dominelli, L. (2012a). *Green social work*. Cambridge: Polity Press.

Dominelli, L. (2012b). Social work in times of disaster: Practising across borders. In M. Kearnes, Klauser, F., and Lane, S. (Eds). *Critical risk research: Practice, politics and ethics*. Oxford: Wiley-Blackwell Publishers. 197–218.

Dominelli, L. (2012c forthcoming). Gendering climate change: Implications for debates, policies and practice. In M. Alston and Whittenbury, K. (Eds). *Women and climate change*. New York: Spring.

Gallopin, D.C. (2006). Linkages between vulnerability, resilience and adaptive capacity, *Global Environmental Change*, *16*, 293–303.

Grande, S. (2004) *Red pedagogy: Native American and political thought*. Lanham, MD: Rowman & Littlefield.

Greenough, P. (2008). Burden of disease and health status among Hurricane Katrina displaced persons in shelters: A population-based cluster sample. *Annals of Emergency Medicine*, *51*(4), 426–432.

Hanson, L. (2009). Environmental justice as a politics of place: An analysis of five Canadian environmental groups' approaches to agro-food issues. In J. Ageyman, Cole, P., Haluza-Delay, R., and O'Riley, P. (Eds). *Speaking for ourselves: Environmental justice in Canada*. Vancouver, BC: University of British Columbia Press. 203–218.

Hoff, M.D., and McNutt, J.G. (Eds). (1994). *The global environmental crisis: Implications for social welfare and social work*. Brookfield, VT: Ashgate.

Jones, P. (2010). Responding to the ecological crisis: Transformative pathways for social work education. *Journal of Social Work Education*, *46*(1), 67–84.

Kasperson, R.E., Kasperson, X.J., and Turner, B.L. (Eds). (1995). *Regions at risk: Comparisons of threatened environments*. Tokyo: United Nations University Press.

Liebenthal, A. (2005). *Extractive industries and sustainable development*. Washington, DC: World Bank.

Maquire, B., and Cartwright, S. (2008). *Assessing a community's capacity to manage change: A resilience approach to social assessment*. Canberra: Bureau of Rural Science Publishers.

McKinnon, J. (2008). Exploring the nexus between social work and the environment. *Australian Social Work*, *61*(3), 268–282.

Mercer, J., Kelman, I., Taranis, L., and Suchet Pearson, S. (2010). Framework for integrating indigenous and scientific knowledge for disaster risk reduction. *Disasters*, *34*(1), 214–239.

Moser, S. (2008). *Resilience in the face of global environmental change*. Santa Cruz, CA: University of California, Santa Cruz.

Perez, E., and Thompson, P. (1994). Natural hazards: Causes and effects. *Pre-Hospital Disaster Medicine*, *9*(1), 80–88.

Pittaway, E., Bartolemei, L., and Rees, S. (2007). Gendered dimensions of the 2004 tsunami and a potential social work in post-disaster. *International Social Work*, *50*(3), 307–319.

Pyles, L. (2007). Community organising for post-disaster social development: Locating social work. *International Social Work*, *50*(3), 321–333.

Ramon, S. (Ed.). (2008). *Social work in the context of political conflict*. Birmingham: Venture Press.

Rogge, M.E. (1994). Environmental justice: Social welfare and toxic waste. In M.D. Hoff and McNutt, J.G. (Eds). *The global environmental crisis: Implications for social welfare and social work.* Brookfield, VT: Ashgate. 53–74.

Rogge, M.E., and Combs-Orme, T. (2003). Protecting children from chemical exposure: Social work and US social welfare policy. *Social Work, 48*(4), 439–450.

Rogge, M.E., and Darkwa, O.K. (1996). Poverty and the environment: An international perspective for social work. *International Social Work, 39*, 395–409.

Rosenhek, R. (2006). Earth, spirit and action: The deep ecology movement as spiritual engagement. *The Trumpeter: The Journal of Ecosophy, 22*(2), 90–95.

Seballos, T., Tanner, M., and Gallegos, J. (2011). *Children and disasters: Understanding impact and enabling agency.* Brighton, UK: Save the Children, UNICEF.

Sherraden, M., and Fox, E. (1997). The great flood of 1993: Response and recovery in five communities. *Journal of Community Practice, 4*(3), 23–45.

Soliman, H.H., and Rogge, M.E. (2002). Ethical considerations in disaster services: A social work perspective. *Electronic Journal of Social Work, 1*(1), 1–23.

Swift, K., and Callahan, M. (2010). *At risk: Social justice in child welfare and other human services.* Toronto, ON: Toronto University Press,

Ungar, M (2002). A deeper, more social ecological social work practice. *Social Service Review , 76*(3), 480–497.

United Nations Division for the Advancement of Women (UNDAW). (2000). *Sexual violence and armed conflict: United Nations response.* New York: United Nations.

United Nations International Strategy for Disaster Reduction (UNISDR). (2005). *The Hyogo Framework for Action 2005–2015: Building the Resilience of Nations and Communities to Disasters.* New York: United Nations.

Van Wormer, K., and Besthorn, F.H., (2011). *Human behavior and the social environment: Groups, communities and organizations* (2nd ed.). New York: Oxford University Press.

Zakour, M.J. (1996). Disasters and social work. *Journal of Social Services Research, 22*(1), 7–25.

Zapf, M.K. (2005). The spiritual dimension of person and environment: Perspectives from social work and traditional knowledge. *International Social Work, 48*(5), 633–643.

Zaviršek, D. (2008). Social work as memory work in times of political conflict. In S. Ramon (Ed.). *Social work in the context of political conflict.* Birmingham: Venture Press.

Conclusion

Mel Gray, John Coates, and Tiani Hetherington

> As a profession, we need to intentionally redefine 'person-in-environment' to incorporate [the] natural environment … then it will become more apparent to us what we need to do locally, nationally, and internationally. The [natural] environment needs to be infused into every aspect of everything social work professionals do, across the micro–macro practice spectrum (Rogge, in Skwiot, 2008: 26).

There is no doubt that ecological justice is firmly on the social work agenda and it is fitting that our opening chapter by Fred Besthorn foregrounded the urgency of social work's environmental responsibilities. But as we ponder the implications of the 'new paradigm' advocated in the preceding chapters, it might be helpful to begin this concluding chapter with an overview of the 'old paradigm' which is being extended and transformed, namely, the ecosystems perspective as it has developed in social work.

The person-in-environment: Revisiting the ecosystems perspective

Historically, ecological systems theory, commonly known as the ecosystems perspective in social work, stemmed mainly from the USA and was embraced by the profession at a time when a unitary framework for practice was being sought (Allen-Meares and Lane, 1987; Siporin, 1980; see Payne (1991) for an account of its uptake in the UK). This came at a historical juncture when diverse fields, like hospital social work and family therapy, and methods of practice, such as casework, group work, community work, and social policy, were spawning their own theories and bodies of literature making social work appear a rather splintered and disjointed profession. The 'person-in-environment' – the signature for ecological systems theory – was born out of the profession's quest for a 'common base' (Bartlett, 1970) or 'unitary approach' to practice (Goldstein, 1973) to bring clinical social workers into a single fold with community-oriented practitioners. This dual purpose had conceptualized social workers' engagement in both micro and macro social change activities. However, what resulted was a dividing of the profession into distinct levels of practice each with its own skills and specializations. Challenges to these silos commenced by the 1950s when Harriet Bartlett pointed to the importance of the 'interaction' between the person and the environment. She was among the first to articulate social work's domain as Person-Interaction-Environment (Bartlett, 1970), later shortened to the now familiar Person-In-Environment (PIE). Hollis' (1964) psychosocial approach was based on social work's dual focus on psychological and social factors, which Germain (1973) developed into an ecological perspective focusing on the interrelationship between individuals and the environment. Germain and Gitterman's (1980) 'life model' reconceptualized practice to reflect 'the continuous transactions among individual, collective, environmental, and cultural processes in human development and functioning' (Germain and Gitterman, 1996: ix). Though the US National Association of Social Workers (NASW, 1980) recognized this overarching perspective in social work practice as early as 1980, over the years, social work has struggled to maintain a balance between the person and environment as social work interventions have focused mainly on changing individual behaviour rather than modifying the social environment (Germain, 1979a, 1979b).

Three theoretical frameworks offered an opportunity to unite these diverse areas of practice: the first came from sociology in the form of Parsons' social systems theory and the second two came from biology in the form of von Bertalanffy's (1971) general systems and ecological theory. The systems-based unitary framework was introduced to the profession simultaneously in three key texts: Pincus and Minahan (1973), Goldstein (1973), and Germain (1973) in which ecological general systems theory was applied to social systems in various ways drawing on Perlman's (1957) earlier work on social work as a problem-solving *process*. Barring Germain (1973), whose early work still adhered to a medical model and, as with Perlman, drew heavily on ego psychology, these writers – and those following in this direction – laid 'the groundwork for a new way of looking at social work practice' (Pardeck, 1988: 133). Importantly, they gradually changed the language of social work from the medically oriented diagnosis and treatment to assessment and intervention focusing on people's social functioning within various systems in their immediate social environment. The healthy functioning of systems was seen to be essential to human and environmental well-being.

However, as Siporin (1980) demonstrated, concern for person and circumstance has a long history in social work dating back to Mary Richmond but situation theory was supplanted by psychoanalytic thinking until Hamilton, Hollis, and Perlman forged what became known as the psychosocial approach to practice with attention to internal psychological and external social factors impinging on the client's situation. This concern to put the 'social' back into social work arose with the influence of social systems theory and the structural-functionalist models of Parsons and

Merton in sociology when it played a major role in the development of the family therapy and community mental health movements in the 1950s and 1960s (Siporin, 1980). Social systems theory influenced Pincus and Minahan's (1973) delineation of three kinds of systems:

1   *Informal or natural systems,* such as family, friends, neighbours, and colleagues.
2   *Formal or organizational systems,* such as community groups and trade unions.
3   *Societal or bureaucratic systems,* more commonly known as social institutions, such as hospitals and schools.

From this began the language of access to and availability of the helping *systems* people needed to live full and flourishing lives. Problems were said to arise when these systems were absent or inaccessible as occurs when people may not know about or want to use them, or when the system's policies created further barriers, or where systems conflicted with one another. The social worker's task then became one of analysing the interactions between clients and their social situation, which comprised a range of interacting systems, in order to identify where system malfunctioning was leading to personal and social problems. Pincus and Minahan (1973) introduced the language of 'change agent systems', 'client systems', 'target systems', and 'action systems' to further delineate the interacting roles and tasks involved in systems change or maintenance.

Systems thinking opened the profession to non-psychological *social* ideas about the diverse influences present in any given situation and how these together impact upon human behaviour. It diverted attention away from intrapsychic processes to the interconnections between the various 'subsystems' of which people were a part. It introduced a relational mode of thinking about systems as greater than the sum of their individual parts, giving rise to the first ideas about holism in social work. As a result, social workers conducted systems analyses using the language of levels of systems with micro, meso or mezzo, and macro levels of analysis at the core of their deliberations. Each level referred to its distance from the individual client with micro, mezzo, and macro mirroring Pincus and Minahan's (1973) informal, formal, and societal systems. Social workers could intervene in any one of these systems with each level suggesting particular methods of practice: casework and group work at the individual level, and community work at the meso level, for example. Significantly, systems thinking offered a framework for analysis but did not prescribe practice interventions. It appeared to provide a largely apolitical view of adaptive and maladaptive functioning and system interaction devoid of any critical or structural analysis, such as class and gendered privilege.

As Pincus and Minahan (1973) introduced social systems theory to social work, Carel Germain (1973) introduced the ecological perspective to address the failures of the person-in-environment to go beyond intrapsychic and interpersonal processes. Most if not all work with the 'environment' concerned gathering information about clients from family members, teachers, employers, friends, and neighbours. While Pincus and Minahan (1973) had drawn on insights pertaining to systems interaction, Germain (1973) saw the organism–environment relations as offering an understanding closer to common human experience, an understanding which led to a simultaneous focus on the person and environment and their reciprocal relationship. As with social systems theory, the goal was a better understanding of the factors promoting individual and family well-being and healthy social functioning. In Germain's (1979a) words, 'The perspective is concerned with growth, development, and potentialities of human beings and with the properties of their environments that support or fail to support the expression of human potential' (pp. 7–8). The ecological perspective drew heavily on developmental theory, establishing normative functioning through various stages of the human 'life course', and held an Aristotelian focus on human functioning or flourishing (Gray, 2011); it came to be referred to as the 'life model' approach to practice (Germain, 1979; Germain and Gitterman, 1980, 1987).

Underlying the ecological systems framework are systems' concepts of equilibrium and disequilibrium. The social worker, as part of a change agent system, could intervene in any area of the system which would result in compensatory changes as the system sought to acquire a new equilibrium. Recognizing that equilibrium could promote adaptive or maladaptive functioning, it is important for the new equilibrium to promote the clients' well-being. Key to systems thinking was the idea that the client and the environment were not necessarily the source of the problem. Rather the problem arose from the interaction between them – at the interface between the person and the social environment. The social worker's goal was to help people to perform essential life tasks to alleviate their distress and achieve the aims and value positions which were important to them. Social workers then became engaged in helping people to use and improve their capacities and abilities to solve problems and build new connections with parts of the system which would help and support their achievement of well-being. Frequently interventions focused on helping people to modify their interactions with significant people in their social systems or access resource systems providing practical help to enable them to do this. Systems thinking fit well with the preceding functional theory in social work typified in Perlman's problem-solving approach wherein the person with a problem comes to a place where he or she is helped by a professional with particular knowledge and skills.

However, as with prior theories of casework, ecological thinking was individualistic and focused on the person's capacity for growth and change, noting the importance of positive self-esteem, personal competency, self-awareness, self-direction, and self-responsibility. Its normative life-stage model focused on individual capacities to make age-appropriate decisions and take purposive action. While it acknowledged issues of power, a broader structural understanding would only emerge later in social work in response to criticisms of the shortcomings of ecosystems understanding in social work (Middleman and Goldberg-Wood, 1989; Moreau, 1979; Mullaly, 1997).

Germain's (1973, 1976, 1978, 1979a, 1979b, 1984, 1985, 1987) work was important to early understanding in social work of the interplay of the physical or natural and social environments. Biotic communities or a species' unique place in the web of life provided a metaphor for the adaptive fit suitable for human flourishing and implied, in Aristotelian terms, a teleological understanding of humans' propensity for self-actualization. Applications of the ecosystems perspective proliferated (Allen-Meares, Washington, and Welsh, 1986; Carlson, 1991; Coulton, 1981; Cox, 1992; Early, 1992; Freeman, 1984; Gitterman, 1991; Guterman and Blythe, 1986; Howard and Johnson, 1985; James and Studs, 1988; Kelley, McKay, and Nelson, 1985; Lee, 1989, 1994; Libassi and Maluccio, 1982; Meyer, 1983; Milner, 1987; Patterson, Memmott, Brennan, and Germain, 1992; Rothman, 1994; Simon, 1994; Wells, Singer, and Polgar, 1986). Noting the more frequent embrace of ecosystems theory than in other professions, Siporin (1980) speculated this was likely:

> because social workers like to think of themselves as being more 'down to earth,' and they feel more partial to the 'earth-consciousness' of an ecological view. Perhaps also, this model is congenial to the self-image as 'earth mothers' held by many social workers ... [referring as it does] to a conceptual system about mind–body-environment in transactional relationships. People and their physical-social-cultural environment are understood to interact in processes of mutual reciprocity and complementary exchanges of resources, through which processes the systemic functional requirements are met, dynamic equilibrium and exchange balances are attained, and dialectical change takes place (p. 509).

Social work brought a dynamic, humanistic perspective to general and social systems theory with its focus on the interaction between people and systems. Germain and Gitterman's (1980) life model of social work practice represented the application of ecosystems theory to direct practice patterned not on remediation but on developmental 'life processes' directed to:

1   enhance people's strengths and their innate push toward health, continued growth, and release of potential;
2   modify environments, as needed, so they might sustain and promote human well-being to the maximum degree possible; and

3   raise the level of person-in-environment fit for individuals, families, groups, and communities.

Germain and Gitterman (1980) supplanted earlier concepts of life space and problems in living with a more encompassing paradigm of life stressors and coping within a particular sociocultural context. They attempted to embrace a range of theoretical developments in social work relating to empowerment and culturally sensitive practice, while drawing on social work knowledge and skills in practice at different levels (as already outlined); relationship-centred practice; and later postmodern notions of clients as experts of their own lives.

A 'new ecological' perspective for social work

The new ecological perspective emerging in social work concerns itself mainly with broadening the notion of environment to include the natural world. While the ecosystems perspective was largely anthropocentric and lacking in political analysis, the new ecological paradigm seeks an ecocentric focus. Several authors have sought to find ethical grounds for social work's commitment to the natural world (Besthorn, 2011; Gray and Coates, 2011; Lysack, 2011; Tester, 1994). Perhaps the most innovative aspect of this new ecological approach is its ecocritical focus. Närhi and Matthies (2001) see the main focus of critique being the entire modernization project. The approach has promoted a critical awareness of ecological crises and environmental questions now 'connected to the very fundamentals of society: its structures, its ways of life and values' (p. 46). According to Peeters (2011), this critical orientation centres 'on a fundamental critique of modern Western culture urging the need for a paradigm shift toward a "holistic" understanding of the human–nature relationship with focused attention on spirituality as a vital component' (p. 3).

For Coates (2003) the new paradigm builds on the acceptance of the wisdom of nature that has evolved over the billions of years of experimentation, development, and adaptation and produced a planet replete with complex life-forms and a 'sophisticated, interdependent, self-regulating, and self-healing system' (p. 80) (see also Lovelock, 1979). Even with tsunamis, asteroids, and harsh winters, nature's fecundity has resulted in a complex and efficient exchange of resources among millions of life forms and billions of creatures of various kinds, so much so that the irreversible process of evolution continues. The new paradigm involves a transition in human thinking away from the mandate of self-serving control so central to frontier and modern industrial cultures, to one which follows the innate tendencies of the Universe (see Swimme and Berry, 1992). Well-being exists within the limitations of nature which should predominate even when humans do not understand the full complexity of the interactions and processes among organisms.

The new paradigm is a shift to a different worldview – what Mezirow (1978, 1990) refers to as a perspective transformation. It is much more than adding another concept or theory – it is a quantum shift in consciousness. Thus expansion of the person-in-environment is a first step to incorporating a larger diversity of stressors, supports, and impacts – for example, the needs of other people, political realities, and the local, regional, and global environments where appropriate. Environmental social work cannot be covered adequately in a single class or a course (see Chapter 11). It is a new framework that requires a transformation from anthropocentrism to ecocentrism, from mechanistic to organic understandings of Earth, from dualism to holism, and from linear to organic determinants of change. It may take many years for mainstream practice to make the transition from considering environmental issues as an additive factor to a full embrace of an all-inclusive ecosocial work perspective. It may take even longer to fully operationalize this new framework, in light of the political and economic resistance of many Western governments and corporations.

One of the major tenets of the new paradigm is the connectedness of individuals and communities to the rest of nature. This understanding develops from acceptance of interdependence and the unity of all things (Berry, 1998; Macy, 2007; Swimme and Berry, 1992) and can take the form of holistic thinking in practice. People are always in relationship not only with their partners, families, and local community, but also, for example, with people who help to produce the clothes they wear, and to the environments impacted by the industrial practices, such as mining and smelting, that produce the metals used in our kitchen appliances. Further, the sense of being in relationship alters the understanding of individualism that is so central to Western thinking and modern social work. Our sense of self is expanded and altered such that one's identity is always in relationship to others in community, and is no longer that of an isolated individual maximizing personal benefit. The sense of personal responsibility expands as we realize more clearly the full consequences of how we live (see also Sinclair, Hart, and Bruyere, 2009).

Further, the social and physical environments in which we grew up and live are seen not only to shape our sense of self, but also to be part of our identity. This is similar to the importance of harmony and place in many Indigenous cultures (see Hart, 2002; Sinclair et al., 2009; Zapf, 2009). This expanded sense of self – ecological self (Macy, 2007) or ecological consciousness – leads one to overcome attitudes that threaten the environment and to feel personally affronted when ecosystems are damaged, and perhaps a sense of social empathy similar to what humans so often feel when they learn about the realities of major disasters such as hurricanes, floods, and droughts. Mische (1982/1998) argued that a thriving Earth is a 'pre-condition for the full development of the human' (p. 12).

A second prominent tenet that flows from the interconnectedness of all things is awareness that human well-being is affected by the well-being of others and the rest of nature. Since humans exist in relationship and grow through relationships and community (see, for example, Berry, 1988; Kegan, 1982), an individual's ability to become self-actualized depends on other people having that same opportunity. Similarly, living within a thriving and healthy Earth is essential for human health and well-being. Cities infested with constant smog will not have healthy citizens. At a more basic level, if, as Maslow pointed out, our basic needs for food, shelter, and safety are fundamental to well-being, human well-being logically depends on all people having their basic needs met. Such a situation of widespread human well-being can only occur if a series of interdependent forces align – well-being depends upon the presence of peace, which depends upon justice (equity), which requires equality, and all of these will only be possible when there are healthy environments capable of supporting a healthy population. One of the challenges facing social work is to help create social and community structures that nurture the well-being of all (see Coates, 2003; Russell, 1998).

A third major tenet is the celebration of diversity and inclusivity. Discoveries of evolution (see for example Swimme and Berry, 1992) note the tendency of the universe not only toward connectedness, but also to increasing complexity and diversity. Interdependence thrives as different ecosystems over millennia develop their unique combination of plants, animals, and inorganic elements contributing to the self-regulating systems of Earth. This diversity has enabled life to flourish almost everywhere on the planet. It is visible among the thousands of human tribes, languages, and cultures, and the unique ecosystems throughout Earth, that have developed and fit uniquely within the particular physical context of their home community. Seen in this way, diversity has supported the evolution of humans and continues to do so as each community provides diverse opportunities for identity, belonging, care and personal well-being. This point is wonderfully developed for the modern context by Jean Vanier (1998) and his work with people with 'unique gifts'.

Variations of the new paradigm are discussed by several authors, including Berger and Kelly (1993), Besthorn (2002), and Coates (2003, 2005). Peeters (2011) outlines some additional features including:

1 Recognition of Earth's biophysical boundaries and limited resources necessitating alternative – solar – energy sources.
2 An 'ecological economy' capable of satisfying human needs while protecting the physical environment.
3 A view of the global world system as a complex network of layered systems, with the economy 'embedded' in society and society in the ecosystem Earth.
4 An ecological ethics embracing an ethics of care as complementary to a deontological rights-based ethics. From its relational view of the person, the foundation of rights in the autonomy of the subject has to be reinterpreted from an idea of 'autonomy in connectedness' (Peeters,

2011) which is similar to the Indigenous emphasis on individual in community (Hart, 2002).

The future of the new paradigm is not without its struggles. The application of such a transformative framework will likely encounter a number of hurdles. First, most social workers are employees who carry out mandates of agencies and organizations. As such, the scope of service may be constrained by organizational and bureaucratic practices. This is particularly important in areas such as child welfare where social workers are trained and hired to carry out this work, but the mandate is held by the agency not the profession. Services that have legislated mandates may be reluctant to reconceptualize services or revise practices in light of this new framework. Second, research on the efficacy of new interventions will take time to be demonstrated. In the interim pressure to use previously established best practices or to follow evidenced-based models may delay research on alternative interventions. Third, social work may have difficulty being accepted for its contribution by professionals and groups that have already established a role for their profession in addressing environmentally related problems. Social work is late into this field, and other professionals, and some social workers, have not fully accepted that there is a relevant role for social work in environmentally oriented practice. Fourth, social work, despite its often expressed claim to be an agent of change, has been very slow to accept theoretical developments – for example, feminist and structural approaches struggled to be recognized and a similar struggle can be foreseen for environmental approaches. The new paradigm may be even more difficult to embrace than work with diverse groups such as the disabled, as it is more than a new area of service. It is a new framework that demands a shift in the social worker's values and ideals. Further, the individualist focus that permeates modern social work is very entrenched and stands as a barrier. Finally, major resistance may come from critical thinkers and scholars who are unable to depart from the centrality of anthropocentrism to mainstream social work.

Environmental social work practice: Redefining and refocusing the social work profession

While the shape of environmental social work practice will ultimately be determined in response to many challenges and opportunities, the contributors to this book believe that, given the increasing public awareness and social work interest in environmental issues, this aspect of practice will grow quickly. To return to the typology for practice shown in Figure I.1 in the Introduction, a number of emerging areas for environmentally related engagement are now discussed. While we here draw attention to how social work can be involved, both directly and indirectly, with a number of environmental challenges, it will be important to social workers in direct practice and traditional settings and areas of practice to develop an expanded framework for practice that is sensitive to environmentally related concerns, predicaments, and interventions. We anticipate that an increasing number of issues will require that social workers employ a critical lens that links social, economic, and ecological realities.

Addressing the destruction of natural resources

First is the need to enhance awareness of the finite nature of Earth's resources which, it is hoped, will lead to attitudinal and lifestyle changes to curb humans' profligate energy use, environmentally destructive mining, forestry, industrial and agricultural practices, and greed-driven consumerism. At the micro level, social workers can work to change people's consumption-oriented values and intervene in crises such as when drinking water is, or is at-risk to be, contaminated by industrial practices, or consult with large corporates on appropriate corporate social responsibility programs (Brueckner and Ross, 2010; Ross, 2009, see Chapter 10). At the mezzo level, social workers can run educational programs to teach people about the scarcity and fragility of environmental resources and the dangers of environmental destruction. Social workers can support the development of conservation and recycling programs, as well as environmental restoration initiatives (see Chapter 9). At the macro level social workers can engage in sustainable community development programs, and initiate and monitor policy change and enforcement to protect and restore natural resources.

We think that social workers will be most active and effective when addressing issues related to local resources that impact people directly. It is at the local level where the intimate knowledge of regional resources and the peculiarities of ecosystems held by farmers, fishers, woodlot owners, and birders, for example, can be taken advantage of in developing sustainable practices. Further, this local emphasis can foster the use of technology that supports local control of local resources for local benefits (see Coates, 2003; Schumacher, 1973).

Global warming and climate change

Human dependence on fossil fuels – oil, gas, and coal – for energy is widely argued as a major source of carbon in the atmosphere and reducing human dependence on them is imperative for mitigating climate change: 'The debate about the limits of the world's fossil fuel resources is of great consequence for climate change' (Giddens, 2009: 38). At the micro level social workers find themselves engaged in health interventions for such issues as skin cancer and other sun-related diseases, and families coping with asthma and other lung ailments resulting from smog, and where natural disasters ensue. Social workers might be involved directly in the provision of services and resources to individuals and families, and be involved in community-level interventions that target secondary prevention, and also tertiary prevention addressing the broader causes of the global warming. Other areas include crisis intervention and recovery assistance for victims of floods, tornados, and other climate-related disasters, such as drought and bushfires (Alston, 2007, 2009; Stehlik, 2003a, 2003b, 2005, see Chapters 7 and 15). At the mezzo level, social workers might be involved in education programs to raise awareness of the short- and long-term dangers of global warming and climate change and behaviour changes needed to mitigate the impacts (see for example, McKenzie-Mohr, Lee, Schultz, and Kotler, 2011; Climate Change Conference, 2012). They might work alongside local government councils to advise on the integration of low-income housing into urban designs that reduce fossil fuel consumption; and be involved in developing organic community gardens, tree planting, and reforestation programs that have therapeutic, social, and biophysical benefits (see Chapters 6 and 9). At the macro level, they might support bicycle- and pedestrian-friendly urban zones, serve on committees concerned with monitoring the enforcement of policy changes on pollution emissions and drought prevention (see Chapter 7), as well as develop and support public education programs, such as Earth Hour. These direct and community level interventions can take place in cooperation with other professions and community activists (Lysack, 2010; Tester, 1997). To enhance effectiveness of these efforts social work education can incorporate learning about the use of media and communication strategies that serve to mobilize public opinion and action. Lobbying local politicians and countering the impact of government passivity and corporate 'green-washing' will be necessary skills.

Toxic materials production and waste disposal

The exposure of low-income, marginalized, and racialized communities, especially their children, to toxins is well known (see Chapter 2). Social workers might intervene at the micro level, offering crisis intervention for stressed families, be involved in advocating for and providing material emergency services (see for example Bertell, 1998), and fact-finding for workplace-based illnesses. At the mezzo level, they might engage in educational programs on the dangers of toxic materials and safety precautions and on the use of alternative, non-toxic materials (i.e. environmentally safe household cleaning products); the coordination of health and social interventions around hazards; community relocation and community development for victims of hazardous waste accidents or irremediable sites. In rural areas, such as northern Canada, where populations are more dispersed, the need for competent and engaged practitioners will be no less needed. For example, in agricultural areas social workers may wish to join or support organizations and government policies regarding the safe use of pesticides and herbicides, and advocate for the safe working conditions for migrant workers. In rural areas the preservation of natural resources such as groundwater, aquifers, and the introduction of water restoration practices may be warranted. A major challenge will be to carry out Social Impact Analyses of sites for production and to find sustainable policies and practices that follow the precautionary principle and address economic needs. It is also primarily in rural areas where work with Indigenous people can take place to support their efforts to protect their traditional lands from unwanted development, or to assist with training and education so members are able to take advantage of sustainable industrial development in their regions.

At the macro level, social workers might serve on committees examining policy and the enforcement of workplace safety standards and advocate for research on the development of non-toxic products for workplace and home, and for monetary compensation and psychological recovery programs for victims of toxic waste, or the misuse of pesticides and herbicides (see, for example, Colborn, Dumanoski, and Myers, 1997).

Air, soil, and water pollution

Health-related issues are seen to result directly from or be exacerbated by air, soil, and water pollution in addition to their contribution to global warming. At the micro level, social workers might engage in crisis interventions and other mental health intervention for stress caused by exposure (e.g. support groups for asthma sufferers) or conduct health assessment and interventions aimed at children (e.g. to determine lead levels). Individual and family assessments can incorporate the exploration of employment and residence histories to explore exposure to toxins and pollutants. This may be particularly relevant in work with marginalized groups (see for example Bullard, 1994); as environmental sensitivities increase social workers may be one of the professions called upon to educate and develop intervention plans for families impacted. At the mezzo level, social workers might work in multidisciplinary teams offering health services for persons with acute or chronic illnesses (e.g. asbestos-related diseases) or be involved in the development of public education programs about the dangers of air and water pollution and citizen involvement in clean-up campaigns. At the macro level, they could advocate for improved public monitoring and enforcement of air, soil, and water quality standards; promote and enforce policy change to reduce air, soil, and water pollution; develop advocacy programs for victims of air, soil, and water pollution (especially in low-income communities); and support research and social impact analysis.

Species extinction

Biodiversity is essential for ecosystem health and overall planetary well-being. If species are eliminated this can weaken the ecosystem, reducing both its productivity and its ability to adapt to change. Extinctions are occurring in response to climate change, but perhaps more so due to unrestrained human behaviour, such as overharvesting of renewable resources, habitat destruction, deforestation and tree farms, monoculture and profit-motivated industrial agriculture, the use of pesticides and herbicides, and even the impact of the policies of the World Bank (WB), International Monetary Fund (IMF), and World Trade Organization (WTO) (see for example Chossudovsky, 1998; Hofrichter, 1993; Lewis, 2005). Examples of overharvesting include the Atlantic salmon and cod fisheries, while the impacts of pollution are well documented in Colborn *et al.* (1997). At the micro level, social workers might be engaged in mental health, personal growth initiatives and lifestyle analysis directed toward changing consumer-oriented values and consumption patterns endangering species. At the mezzo level they might be part of educational initiatives to teach about ecological science (species interdependency) and sustainability; the development of habitat conservation programs; and support Indigenous Peoples' involvement in and benefit from conservation initiatives on their traditional lands. At the macro level, social workers might participate in sustainable economic development initiatives with communities to support species preservation; community and family-based sustainable agriculture (research and policy on community-based food systems); educational initiatives and improved policy measures to support endangered species and habitat; and groups for the preservation of agricultural seed diversity and public education on the dangers and social injustices of corporate patenting of life forms. An important area where people in the Global North can become involved is in partnering with and supporting NGOs and local groups throughout Earth who are engaged in direct and indirect conservation efforts.

Sustainable development and food security

Development that meets the needs of the present without compromising the ability of future generations to meet their own needs – a core tenet of sustainability – requires attention to food security, water management, and sustainable agricultural practices. Social workers might become involved in such initiatives at the mezzo level through community gardens in low-income neighbourhoods (Stocker and Barnett, 1998) and educational initiatives around food consumption and transportation patterns, as well as social and environmental justice efforts to confront the ill effects of globalization by supporting, for example, the sale of locally grown fresh produce and farmers' markets. Significant contributors to loss of biodiversity include the extremes of poverty and wealth where scavenging for survival and extravagant lifestyles contribute disproportionately to environmental destruction and pollution. A major contribution by social workers can be in the areas of poverty reduction and more equitable tax policies can serve to promote sustainability (see Chapter 3).

At the macro level, social workers might be involved in groups promoting urban and community-supported agriculture to create employment, sustainable livelihoods, and food security; national and international policies that enable poverty reduction and food security in less developed countries; and protests against investments by food-deficient, but wealthy countries and corporations in the farming systems of poorer countries (Polack, Wood, and Bradley, 2008). A significant benefit could be gained if policies of the WB, IMF, and WTO shifted to support sustainable agricultural practices of local and subsistence farmers. There are substantial biophysical advantages to local agricultural initiatives that enable local farmers to have viable and sustainable livelihoods. Even in the Global North more humane and environmentally safe and sustainable practices could be found if people consumed less meat or switched to more pasture-fed and free-range cattle and poultry. A change in diet by a large number of people could reduce the atrocities of factory farming, meat processing, and the run-off from large feed-lots (see, for example, Schlosser, 2001). Changing food habits, especially in the Global North, can have significant personal and ecological benefit (see, for example, SustainableTable, n.d.).

Responses to natural disasters and traumatic events

Disasters, such as drought, mudslides, floods, hurricanes, and environmental refugees, are seen to be influenced by climate change on a planet substantially altered by human activities such as globalization, deforestation, pollution, industrial agriculture, and dam construction (see Chapters 5 and 15). Social workers might be involved at the micro level in disaster response teams providing crisis intervention disaster relief services for survivors (Mathbor, 2007; Pawar, 2008a, 2008b, 2008c, see Chapter 15). At the mezzo level they might be part of community educational initiatives that inform people about the causes and consequences of disasters and of appropriate responses to them. Further, in many areas educational initiatives can help prepare for an emergency, by having a safe evacuation plan, and emergency survival kits. At the macro level, social workers might be part of multidisciplinary disaster response teams planning for the reception of environmental refugees and supporting alternatives to such damaging practices as dam construction, deforestation, and industrial agriculture.

The message from this book is clear. Environmental interventions are multidisciplinary. While individual actions, like boycotting products made in sweatshops, can have a powerful effect, and every little thing we do to save electricity or recycle waste helps, for the most part, real change will come from the alignment of diverse groups in society promoting myriad programs to increase environmental awareness, engaging in environmental restoration, reforming government policy and industrial practices, or assisting people dealing with the fallout of environmental hazards or disasters. Ultimately, social work is context-based and most of the contexts in which social workers are formally employed do not have biophysical concerns as a major focus, but environmentally aware social workers ask questions in health contexts about the physical environments in which people live. They know those communities linked with certain illnesses, such as coalmining communities, or those about to lose their livelihoods through mining development (see Chapter 10). They know the communities affected by drought (see Chapter 7) and so on. All the chapters in this book appeal for social workers to broaden their concerns beyond the profession's humanistic and anthropocentric focus to embrace environmental issues and concerns. All call upon the profession to extend its focus beyond social to ecological justice and environmental sustainability; to work with marginalized populations most likely to be affected by climate change and to see climate change as a human rights issue; to work with drought-affected families; to include pets in family assessments and interventions; to appreciate and harness the healing powers of the environment; to see the potential for community organizing and environmental activism in building community gardens and urban green spaces, that too have healing or stress-reducing properties; to see the terrain of environmental restoration as one of promise for the rehabilitation of young offenders; to become part of corporate social responsibility programs at the corporate or community level; to engage in social work education as a domain of practice to transform the curriculum; to challenge students to develop an ecological consciousness, respond to environmental issues, engage in environmental advocacy, and learn to work in multidisciplinary response teams, especially in disaster relief work. Such is the broad and diverse terrain of environmental social work.

This book has introduced an array of environmental issues engaging social work students and practitioners around the world, giving them the brief to become active concerning issues that arise in their social work practice. It is likely, however, that embracing environmental issues also means working in new and diverse contexts. Some aspects of this work can be an extension of conventional social work practice in those contexts already close to the issues. For example, social workers working with mentally ill, disabled, or elderly people with dementia or Alzheimer's are more likely to use animals to enhance communication, engage with clients, and build relationships than those working in highly regulated, bureaucratic contexts (Churchill, Safaouli, McCabe, and Baun, 1999; Risley-Curtiss, 2010; Turner, 2005, see Chapter 8). Social workers in rural contexts are more likely to engage in drought- or flood-related issues, especially with marginalized communities likely to be affected by these natural disasters, among others. Those working in industry or large corporations are more likely to become involved in corporate social responsibility programs. The point is that it will be more difficult for social workers to remodel existing and traditional contexts of practice to embrace environmental concerns than to move into new contexts. Ecologically aware social workers might begin to expand their thinking in ways not currently accessed as boundaries open and 'thinking outside the box' becomes standard. Asking questions about environmental and employment histories, recreational activities, and special or sacred places in their assessments, and building on people's current engagement with nature, are examples of places to start. But social work practice will probably change slowly. Like Tom in Hayward *et al.*'s example (see Chapter 13), it is more likely that social work graduates will begin to seek out new contexts of practice. It is also highly likely that the work they engage in will be multi- or interdisciplinary and involve community-based interventions or community engagement of some sort (see Chapter 14). Elsewhere Heinsch (2011) wrote about her engagement as a student in a nature-based intervention with children. Social workers working in faith-based contexts are more likely than those in public services to engage in environmentally related practice, as Lysack's chapter shows (see Chapter 12). Lysack's work involves harnessing opportunities for capacity building within faith communities to take a lead in and advocate for the protection of the climate and environment.

These chapters collectively attest the growing importance of ecological justice in social work as the profession's scholars, researchers, and practitioners work to develop theoretical understanding and practical interventions for social workers around the world grappling with their environmental responsibilities. The dialogue has begun and it is hoped these chapters have furthered the discussion and provided some pointers to practical ways in which social workers might engage in pressing environmental issues and concerns.

References

Allen-Meares, P., and Lane, B.A. (1987). Grounding social work practice in theory: Ecosystems. *Social Casework, November,* 515–521.

Allen-Meares, P., Washington, R.O., and Welsh, B.L. (1986). *Social work services in schools.* Englewood Cliffs, NJ: Prentice Hall.

Alston, M. (2007). It's really not easy to get help: Services to drought-affected families. *Australian Social Work, 60*(4), 421–435.

Alston, M. (2009). Drought policy in Australia: Gender mainstreaming or gender blindness? *Gender, Place & Culture: A Journal of Feminist Geography, 16*(2), 139–154.

Bartlett, H.M. (1970). *The common base of social work practice.* New York: National Association of Social Workers.

Berger, R., and Kelly, J. (1993). Social work in the ecological crisis. *Social Work, 38,* 521–526.

Berry, T. (1988). *The dream of the Earth.* San Francisco: Sierra Club.

Berry, W. (1998). *A timbered choir.* Washington, DC: Counterpoint.

Bertell, R. (1998). Environmental Influences on the health of children. Paper presented at the *International Conference on Children's Health and the Environment,* Amsterdam, Holland. Retrieved January 23, 2012 from http://iicph.org/children_health.

Besthorn, F.H. (2002). Expanding spiritual diversity in social work: Perspectives on the greening of spirituality. *Currents: New Scholarship in the Human Services, 1*(1). Retrieved January 27, 2012 from http://fsw.ucalgary.ca/currents/fred_besthorn/besthorn.htm.

Besthorn, F. (2011). Deep Ecology's contributions to social work: A ten-year retrospective. *International Journal of Social Welfare, 21,* 1–12. Article first published online: 9 DEC 2011 | DOI: 10.1111/j.1468-2397.2011.00850.x.

Brueckner, M., and Ross, D. (2010). *Under corporate skies: The struggle between people, place and profit.* Western Australia: Fremantle Press.

Bullard, R. (Ed.). (1994). *Unequal protection.* San Francisco, CA: Sierra Club Books.

Carlson, B.E. (1991). Causes and maintenance of domestic violence: An ecological analysis. *Social Service Review, 58,* 569–587.

Chossudovsky, M. (1998). *The globalization of poverty: Impacts of the IMF and World Bank reforms.* Halifax, NS: Fernwood.

Churchill, M., Safaouli, J., McCabe, B.W., and Baun, M.M. (1999). Using a therapy dog to alleviate the agitation and desocialisation of people with Alzheimer's disease. *Journal of Psychosocial Nursing & Mental Health Services, 37*(4), 16–22.

Climate Change Conference. (2012). *Fourth International Conference on Climate Change: Impacts and responses.* University of Washington, July 12–13, 2012. Online at http://on-climate.com/conference-2012/.

Coates, J. (2003). *Ecology and social work: Toward a new paradigm.* Halifax, NS: Fernwood Books.

Coates, J. (2005). Environmental crisis: Implications for social work. *Journal of Progressive Human Services, 16*(1), 25–49.

Colborn, T., Dumanoski, D., and Myers, J. (1997). *Our stolen future.* New York: Penguin.

Coulton, C. (1981). Person–environment fit as the focus in health care. *Social Work, 26,* 26–35.

Cox, C. (1992). Expanding social work's role in home care: An ecological perspective. *Social Work, 37,* 179–183.

Early, B.P. (1992). An ecological–exchange model of social work consultation within the work group of the school. *Social Work in Education, 14,* 207–214.

Freeman, E. (1984). Multiple losses in the elderly: An ecological approach. *Social Casework, 65,* 287–296.

Germain, C.B. (1973). An ecological perspective in casework practice. *Social Casework, 54,* 323–330.

Germain, C.B. (1976). Time: An ecological variable in social work practice. *Social Casework, 57,* 419–426.

Germain, C.B. (1978). Space: An ecological variable in social work practice. *Social Casework, 59,* 512–522.

Germain, C.B. (1979a). Introduction: Ecology and social work. In C.B. Germain (Ed.). *Social work practice: People and environments.* New York: Columbia University Press. 1–22.

Germain, C.B. (Ed.). (1979b). *Social work practice: People and environments.* New York: Columbia University Press.

Germain, C.B. (1984). *Social work practice in health care: An ecological perspective.* New York: Free Press.

Germain, C.B. (1985). The place of community work within an ecological approach to social work practice. In S.H. Taylor and Roberts, R.W. (Eds). *Theory and practice of community social work.* New York: Columbia University Press. 30–55.

Germain, C.B., and Gitterman, A. (1980). *The life model of social work practice.* New York: Columbia University Press.

Germain, C.B., and Gitterman, A. (1987). Ecological perspective. In A. Minahan (Ed.-in-Chief). *Encyclopedia of social work, vol. 1* (18th ed.). Silver Spring, MD: National Association of Social Workers. 488–499.

Germain, C.B., and Gitterman, A. (1996). *The life model of social work practice* (2nd ed.). New York: Columbia University Press.

Giddens, A. (2009). *The politics of climate change.* Cambridge: Polity Press.

Gitterman, A. (1991). Introduction to social work practice with vulnerable populations. In A. Gitterman (Ed.). *Handbook of social work practice with vulnerable populations.* New York: Columbia University Press. 1–34.

Goldstein, H. (1973). *Social work practice: A unitary approach.* Columbia, SC: University of South Carolina Press.

Gordon, W.E. (1969). Basic constructs for an integrative and generative conception of social work. In G. Hearn (Ed.). *The general systems approach: Contributions toward an holistic conception of social work.* New York: Council on Social Work Education. 5–12.

Gottlieb, B. (Ed.). (1986). *Marshalling social support: Formats, processes, and effects.* Newbury Park, CA: Sage Publications.

Gray, M. (2011). Back to basics: A critique of the strengths perspective in social work. *Families in Society: The Journal of Contemporary Human Services, 92*(1), 5–11.

Gray, M., and Coates, J. (2011). Environmental ethics for social work: Social work's responsibility to the non-human world. *International Journal of Social Welfare, 21.* Article first published online: 13DEC2011 | DOI: 10.1111/j.1468-2397.2011. 00852.x.

Guterman, N., and Blythe, B. (1986). Toward ecologically based intervention in residential treatment for children. *Social Service Review, 60,* 633–643.

Hareven, T. K. (1982). Preface. In T.K. Hareven and Adams, K.J. (Eds). *Aging and life course transitions: An interdisciplinary perspective.* New York: Guilford Press. xiii–xvi.

Hart, M.A. (2002). *Seeking mino-pimatisiwin: An Aboriginal approach to helping.* Halifax, NS: Fernwood Publishing.

Hartman, A. (1994). *Reflection and controversy: Essays on social work.* Washington, DC: NASW Press.

Hartman, A., and Laird, J. (1983). *Family-centered social work practice.* New York: Free Press.

Heinsch, M. (2011). Getting down to earth: Finding a place for nature in social work practice. *International Journal of Social Welfare, 21.* Article first published online: 9 DEC 2011 | DOI: 10.1111/j.1468-2397.2011.00860.x.

Hofrichter, R. (Ed.). (1993). *Toxic struggles: The theory and practice of environmental justice.* Philadelphia, PA: New Society.

Hollis, F. (1964). *Casework: A psychosocial therapy.* New York: Random House.

Howard, T.U., and Johnson, F.C. (1985). An ecological approach to practice with single-parent families. *Social Casework, 66,* 482–489.

James, C.S., and Studs, D.S. (1988). An ecological approach to defining discharge planning in social work. *Social Work in Health Care, 12,* 47–59.

Kegan, R. (1982). *The evolving self.* Cambridge, MA; Harvard University Press.

Kelley, M.L., McKay, S., and Nelson, C.H. (1985). Indian agency development: An ecological approach. *Social Casework, 66,* 594–602.

Laird, J. (1989). Women and stories: Restorying women's reconstructions. In M. McGoldrick, Anderson, S.M., and Walsh, F. (Eds). *Women in families.* New York: W. W. Norton. 427–450.

Lazarus, R.S. (1980). The stress and coping paradigm. In L.A. Bond and Rosen, J.C. (Eds). *Competence and coping during adulthood.* Hanover, NH: University Press of New England. 28–74.

Lazarus, R.S., and Folkman, S. (1984). *Stress, appraisal and coping.* New York: Springer.

Lee, J.B. (Ed.). (1989). *Group work with the poor and oppressed.* New York: Haworth Press.

Lee, J.B. (1994). *Empowerment practice in social work.* New York: Columbia University Press.

Lewis, S. (2005). *Race against time.* Toronto, ON: Anansi Press.

Libassi, M.F., and Maluccio, A. N. (1982). Teaching the use of ecological perspective in community mental health. *Journal of Education for Social Work, 18,* 94–100.

Lovelock, J. (1979). *Gaia: A new look at life on Earth.* New York: Oxford University Press.

Lysack, M. (2010). Environmental decline, loss, and Biophilia: Fostering commitment in environmental citizenship. *Critical Social Work, 11*(3). Retrieved May 24, 2011 from http://www.uwindsor.ca/criticalsocialwork/environmental-decline-loss-and-biophilia-fostering-commitment-in-environmental-citizenship

Lysack, M. (2011). Building capacity for environmental engagement and leadership: An ecosocial work perspective. *International Journal of Social Welfare, 21.* Article first published online: 13DEC2011|DOI:10.1111/j.1468-2397.2011.00854.x.

Macy, J. (2007). *World as lover, world as self: Courage for global justice and ecological renewal.* Berkeley, CA: Parallax Press.

Mathbor, G.M. (2007). Enhancement of community preparedness for natural disasters: The role of social work in building social capital for sustainable disaster relief and management. *International Social Work, 50*(3), 357–369.

McKenzie-Mohr, D., Lee, N., Schultz, P., and Kotler, P. (2011). *Social marketing to protect the environment: What works.* Thousand Oaks, CA: Sage Books.

Meyer, C. (1983). *Clinical social work in the eco-systems perspective.* New York: Columbia University Press.

Mezirow, J. (1978). Perspective transformation. *Adult Education, 28*(2), 100–110.

Mezirow, J. (1990). *Fostering critical reflection in adult life.* San Francisco: Jossey-Bass.

Middleman, R.R., and Goldberg-Wood, G.G. (1989). *The structural approach to social work.* New York: Columbia University Press.

Milner, J.L. (1987). An ecological perspective on duration of foster care. *Child Welfare, 66,* 113–123.

Minahan, A. (Ed.-in-Chief). (1987). *Encyclopedia of social work (18th ed.).* Silver Spring, MD: National Association of Social Workers.

Mische, P. (1982/1998). *Toward a global spirituality* (revised edition). New York: Global Education Associates (Originally published in *The Whole Earth Papers* 1982, 16). http://winonaworks.com/web_documents/Mische.pdf.

Moreau, M. (1979). A structural approach to social work practice. *Canadian Journal of Social Work Education, 5*(1), 78–94.

Mullaly, B. (1997). *Structural social work* (2nd ed.). Oxford: Oxford University Press.

Närhi, K., and Matthies, A.-L. (2001). What is the ecological (self-)consciousness of social work? Perspectives on the relationship between social work and ecology. In A.-L. Matthies, Närhi, K., and Ward, D. (Eds). *The eco-social approach in social work.* Jyväskylä: Sophi, 16–53.

National Association of Social Workers (NASW). (1980). *NASW Code of Ethics.* Washington, DC: NASW.

Pardeck, J. (1988). An ecological approach to social work practice. *Journal of Sociology and Social Welfare, 15,* 133–142.

Patterson, S., Memmott, J., Brennan, E., and Germain, C.B. (1992). Patterns of natural helping in rural areas: Implications for social work research. *Social Work Research and Abstracts, 28*(3), 22–26.

Pawar, M. (2008a). The flood of Krishna river and the flood of politics: Dynamics of rescue and relief operations in a village in India. *Asia Pacific Journal of Social Work and Development, 18*(2), 19–35.

Pawar, M. (2008b). Interventions in disasters. *Asia Pacific Journal of Social Work and Development, 18*(2), 72–83.

Pawar, M. (2008c). Disaster preparedness/management agencies and centers. *Asia Pacific Journal of Social Work and Development, 18*(2), 84–91.

Payne, M. (1991). *Modern social work theory.* Basingstoke: Macmillan.

Peeters, J. (2011). The place of social work in sustainable development: Towards ecosocial practice. *International Journal of Social Welfare, 21,* 1–12. Article first published online: 13 DEC 2011 DOI: 10.1111/j.1468-2397.2011.00856.x.

Perlman, H.H. (1957). *Social casework: A problem-solving process.* Chicago, Il: University of Chicago Press.

Pincus, A., and Minahan, A. (1973). *Social work practice: Model and method.* Itasca, IL: F.E. Peacock Publishers.

Polack, R., Wood, S., and Bradley, E. (2008). Fossil fuels and food security: Analysis and recommendations for community organizers. *Journal of Community Practice, 16*(3), 359–375.

Risley-Curtiss, C. (2010). Social work practitioners and the human-companion animal bond: A national study. *Social Work, 38*(9), 1–12.

Ross, D. (2009). Emphasizing the 'social' in corporate social responsibility: A social work perspective. *Professionals' Perspectives of Corporate Social Responsibility, 4,* 301–318.

Rothman, J. (1994). *Case management: Integration of individual and community practice.* Englewood Cliffs, NJ: Prentice Hall.

Russell, P. (1998). *Waking up in time.* Novato, CA: Origin Press.

Schlosser, E. (2001). *Fast food nation: The dark side of the all-American meal.* Boston, MA: Houghton Mifflin.

Schumacher, E.F. (1973). *Small is beautiful.* New York: HarperCollins.

Simon, B.L. (1994). *The empowerment tradition in American social work: A history.* New York: Columbia University Press.

Sinclair, R., Hart, M.J., and Bruyere, G. (Eds). (2009). *Wichitowin: Aboriginal social work in Canada.* Winnipeg, MB: Fernwood.

Siporin, M. (1980). Ecological systems theory in social work. *Journal of Sociology and Social Welfare,* 7(4), 507–532.

Skwiot, R. (2008). Green dream: Environmental justice is emerging from the shadows. *Social Impact, Fall,* 23–29. Retrieved January 23, 2012 from http://gwbweb.wustl.edu/Pages/SocialImpactF2008.aspx.

Stehlik, D. (2003a). Australian drought as lived experience: Social and community impacts. In L. Botterill and Fisher, M. (Eds). *Beyond drought in Australia: People, policy and place.* Canberra: CSIRO Press. 87–108.

Stehlik, D. (2003b). Summarising research and issues relating to topics as identified by the inaugural NRWC Roundtable. Invited paper presented at the National Rural Women's Coalition (NRWC) *Managing Drought: Managing Solutions Forum.* Dubbo, New South Wales.

Stehlik, D. (2005). Managing risk? Social policy responses in time of drought. In D. Wilhite and Courtney Botterill, L. (Eds). *Drought in Australia.* Dordrecht: Springer. 65–83.

Stocker, L., and Barnett, K. (1998). The significance and praxis of community-based sustainability projects: Community gardens in Western Australia. *Local Environment,* 3(2), 179–189.

Sustainable Table, (n.d.). http://www.sustainabletable.org/home.php.

Swimme, B., and Berry, T. (1992). *The Universe story: From the primordial flaring forth to the ecozoic era – a celebration of the unfolding of the cosmos.* New York: Harper One.

Tester, F. (1994). In an age of ecology: Limits to voluntarism and traditional theory in social work practice. In M. Hoff and McNutt, J. (Eds). *The global environmental crisis: Implications for social welfare and social work.* Aldershot, Hants: Avebury. 75–99.

Tester, F.J. (1997). From the ground up: Community development as an environmental movement. In B. Wharf and Clague, M. (Eds). *Community organizing: Canadian experiences.* Toronto, ON: Oxford University Press. 228–247.

Turner, W.G. (2005). The role of companion animals throughout the family lifecycle. *Journal of Family Social Work,* 9(4), 11–21.

Vanier, J. (1998). *Becoming human.* Toronto, ON: Anansi Press.

Von Bertalanffy, L. (1971). *General systems theory: Foundations, development, application.* London: Allen Lane.

Weick, A., and Vandiver, S.T. (Eds). (1982). *Women, power, and change.* Washington, DC: National Association of Social Workers.

Weiss, R.S. (Ed.). (1973). *Loneliness: The experience of emotional and social isolation.* Cambridge, MA: MIT Press.

Wells, L.M., Singer, C., and Polgar, A.T. (1986). *To enhance quality of life in institutions. An empowerment model in long term care: A partnership of residents, staff and families.* Toronto, ON: University of Toronto Press.

Zapf, M.K. (2009). *Social work and the environment: Understanding people and place.* Toronto, ON: Canadian Scholars Press.

Glossary

Anthropocentric   Human centred.

Anthropocentrism   The belief that human interests are central in environmental matters, specifically the inclination of the human species to regard itself as the dominant and most important entity in the universe. It is the evaluation of all reality and all action through an exclusively human perspective.

Anthropogenic   Human-caused or pertaining to human causes.

Artificial environment   One that has been created by humans rather than nature.

Biocentric   Literally, biology-centred or centred on the biological or natural world and denotes a commitment to the equality of species.

Biodiversity   There is variation in understanding this term. It often refers to the variety of life forms in a specific area, where a decline in biodiversity is used frequently as an indicator of ill-health. However, biodiversity has also been referred to as the study of the processes that maintain diversity and this can include genetic diversity, the diversity of species, and the diversity of ecosystems (see for example Canadian biodiversity website, n.d.).

Biophysical environment   Includes all that is within the biosphere and is a useful synonym for the terms nature and natural environment, especially when one wants to avoid the ambiguity around the terms human and nature (when humans are part of nature).

Biosphere   Includes all the living organisms and all that has been produced by them over the course of time. It can also be understood as the top crust of the Earth (minerals, coal, oil, forests and mountains, water, land, ice, and so on) along with the thin layer of air (atmosphere) within which all the biological processes of the planet take place (Encyclopedia of Earth, n.d.).

Biotic community   A phrase popularized by US naturalist Aldo Leopold to describe the interacting effect of organisms living together in a habitat or ecosystemic community.

Built environment   Refers to the settings that have been constructed to accommodate human activity; included are buildings, civic projects, highways and dams. A major portion of modern life takes place in built environments, and there are efforts in the areas of architecture and urban design to build environments that are in greater harmony with nature.

Climate change   Usually refers to long-term changes in the Earth's climate, most recently due to an increase in average temperature. Global warming is a type of climate change, referring to a long-term shift in weather patterns that is the result of changes in the chemical composition of the atmosphere. Human activity and natural events contribute to climate change but most recent scholarship has focused on the impact of human activity, such as pollution, deforestation, and the release of carbon dioxide.

Corporate social responsibility   In general, corporate social responsibility refers to the various ways that public and private sector organizations can integrate social and environmental concerns with their economic realities. CSR involves any number of practices, such as charitable donations, fair labour practices, and environmental considerations in managing purchasing and waste. An example is the voluntary guideline (ISO 26000) adopted in 2010 by the International Organization for Standardization involving principles for seven core areas – organizational governance, human rights, labour practices, environment, fair operating practices, consumers, and community involvement and development (ISO, 2010).

Deep Ecology   Is (i) a formal philosophical system developed in the early 1970s by late Norwegian philosopher Arne Naess and (ii) a broad sociopolitical, environmental movement focused on humanitiy's deeper (ontological and experiential) interrelationship with the natural world as a starting point for a balanced and just response to critical ecological concerns.

Deep justice   A term used by supporters of radical environmental thought to describe a broadened and ecocentric concept of justice whose focus is primarily on the fact that non-sentient beings and natural systems have equal moral standing. The human species is not privileged in considerations of moral action.

Distributive justice   An ethical theory which concerns the allocation of scarce social benefits and harms in a society in a socially just manner.

Ecocentric   Is a nature-centred system of values (versus human centred) that sees all things as interconnected and the human as inseparable from nature. All life forms have intrinsic value, and human needs are not seen as superior to those of other life forms.

Ecocentrism   A term used to denote a nature-centred, as opposed to human-centred, system of values. Supporters of ecocentrism deny that there are any essential or necessary divisions between human and non-human nature and that all entities in the natural world have intrinsic worth or value. Ecocentrism does not deny the importance of social justice and the challenges of social problems, but argues that human concerns must be seen in the larger ecological context.

Ecocide   The 'extensive destruction, damage to or loss of ecosystem(s) of a given territory, whether by human agency or by other causes, to such an extent that peaceful enjoyment by the inhabitants of that territory has been severely diminished' (Higgins, 2010: 63).

Ecological health   The interdependent health of humans, animals, and ecosystems.

Ecological justice   An environmental ethic which seeks to preserve the integrity and beauty of the natural world, its primary focus is the intrinsic worth of the natural world irrespective of its use or utilitarian value to human welfare. It posits that meaningful efforts to protect nature must begin with a firm commitment to the inherent value of all aspects of the natural world.

Ecological literacy or ecoliteracy   Refers to a deep understanding of the operation of natural systems and humans' place in these systems. Beyond common human associations with reading and writing, literacy refers to competence or knowledge in a specific area. *Environmental literacy* therefore entails an understanding of the features of the environment – being able to identify endemic species, or understanding the water cycle, for example. *Ecological literacy* includes this environmental dimension but goes beyond such instrumental knowledge to focus not just on the operation of natural systems but also on the relationships between and within such systems. Particular emphasis is placed on recognizing the interrelationships and interdependencies between human and non-human systems.

Ecological self   Refers to the core connection that people have toward other species and the Earth itself such that we react to their interests as if they were our own (Naess, 1985). Other writers, such as Freya Mathews (1991), see that while humans have a sense of individuality each of us is part of the life process and is intimately connected to the cosmos. It is not just a consciousness but is also a deep connection to all life. Individuality and the Ecological Self are mutually supportive, not in opposition (see Clarke, 2008).

Ecology   Most commonly understood as the relationship of organisms to their environments, in social work it has come to refer to the relationship of humans to their social and physical environments, and involves concern and responsibility for the short- and long-term impacts of human behaviour on other people and on the physical environments of which we are a part, both social and natural. Ecology and ecological are used in an expanded manner, to refer to the holistic, complex set of interdependencies and interrelationships between all organisms, human and non-human, and their total environment.

Ecosocial   A conflation of ecological and social, *ecosocial* is a shorthand way of indicating issues or approaches where the traditional human–nature dichotomy is rejected and explicit recognition is given to the interrelatedness and interdependence between humans and the non-human world. An ecosocial orientation would argue that both the ecological and the social are inextricably related and cannot be considered in isolation from one another.

Ecosphere   The part of a planet and the ecosystems in it that is capable of supporting life – the biosphere.

Ecospiritual   An approach to social work that develops from the assumption that the Earth and all on it are sacred. Based on this both social justice and ecological justice are primary values, and there is an inherent responsibility for humans to manage their activities (economic and social) with regard to the well-being of all things. Ecospirituality is holistic, and recognizes the interdependence and connectedness of all things, and that evolutionary processes are in place.

Ecosystems   An ecosystem is the whole complex of living organisms that interact and comprise an ecological community. When an ecosystem is healthy, organisms that form the ecosystem are able to reproduce in a balanced and sustainable manner. They vary in size and smaller ecosystems can be elements in larger ecosystems.

El Niño   A commonly used term to describe a climate pattern within the nations of the Pacific including Australia that has a direct effect on Australia's weather patterns. Usually El Niño signifies a drier Australian eastern seaboard.

Environment   In a general sense, usually refers to the aggregate of surrounding things so it is possible to speak of a person's social environment, which might include the family, employment, relations to organizations, and so forth. Human beings live in the environment and are elements of the environment. Some use an anthropocentric view of environment as the '*non-human natural* conditions and surroundings [around people]' (Sutton, 2007: 1, original emphasis).

Environmental   Refers to issues pertaining to the natural world, as in the elements – air, water, minerals, and other organisms – that might surround any given organism.

Environmental crisis   Refers to a crisis unfolding in the natural world and, in particular, where that crisis has been precipitated by human activity, i.e. it is anthropogenic in nature.

Environmental degradation   The belief and observation that harm to the environment is a major consequence of human intervention, to the point that the damage is becoming irreparable.

Environmental justice   An environmental ethic which is an extension of the distributional and utilitarian aspects of modern liberal-democratic ideas of social justice. An important element is that risks, harms, benefits, information, participation in decision making, and access to due process, are distributed equally among humans.

Environmental movement A political movement centred on environmental concerns.

Environmental perspective The view that nature includes humans as part of nature: rather than nature being what society is not and separate from society, the environmental perspective holds that there is a symbiotic relationship between nature and society (Sutton, 2007).

Environmental sustainability A discourse that explores 'the relationship among economic development, environmental quality, and social equity' (Rogers, Jalal, and Boyd, 2008: 42).

Environmentalism An ideology centred on the environment.

Global warming A term – backed by collective scientific evidence – to indicate that the world is getting warmer, often centred on the idea that this climatic effect is a result of human interference, though this is an area of much controversy. Climate change has become the preferred term for changes in climatic and weather patterns (see **Climate change**).

Green politics A minority *political* orientation with environmental concerns and sustainable development as central ideas.

Green prison reform Refers to recidivism reduction programs that teach life skills in the context of environmental sustainability and conservation.

Greenhouse effect The trapping and absorbing of radiation in the atmosphere that leads to a warming of the Earth's surface. Many scholars attribute global warming to the greenhouse effect due to the increase of greenhouse gases in the atmosphere.

Greenhouse gases Water vapour, carbon dioxide and other gases that build up in the atmosphere (largely due to the burning of fossil fuels) and trap radiation, resulting in global warming.

Human exceptionalism The belief that humans have a special status in nature based on their unique capacities, which provides the grounding for some naturalistic concepts of human rights.

Human exemptionalism The attitude that humans are exempt from natural ecological limits.

Intergovernmental Panel on Climate Change (IPPC) The IPCC seeks to evaluate the state of climate science, as described in scholarly literature, in order to inform policy. It was established by the World Meteorological Organization and the United Nations Environmental Programme. The fourth assessment report (IPCC, 2007) reviewed 928 papers published between 1993 and 2003.

Intrinsic value An ethical proposition suggesting that a person or thing has in itself or for its own sake an intrinsic or inherent worth. An object or person with intrinsic value may be regarded as an end in itself, irrespective of its use-value to others.

La Niña A commonly used term to describe a climate pattern within the Pacific Ocean that has a direct affect on Australia's weather patterns. Usually La Niña signifies a wetter than average eastern seaboard of Australia.

Living democracies   In a living democracy the citizenry actively claims the rights and responsibilities for the community and society (Shiva, 2005). It is 'a way of life, a civic culture in which people creatively participate in public life' (Atlee, 1992: 1).

Living economies   Are nonviolent economies (Shiva, 2005). In a living economy 'communities of people [are] engaged in the business of creating just, sustainable, and fulfilling livelihoods for themselves while contributing to the economic health and prosperity of the community' (Korten, 2002: 1).

Modernity   The post-medieval historical period, characterized by Enlightenment philosophy, capitalism, industrialization, secularization, and the rise of the nation-state.

Natural environment   More commonly refers to '*the non-human world within which human societies and their products exist*' (Sutton, 2007: 4; original emphasis). Even cities and buildings – the artificial or built environment – are part of nature built from natural materials and constitute part of human beings' manipulation of the natural environment (Sutton, 2007) (see **Environment**).

Nature   The natural as distinct from the human world, all that surrounds us, of which we are part.

New Ecological Paradigm (NEP)   Emerged as a counter to the human exemptionalism that considered humans as 'exempt' from environmental relationships and the anthropocentrism, dualism and determinism that are characteristic of modernity and western thinking. The NEP considers humans as connected with, and subject to, the laws of nature, and that humans must consider the impact of their economic activity on the ecosystems of the planet. While recognizing the unique abilities of the human species the NEP argues that humans must live within the limits of nature (see Catton and Dunlap, 1980).

Person-in-environment   A social work-theoretical and practice perspective based on the notion that an individual cannot be understood fully without consideration of the various interactive aspects of each person's environmental contexts.

Positive peace   Positive peace is the presence of justice and the absence of cultural, structural, and direct violence (Galtung, 2001).

Radical egalitarian ecological justice   An extended environmental ethic stresses that humans are systemically embedded and biologically embodied beings whose ethical responsibilities *emerge from* and *extend to* all non-human beings and entities.

Rehabilitation   Refers to a return to health and applies to both humans and the biophysical environment.

Restoration   The work needed to facilitate rehabilitation of the land and people.

Shallow justice A term used by supporters of radical environmental thought to describe a narrow and often utilitarian and distributive concept of justice whose focus is primarily on the distributive responsibilities existing between members of the human species.

Small Island Developing States Low-lying coastal countries that tend to share similar environmental and sustainable development challenges.

Social capital See **Social value creation**.

Social entrepreneurship Involves engaging entrepreneurial principles to address the social problems that plague our global community, similar to those identified in the United Nations' Millennium Development Goals. Success is measured in social value creation (social capital) rather than profit (economic capital).

Social justice Generally refers to the ethical idea of creating a society that is based on principles of equality and human rights that recognizes the dignity of every human being.

Social value creation A new term used in place of the much-hackneyed 'social capital'. It is a term originating in the USA in the field of philanthropy, where there is a great deal of enthusiasm for applying 'business principles' and 'investment analyses' to decisions about funding nonprofit organizations and programs. These approaches integrate measures of cost in their calculations of the relative benefits of funding a particular program or organization for its 'social value creation' potential (see Tuan, 2008).

Sustainability '[C]reates and maintains the conditions under which humans and nature can exist in productive harmony, that permit fulfilling the social, economic and other requirements of present and future generations' (United States Environmental Protection Agency (EPA), n.d., p. 1). It promotes the wise and sustainable use of natural resources through *inter alia* recycling and curbs on consumption.

Sustainable development A way of talking about and planning for an improved relationship between human societies and the natural environment used by businesses, national governments, and local, national, and international organizations concerned with reducing the human footprint on the natural environment (Sutton, 2007).

Utilitarianism An ethical theory developed in the nineteenth century positing the best ethical course of action is the one that maximizes the most happiness for the greatest number. It is a form of consequentialism suggesting the value of a moral action is determined by its outcome. The most influential contributors to this theory were Jeremy Bentham and John Stuart Mill.

Zoonotic Transmitted from animals to humans as in zoonotic diseases.

References

Atlee, T. (1992). Living democracy. *Thinkpeace, 7*(2&3). Retrieved January 30, 2012 from http://www.co-intelligence.org/CIPol_LivingDemoc.html.

Canadian biodiversity website (n.d.). *Biodiversity*. Retrieved January 30, 2012 from http://canadianbiodiversity.mcgill.ca/english/index.htm.

Catton, W., and Dunlap, R. (1980). The new ecological paradigm for post-exuberant sociology. *American Behavioural Scientist, 24*, 15–47.

Clarke, C. (2008). The ecological self. *Green Spirit Journal, 10*(1), 4–6.

Encyclopedia of Earth (n.d.). *Biosphere*. Retrieved January 30, 2012 from http://www.eoearth.org/article/Biosphere

Galtung, J. (2001). *Peace by peaceful means*. Thousand Oaks, CA: Sage.

Higgins, P. (2010). *Eradicating ecocide: Exposing the corporate and political practices destroying the planet and proposing the laws needed to eradicate ecocide*. London: Shepheard-Walwyn Publishers Ltd.

International Organization for Standardization (ISO). (2010). *ISO 26000 Social responsibility*. Retrieved January 12, 2012 from http://www.iso.org/iso/pressrelease.htm?refid=Ref1366.

International Panel on Climate Change (IPCC). (2007). *Climate change 2007: Synthesis report*. A contribution of working groups I, II, and III to the fourth assessment report of the Intergovernmental Panel on Climate Change. [Core Writing Team, Pachauri, R.K. and Reisinger, A. (eds)]. Geneva: IPCC. Retrieved August 5, 2011 from http://www.ipcc.ch/publications_and_data/ar4/syr/en/contents.html.

Korten, D. (2002). *Living economies for a living planet, Part 1: Introduction*. Retrieved January 30, 2012 from http://livingeconomiesforum.org/i-intro.

Mathews, F. (1991). *The ecological self*. Abingdon, Oxon: Routledge.

Naess, A. (1985). Identification as a source of deep ecological attitudes. In M. Tobias (Ed.). *Deep Ecology*. San Diego, CA: Avant Books. 256–270.

Rogers, P.P., Jalal, K.F., and Boyd, J.A. (2008). *An introduction to sustainable development*. London: Earthscan.

Shiva, V. (2005). *Earth democracy: Justice, sustainability, and peace*. Cambridge, MA: South End Press.

Sutton, P.W. (2007). *The environment: A sociological introduction*. Cambridge: Polity Press.

Tuan, M.T. (2008). *Bill & Melinda Gates Foundation – Impact Planning and Improvement Measuring and/or Estimating Social Value Creation: Insights into Eight Integrated Cost Approaches*. FINAL 12/15/08. Available at: http://www.gatesfoundation.org/learning/documents/wwl-report-measuring-estimating-social-value-creation.pdf.

United States Environmental Protection Agency (n.d.). *What is sustainability?* Retrieved December 8, 2011 from http://www.epa.gov/sustainability/basicinfo.htm.

Index